Physical Management for the Quadriplegic Patient SECOND EDITION

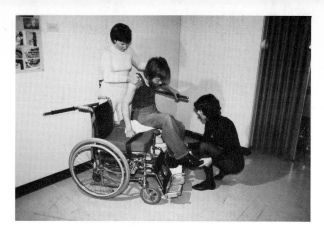 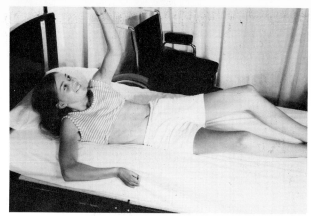

Jack R. Ford, R.G.

Former Department Director, Remedial Gymnastics,
G.F. Strong Rehabilitation Centre, Vancouver, British Columbia

Bridget Duckworth, B.S.R., (O.T.)

Department Director, Occupational Therapy,
G.F. Strong Rehabilitation Centre, Vancouver, British Columbia

Cover photograph by Carol Hussey, B.F.A.

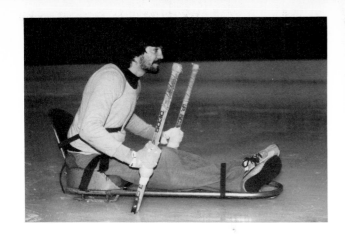
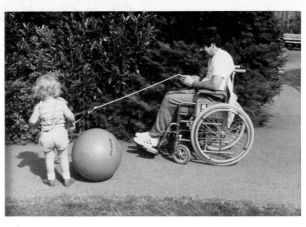

Physical Management for the Quadriplegic Patient *SECOND EDITION*

 F.A. DAVIS COMPANY · Philadelphia, Pennsylvania

Printed in the United States of America.

Cover photograph by Carol Hussey, B.F.A.

96900

Library of Congress Cataloging-in-Publication Data

Ford, Jack R.
    Physical management for the quadriplegic patient.
    Bibliography: p.
    Includes index.
    1. Quadriplegics—Rehabilitation.   I. Duckworth,
Bridget.   II. Title.   [DNLM: 1. Quadriplegia—
rehabilitation.   WL 346 F699p]
RC406.Q33F67   1987   617'.375   87-479
ISBN 0-8036-3676-8

Preface

This manual is written primarily for the use of health professionals: therapists, nurses, and students who work with traumatic quadriplegic patients. It will be found that the methods and information also apply to people with disabilities other than traumatic quadriplegia, such as multiple sclerosis, muscular dystrophy, and Guillain-Barré. Technical terminology has been avoided as much as possible in anticipation that the manual may also be used by the quadriplegic patient and his or her family or attendants. A glossary is included for further clarity.

The style is in note form with steps well illustrated for quick and easy reference. It is designed in this way so that it may be used as a working manual. There is no mention of level of injury in the body of the book; the level often is meaningless in regard to physical ability. The patient with a lower level lesion and many complications may not perform as well as the patient with a higher lesion. For this reason, methods have been put in sequence, outlining the method used by the most able patient and progressing to that used by the less able patient. The methods are interchangeable and may be varied considerably. Clarity and space demand that all variations are not described under each method.

There is a growing population of quadriplegic people. This is due to both an increased accident rate and an increased survival rate. These factors demand that a book of this type be available to aid quadriplegic individuals to realize their maximum capabilities and return them to useful and satisfying lives.

Vocational concerns and possibilities are not discussed, but many of the physical methods that allow a quadriplegic person to work will be found in the body of the book. Writing, typing, managing phones, computers, and driving are all examples of physical abilities that may be needed. The list of possible occupations is endless, and depends on physical and mental abilities, the individual's drive and desire to work, and the availability of suitable work or training. It is realized that work is necessary for the stimulation, social contacts, and standard of living of most people.

The manual is written for those who may be capable of becoming independent, but does not overlook those who will not be able to reach this goal. It is hoped that the chapter on care of the dependent patient will help the latter and their families solve the problems they will encounter.

Although we have not written much about the social and psychological adjustments that must be made by patients and their families, this does not mean that they are regarded lightly. They may well be the most important factors in successful rehabilitation.

We have covered in detail the physical methods of management that have been successfully used by many patients at the G.F. Strong Rehabilitation Centre, Vancouver. British Columbia. Canada.

In many areas of the world quadriplegic patients are now much better off than they were when the first edition of this book was written. Before that time, in most cases, patients had the choice between going to an extended care hospital as dependent patients, or attaining complete independence in their self-care; unless they were fortunate in having families who could look after their needs. Presently, in many areas, there are homemakers and home care nurses available to do some of the care. There are also group homes in some areas, so that several disabled persons may share the cost of housing and the help they require. The result is that many patients will choose independence if it is possible, but some will choose to be dependent even though independence is within their reach. Those who have no choice but to remain dependent are now better served where home services are provided. The feeling of "failure" because independence could not be achieved is greatly minimized when individuals have the means to pay for, and choose attendants, and be in charge of their own affairs.

It is well to advise patients who could become physically independent to attempt to do so. They will have more options later for choice of home, business, and social activities. The more independent the person is, the less reliance must be placed on relatives and friends; help may be accepted, but does not have to be relied upon. When patients are independent they can make a considered choice once they are in the stream of life again. Is it important to sacrifice ten minutes in bed to put on one's own socks? Will people accept help in the bathroom and thus reserve energy for work? Will they maintain range of motion and muscle strength by activities such as dressing and transferring, or do they find it necessary or more desirable to have some other type of maintenance? A wise choice is hard to make until the patient has fitted into the home routine.

Another change since this book was first written is the increased survival rate of high lesion quadriplegics, who must be given the opportunity to lead satisfying lives. With medical progress goes medical responsibility, and it goes without saying that survival is not enough. Fortunately, technical progress has meant that cheaper and more reliable environmental controls are being developed, and more importantly, are available so that those requiring care can maintain some control and independence. Computers may be used by virtually all who wish to use them. Wheelchairs are more versatile and are available with more sophisticated controls, thus allowing mobility for the severely disabled patient.

Attitudes and programs have changed somewhat, and disabled people and their families are now being educated to be more responsible regarding their own needs, and their own care, to be involved in setting their own goals, and to be more knowledgeable about their disability, their psychological adjustment and their families' needs.

There is still a long way to go. In many cultures disabled people are not accepted, in others they are overprotected and not able to reach their potential. Many countries are too poor to give disabled people the opportunities they need, and even in wealthier countries, opportunities for care, education, work, recreation, housing, social participation, and adequate income do not equal those for the nondisabled.

CHANGES IN THE SECOND EDITION

Although we have retained the philosophy and organization of the First Edition that our readers have found so useful, we have made many modifications that reflect changes that have occurred in the intervening years.

All chapters have been extensively updated to present the latest information and thinking on the management of quadriplegic patients.

We have vastly increased the coverage of Chapter 2, "Wheelchairs, Propelling and Mobility"; Chapter 11, "Household Management"; Chapter 12, "Car Transfers and Driving"; Chapter 13, "Housing"; and Chapter 14, "Recreation."

Two new chapters have been added: Chapter 9, "Sexual Management," written by Dr. George Szasz, and Chapter 10, "Parenthood."

We have also added two new appendices covering lesion levels associated with function, sample bathroom and kitchen plans, and home accessibility evaluation.

Finally, over a third of the illustrations are new for this edition.

Acknowledgements

We would like to express our deep gratitude

to Shaughnessy and Pearson Hospitals for allowing us to take photographs in their facilities and for their advice about the respirator dependent patient

to the counsellors with the Canadian Paraplegic Association, B.C. Division, and particularly to Tom Parker, a cheerful and helpful resource in the area for sports and recreation

to our enthusiastic typists Annette Chestnutt and June Mauthe

to the spinal cord staff at G.F. Strong Rehabilitation Centre, Vancouver, Canada, for their active cooperation and encouragement, and for sharing their knowledge with us. In particular we would like to thank:

> Mrs. Higgins, formerly of the Community and Follow-up Service, for sharing her knowledge and for the information she has brought us back from people living in the community

> the Nursing Unit spinal cord wing nurses, and especially Marion Orser, who checked and helped us a great deal with the bladder care information, as did Bill Eisenbock, Chief Orderly

> the Occupational Therapists on the spinal cord service, especially Jill Hall for her patience and for sharing her knowledge and experience, and Katy Tosh and Cathy Brighton, our two willing models

> the Physiotherapy Department and the contributions they have made to the quadriplegic program

> the Remedial Gymnasts on the spinal cord service and especially to John

Borthwick, who has taught so many quadriplegics so much over the years. Many developments and ideas are due to his inventive mind.

the staff at F.A. Davis, especially William Donnelly, Art Director, Susan Ferragino, Department Secretary, Anthony R. Heffron, Production Editor, and Jean-François Vilain, Allied Health Editor; their professionalism and cheerfulness have made our task easier than it might otherwise have been.

We would especially like to thank the many quadriplegic people who have generously given us their time and from whom we learn so much and who kindly demonstrated the methods for the book. Their willing assistance and encouragement made this publication possible.

Contents

1

Introduction and Biomechanical Principles

FACTORS THAT MAY INFLUENCE REHABILITATION	MECHANICAL PRINCIPALS
	Levers
	Pendulum
CORRELATION WITH THE HOME SITUATION	Momentum
	Friction
PROGRESSION	Example Transfer Analyzed

FACTORS THAT MAY INFLUENCE REHABILITATION

Nearly all quadriplegic patients have periods of depression before they can start to accept their disabilities. These may be manifest in many ways, such as apathy, aggression, overcheerfulness, or unrealism. Patients may not be able to apply themselves fully to rehabilitation until they have at least partially accepted their disabilities.

Younger people who were athletically inclined prior to injury will find it easier to learn physical skills than older or nonathletic individuals or those who have medical complications such as cardiac, visual, psychiatric, or psychologic problems. Mild head injury is often masked by the severity of the primary injury. This may be suspected when patients have undue difficulty in learning or retaining techniques; they may also have difficulty in problem solving.

Many patients quickly learn how to avoid medical complications such as skin breakdown or urinary infection, which otherwise would cause frustration and delay rehabilitation.

Type of body build can be an asset or a detriment. Excessive flaccidity of muscles and ligaments, or lack of joint range can greatly interfere with the application of mechanics to movement. Emaciation, obesity, or disproportionate build can also interfere with the application of mechanics.

Although some spasticity can be useful, an excessive amount may require treatment by a physician. Sometimes positioning may be worked out to prevent triggering unwanted spasticity.

Examples of the influence of body build on transfers, together with muscle charts and teaching tips will be found in Appendix I.

CORRELATION WITH THE HOME SITUATION

Early discussion with patients and their families may clarify issues and enable self-care methods to be correlated with the layout of the home. If the methods envisaged and the physical layout of the home are incompatible, the home may be modified or the self-care methods changed.

Patients and families should be shown what the patient may be able to accomplish so that they may have a reasonable estimate of long and short term goals, can feel that they are part of the rehabilitation team, and will also be able to contribute their efforts.

If equipment is required, it should be set up in the home so that it can be used during preliminary weekend and holiday visits by the patient so that confidence and a feeling of growing independence and realism is engendered. These visits also enable patients to retain their place in the family, and to explore their capabilities and needs in the home and community.

Apartments in or near a rehabilitation center can be very helpful for patients and their families prior to discharge so that supervision and help can be obtained and learning and confidence enhanced. An apartment can be helpful for the patient who hopes to be independent, or partially independent in self-care and homemaking; it can also be useful for those who are dependent and whose family or attendants need to learn and gain confidence in care techniques, and to have assistance to adjust to the new circumstances.

A follow-up program after discharge will disclose any previously unforeseen difficulties and should give support during the initial difficult process of adapting to wheelchair living outside the rehabilitation facility.

PROGRESSION

Suggestions and questions by patients should be encouraged. Thus they are involved in their own programs, their interest is aroused, and they learn to solve problems and adapt to situations that may arise later.

When a patient begins self-care training, a considerable amount of equipment may be necessary. As he approaches peak performance, the patient should be encouraged to discard it, and remaining equipment reduced to a minimum so that the patient can be more versatile in differing situations.

All equipment must be safe, stable, and reliable. The helper must be in a position to prevent falls. If the helper has to change position while the patient is transferring, he should first make sure the patient is in a safe position. The patient must have confidence in the helper's ability to prevent him from falling before he can put full effort into self-care training (see Appendix I).

An adequate exercise program to improve strength and balance is a prerequisite to the learning of new skills. Lighter self-care techniques (eating, washing, etc.) should be started as soon as the medical status permits. Encouragement is given at first by establishing easy self-care goals that are sure to be accomplished. Patients should not be asked to attempt an activity unless it is known that they can accomplish at least part of it.

As the condition of the patient improves, both exercise program and self-care program should become more vigorous.

When a task has been accomplished, the patient and his family should be encouraged to continue it as a practical daily activity. This builds up tolerance so that the patient can progress to other demanding skills. As the patient's ability to look after himself increases, the exercise program may be cut back to allow more time for practical application of self-care skills. If a person has accomplished all his self-care, he will find little need for extra exercise. Self-care, in itself, is physically demanding for a quadriplegic patient and, at first, very time consuming. When he has become proficient in self-care, he should have reduced the time required to a practical level, allowing time for work and social activities.

MECHANICAL PRINCIPLES

The body, with all its bones and joints, may be regarded as a series of levers and hinges. Therefore, it is reasonable to apply mechanical principles to create mechanical advantages.

LEVERS

First Class Lever (Fig. 1-1A and B)

When a seated person leans forward, the knees form a fulcrum and the head and shoulders help to counterbalance the weight of the lower trunk and thighs

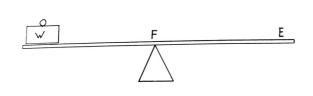

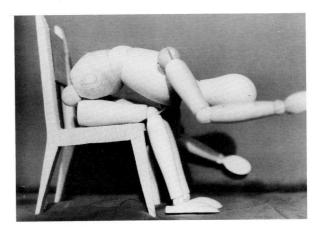

FIGURE 1-1   A   B

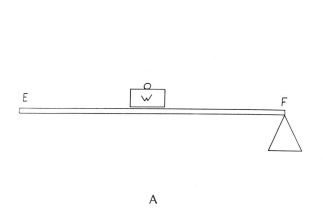

A

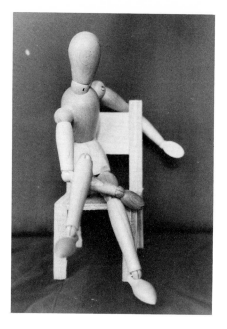

FIGURE 1-2

B

(Fig. 1–1A and B). This reduces the weight of the lower trunk and thighs on the chair by the weight of the chest, head, and shoulders.

Second Class Lever (Fig. 1-2A and B)

To reduce the effort required to lift a weight, a fulcrum may be utilized. The manikin has placed an arm under one leg with the wrist resting on the other knee as a fulcrum (Fig. 1-2A and B). "Effort" or straightening the arm will lift the leg. A patient may use this leverage to cross his legs.

Third Class Lever (Fig. 1-3A and B)

The hip joint forms the fulcrum, the leg forms the lever, and the effort is applied by the arm to lift the weight of the lower leg (Fig. 1-3A and B). This is the least efficient of the three levers.

Example One in the Use of Levers (Fig. 1-4A, B, C, and D)

In Figure 1-4 the wheelchair can be regarded as a first class lever, or balance scale, with the castors forming the fulcrum (Fig. 1-4A). With a 150-pound (68 kilograms) man in the chair, if the castors are turned back, 40 pounds (18 kilograms) of weight placed on the footrest will tip the chair (Fig. 1-4B). With the castors turned forward, the fulcrum is about four inches further forward (Fig. 1-4C), and a 210-pound (95.3 kilograms) man can stand upright on the footrests

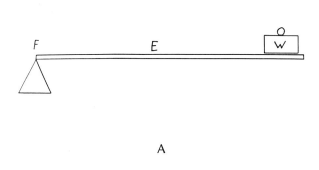

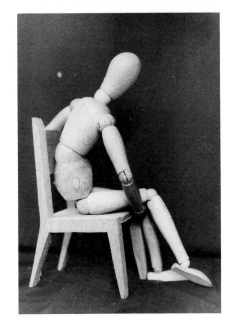

A

FIGURE 1-3

B

without tipping the chair forward (Fig. 1-4D). For this reason castors must be turned forward for stability in transfers, or for leaning forward in the chair while the feet remain on the footrests.

Example Two in the Use of Levers

Because many people will use a lift which may be almost instinctive, and which is not necessarily the most efficient, a weighing scale was set up to compare the amount of effort used to move a patient using two different methods, one of which is often used instinctively, and another which makes extensive use of levers. The results demonstrate the advantage of working out the mechanics before attempting any move.

A platform was made with a cutout to accommodate a scale of the same height (Fig. 1-5). The wheelchair was placed on the platform. The helper stood on the scale to obtain and compare the effort used for the two following methods of moving a patient back in the chair.

In Figure 1-6A the helper slides her hands under the patient's axillae, and holds the patient's wrists. She now lifts and pulls the patient to slide her back in the wheelchair. The weight registered on the scales is 230 pounds (105 kilograms) (Fig. 1-6B).

In this move the helper's back is hyperextended because a good deal of lift is lost in elongating the patient's back and elevating her shoulder girdle. The patient cannot be moved properly in the wheelchair because the top of the wheelchair back acts as a fulcrum and tends to hold her forward. This lift is not only difficult for the helper; it may be quite uncomfortable for the patient, particularly if she has a weak shoulder girdle.

5

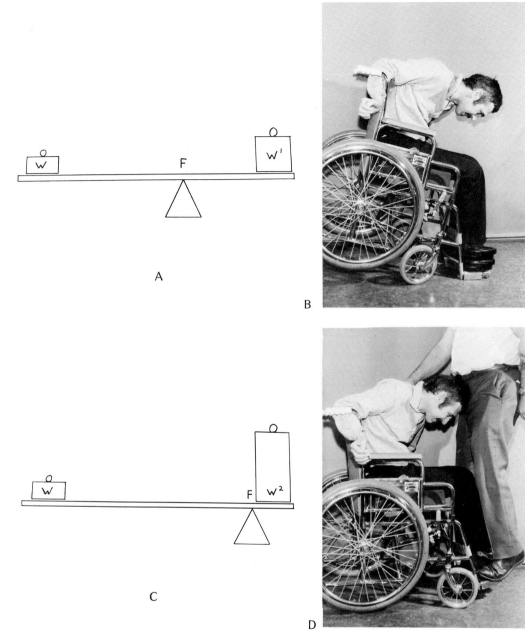

FIGURE 1-4A.   First-class lever
FIGURE 1-4B.   With castors turned back, 40 pounds (18 kilograms) on the footrest will tip the wheelchair.
FIGURE 1-4C.   With castors turned forward, the fulcrum is moved forward.
FIGURE 1-4D.   Thus 210 pounds (93.3 kilograms) on the footrest will not tip the chair.

6

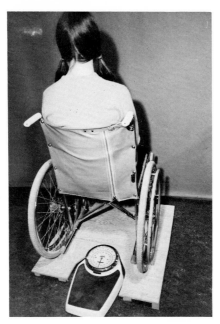
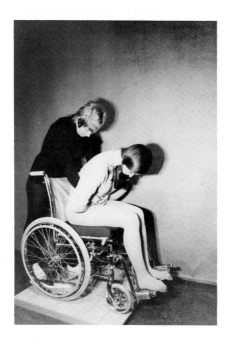

FIGURE 1-5.   Platform and Scale

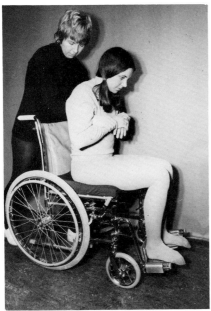
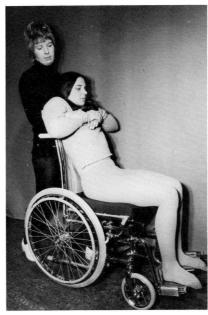
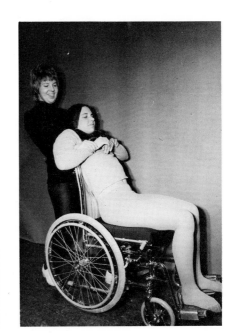

FIGURE 1-6A.   "Instinctive" Lifting Method

7

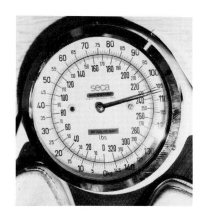

FIGURE 1-6B.   Weight Registered During Lift

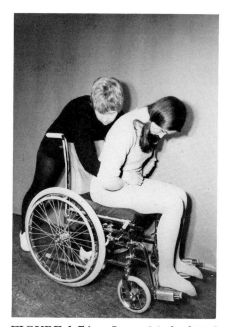 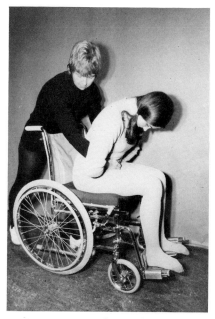 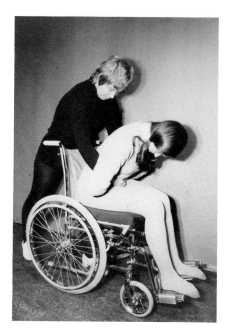

FIGURE 1-7A.   Lever Method Utilizing Maximum Mechanical Advantage

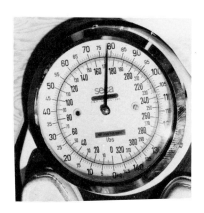

FIGURE 1-7B.   Weight Registered

In Figure 1-7A the helper places the patient's hands over her lower abdomen. The helper's hands are placed over the patient's hands, with her forearms under the patient's rib cage. The patient is flexed forward. The fulcrum of the lever is the point where the forearms hug under the rib cage. The effort is exerted at the helper's upper arm by a shrug of her shoulders and the pressure is applied at the symphysis pubis as the helper's arms straighten and force the patient back. This is a most effective first class lever as shown by the pressure on the scale of 170 pounds (78 kilograms) (Fig. 1-7B).

PENDULUM

Pendular movements may be used to advantage, the result being dependent on the placement of the fulcrum. In Figure 1-8B the patient swings beyond the

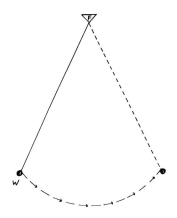

FIGURE 1-8A

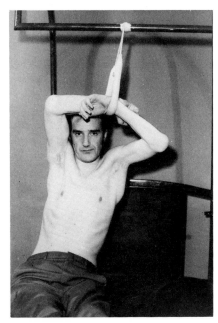
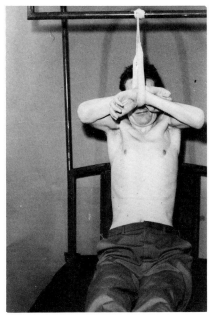
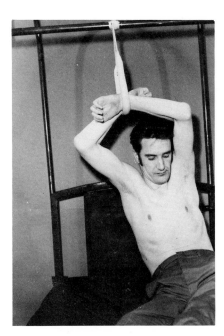

FIGURE 1-8B

9

point beneath the fulcrum by taking advantage of the placement of the fulcrum. The lift must be high enough to clear at the low point of the arc if the pendulum is used on a flat surface. In this instance the feet are moved across first so that they assist rather than retard the swing.

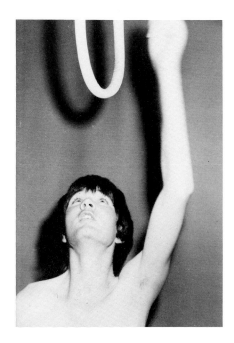
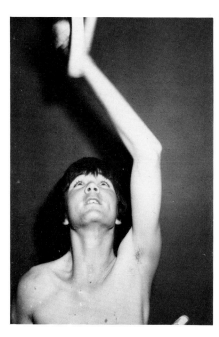

FIGURE 1-9A.   Fast Movement.

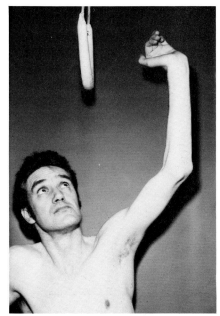
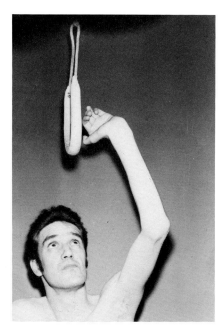
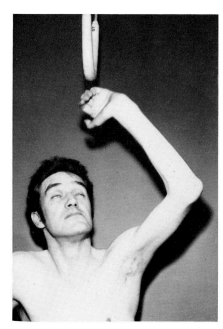

FIGURE 1-9B.   Slow Movement

10

MOMENTUM

Momentum also can be used to advantage. An example is the attempt to throw a forearm into a sling when the triceps muscle is not working. In Figure 1-9A the arm is flung into the sling so that the elbow has no time to bend. If a patient reaches for the sling slowly his forearm drops before his hand is in position (Fig. 1-9B). Because of his momentum, a patient moving fast with vigor will move easily.

FRICTION

As shown in Figure 1-10 a great deal less weight or effort is required to move an object sliding on a smooth surface, such as nylon, than is required on a rough surface, such as cotton. Therefore, nylon draw sheets and cushion covers are frequently used, and patients are advised to wear nylon-cotton pants rather than corduroy or jeans when learning transfer techniques. Many patients prefer to be in the fashion and must have nylon patches sewn to the seat of non-slippery pants to reduce friction. If hands should slip when pushing on a slippery surface, friction may be increased by using pusher mitts with a non-slip material.

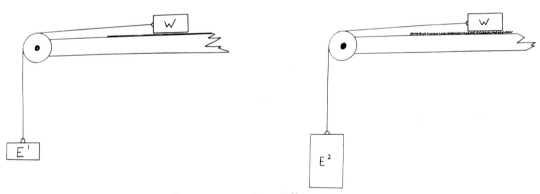

FIGURE 1-10.   Smooth Surface Requires Less Effort
Rough Surface Requires More Effort

EXAMPLE TRANSFER ANALYZED

One dependent transfer, the "thigh pivot slide transfer", is analyzed in detail to illustrate the application of mechanics to a transfer where a twelve-year-old boy is moving a 210 pound (95.3 kg) man (see Chapter 15, Figures 15-42, 15-77 and 15-85).

A human being can be visualized as a series of levers, joined by hinges (Fig. 1-11).

A first class lever is the most efficient lever, and is best shown as a teeter-totter or see-saw. The teeter-totter is shown superimposed over the figure of the person (Fig. 1-12); this illustrates the point of the fulcrum at the person's knees, and

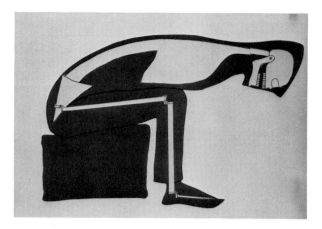

FIGURE 1-11

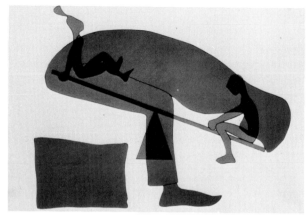

FIGURE 1-12

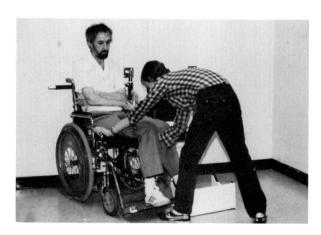

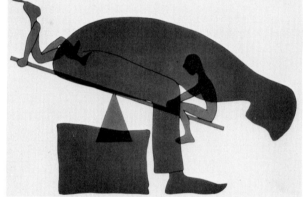

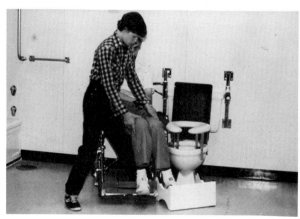

FIGURE 1-13

shows how the head and shoulders counterbalance the buttocks and lower trunk. During the transfer, a combination of a pull down on the shoulder and a lift on the buttocks activates the teeter-totter.

In this transfer the fulcrum can be moved even further back, taking more weight off the buttocks. To do this, the boy pulls the man forward to allow himself room to place his leg in position under the man's thigh. The fulcrum is thus the point where the boy's leg is against the man's thigh (Fig. 1-13).

The man is levered onto the toilet or bed by using the helper's front leg as a lever and the back leg as the force. The front leg can be used to lift slightly if the helper rises onto the ball of his foot as he pushes (Fig. 1-14).

In this same transfer a person can be visualized from above, with his trunk lying over his knees (Fig. 1-15). The fulcrum point is again at mid thigh where the boy's leg is under the man's thigh.

When the teeter-totter is superimposed over the figure, it can be seen that a pull on the shoulder and a push on the buttocks utilizes a second first-class lever to pivot the buttocks over onto the toilet.

These moves must all be synchronized into one smooth movement.

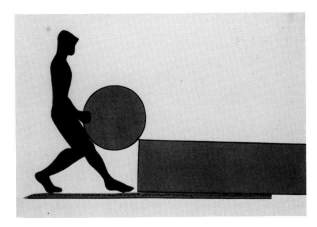
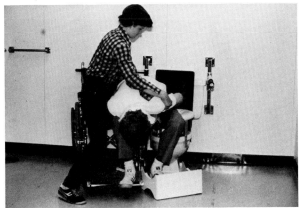
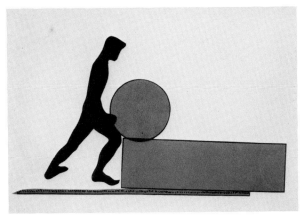
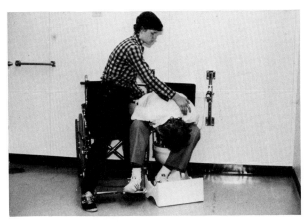

FIGURE 1-14

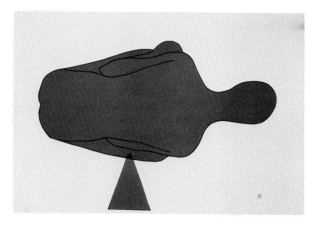 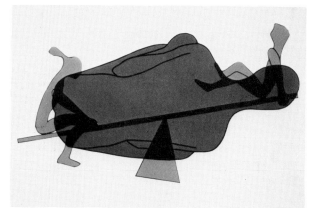

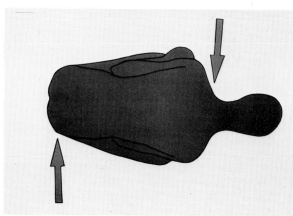 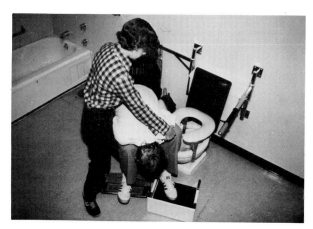

FIGURE 1-15

This example shows that thought must be given to each transfer to analyze the mechanical advantages and disadvantages, so that optimum methods can be worked out and applied.

If these basic mechanical principles are understood, the reasons underlying the methods explained in the manual will be clear, and variations, combinations, and new methods will evolve more easily.

2

Wheelchairs, Propelling and Mobility

WHEELCHAIR SELECTION
  Frame Type
  Seat Width
  Seat Depth
  Seat Tilt
  Leg Rests
  Foot Plates
  Leg Straps
  Backs
  Wheels
  Castors and Castor Locks
  Retainer Straps

Cushions
Accessories
Brakes
Braking
Getting In and Out of the Chair
   to the Floor
Electrically Powered Wheelchairs
Self Positioning
Weight Relief
Maintenance

The wheelchair has gradually become more sophisticated over the years, with the advent of the tubular metal frame, which reduced its size, permitted folding, and provided better mobility. The tubular metal frame lent itself to easy modification. First, the large wheels were moved from the front to the rear, which improved maneuverability and allowed removable arms to be used. The next major changes provided brakes, then elevating leg rests, swing away leg rests, castor locks, and adjustable height backs.

Improved wheelchairs permitted people to have a more active role in sports, along with a greater desire by the disabled to become more active in all aspects of living. Increased participation in sports has snowballed and has had a direct effect on the latest improvements in wheelchair design. They are becoming lighter, easier to operate with precision bearings in all four wheels, and they are becoming more adjustable to the individual.

Despite the fact that there are excellent models now in production, wheelchair design must be closely monitored in the future to make sure that the most efficient wheelchair is recommended to the patient.

WHEELCHAIR SELECTION

Function, management, balance, and safety of the quadriplegic patient must be considered when selecting a wheelchair.

Patients must be involved in the process of selecting a wheelchair so that their ideas and desires are included and so that they learn about the considerations involved in wheelchair prescription and will be able to make educated selections in the future. These considerations will include balance and safety, propulsion, transfers and future plans, such as sports activity, and vocation.

Very early selection of a wheelchair is not always indicated because balance, strength, and extent of possible recovery is not always known. For example, some patients may require a tall back in the early stages which later may not be required, and which will interfere with their wheeling ability.

It is desirable to have a selection of wheelchairs available for loan so that

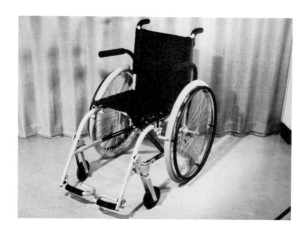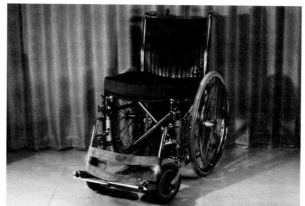
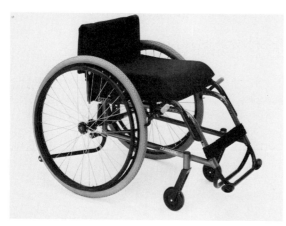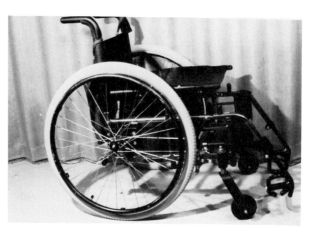

FIGURE 2-1

patients may experience the difference between various types, and may progress from one style to another as they become more adept (Fig. 2-1).

FRAME TYPE (FIG. 2-1)

Generally, a totally rigid design is not desirable since it is possible for a wheel to lose contact with the ground. If one of the large drive wheels loses contact with the ground, the chair can be immobilized. A rigid frame made of a flexible metal may partially solve the problem, but frequent flexing may cause metal fatigue. A single X frame type wheelchair is flexible and will ride well over rough ground and allow all wheels to be in contact with the surface at all times. Since the cross bars of the X frame are a mechanical link between two separate frame halves, metal fatigue will no longer be a problem, but because tubes slide one inside the other, care must be taken to insure the frame is not bent. The extra material required in this frame will add weight to the wheelchair.

Special purpose apparatus such as stair climbing wheelchairs, standing wheelchairs, or mobile standing aids must be carefully evaluated for the individual, preferably with a trial period with the equipment. Frequently, to add a desired feature, some other feature must be sacrificed. For instance, a stair climbing wheelchair may be heavier, or larger, and this must be weighed against the advantages. A standing mobility aid may be ideal for a receptionist who likes to be able to talk to people at a standing level, but getting into it unaided may be a problem. Working in a kitchen may seem to be ideal in a standing mobile aid, but the potential user must check that a hand is left free for carrying, and that counters are accessible, as well as high cupboards. As new equipment comes on the market, it must be monitored for usefulness, durability, and cost.

SEAT WIDTH

This is measured from the outside of the seat rails. The width should allow room for the patient to twist in the chair when changing position, and should allow room for winter clothing. The patient may also need room to place his hands on the cushion to change position, do a push up or initiate a transfer. If he is dependent, room will be required for a helper's hands to adjust his position, clothing, and so forth. In addition, a wider wheelchair may be easier for some patients to push because of the "hugging" action used by patients lacking active elbow extension. The advantages of a narrow chair for access through doorways is so obvious that sometimes this necessity for room in the chair is overlooked. Generally, when assessing a wheelchair for width, a flat hand should slip easily between the patient's hips and the wheelchair arms. If necessary at a later date, the width and height of the wheelchair may be changed by exchanging the cross frames and the upholstery. This may obviate the purchase of a new wheelchair.

If a wheelchair requires narrowing temporarily, for instance for a narrow doorway, a wheelchair narrower may be used. A lever type narrows the wheelchair with one movement (Fig. 2-2A). A screw type takes some time to wind, and is more difficult to manage than the lever type (Fig. 2-2B). A belt strapped around the pushing handles or the tipping levers is an excellent temporary narrower if it can be applied before the patient sits in the wheelchair (Fig. 2-2C).

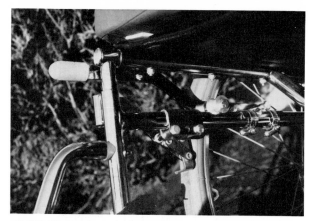

FIGURE 2-2A   Normal Position

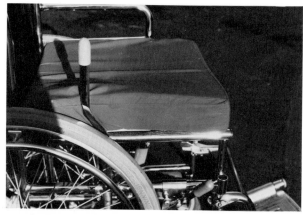

Narrowed Position

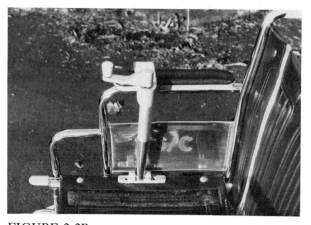

FIGURE 2-2B

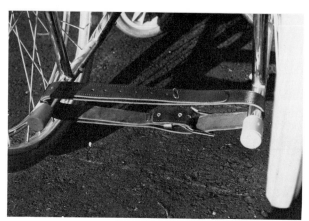

FIGURE 2-C

SEAT DEPTH

A standard wheelchair is 16 inches (40.64 cm) deep, which will accommodate to most adults. The person with a longer thigh may require a sports model with a 17-inch (43.18 cm) depth. Although this is not a critical measurement, the width of a fist between the back of a patient's knees and the seat front will allow enough length of cushion to support the thighs adequately, while allowing the person to twist or maneuver in the wheelchair. The edge of the seat should not contact the back of the knees. It is seldom necessary to purchase a custom built wheelchair to accommodate thigh length, as some variation in the length of the thigh touching the seat is permissible.

SEAT TILT

It should be noted that the back of the seat of a standard wheelchair is approximately 1 inch (2.54 cm) lower than the front. If an increased tilt is desired

18

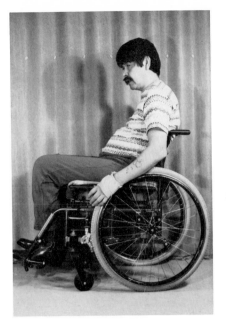 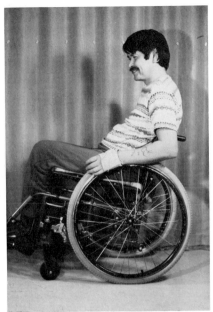

FIGURE 2-3A   FIGURE 2-3B

because of the patient's spasticity, positioning, or because he slides forward, a wedge cushion may be used.

The tilt of sport wheelchairs may be adjusted to the individual. In the first example shown, minimal tilt (Fig. 2-3A) suited the individual because of his build and balance ability; in the more reclined position (Fig. 2-3B) he had the feeling that he was falling backwards, and was not stable.

The natural sag of the wheelchair seat sometimes causes the knees to slide together (Fig. 2-4). This is not desirable because it disturbs balance. A ¼ inch (.635 cm) tempered hardboard rectangle may be placed under the cushion inside

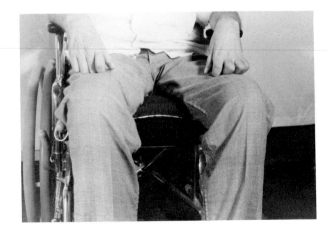 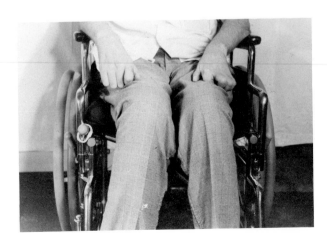

FIGURE 2-4

the cover. This must be about 1–1/2 inches (3.81 cm) inside the seat rail on either side to avoid interfering with the flexibility of the wheelchair. Alternatively, a firm contoured material may be used to level out the sag in the wheelchair seat. If this is not enough correction, a saddle may be formed by placing a wedge of foam rubber under the center front of the cushion. As a temporary measure, or for assessment, a roll of towelling will suffice.

LEG RESTS

The standard swing away removable leg rest is convenient for the patient who transfers to the bathtub. It is also convenient for close approach to bed or toilet, for easy stowing in the trunk of a small car, or for negotiating tight corners on occasion. The helper of a dependent patient may need to remove a leg rest to get close enough to ease the transfer.

A locking lever mechanism is usually operable by a person who is capable of removing a leg from the footrest to allow the leg rest to swing out. Occasionally the lever must be lengthened or curved out to make it easier to reach.

Some patients must have elevating leg rests, usually because of persistent edema, or because they are using power recliner wheelchairs. Elevating leg rests elongate the wheelchair, reducing maneuverability. The type of elevating leg rest that accommodatess the patient's leg length as it is raised must be hinged from a point above the seat, level with the patient's knee joint; but this leaves a raised portion, impeding safe transfers. If the leg rest does not swing from this high point, it does not adjust to the patient's leg length in all positions. For these reasons elevating leg rests should only be ordered when absolutely necessary.

FOOT PLATES

These are available in several sizes, or as adjustable foot plates (Fig. 2-5) that allow the foot to be positioned in dorsi or plantar flexion. Since the width of the foot plate is dependent on the width of the wheelchair, an adjustment to the wheelchair's width may therefore necessitate a change of foot plate size. The

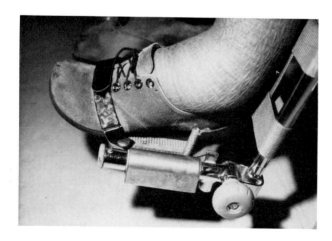

FIGURE 2-5

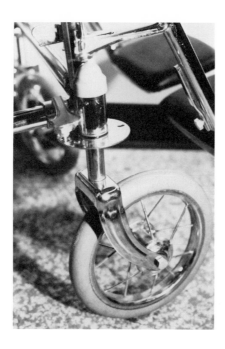

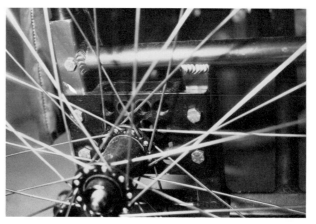

FIGURE 2-6B

FIGURE 2-6A

length of the foot plate is standard on the swing away leg rest, but longer on the elevating leg rest. A person with a large foot, who is unable to keep his feet on the standard foot rest, may exchange a standard foot plate for one from an elevating leg rest.

The height of the foot plates is critical for the positioning of the patient. The rule of thumb is that a flat hand can be inserted under the thighs easily. The object is to have even pressure along the length of the thighs, thus relieving some pressure from the buttocks. If the foot rests are too high, too much weight is placed on the buttocks, and if they are too low, circulation to the lower leg may be impeded, or the weight of the legs beyond the front edge of the cushion may tend to lever the patient out of the wheelchair.

If, when the foot plates are correctly adjusted, they do not provide adequate clearance from the ground, a higher model, or a custom wheelchair may be required. If it is to the patient's advantage to be slightly reclined to improve his balance, the castor spindle may have a bushing sleeved over it to elevate the front part of the wheelchair slightly (Fig. 2-6A). If there are multi positions on the wheelchair for the rear wheel axles, the axles can be placed in a higher position. This also tilts the wheelchair back and raises the foot rests (Fig. 2-6B).

LEG STRAPS

One or two detachable leg straps (Fig. 2-7A), or an H-strap (Fig. 2-7B) may be fastened with velcro or a post and loop, one strap behind the heel and another optional one at about midcalf. These prevent the feet from becoming caught behind the foot rests. Individual heel straps are not recommended for the quadriplegic patient because the metal uprights which retain the heel straps are hazardous.

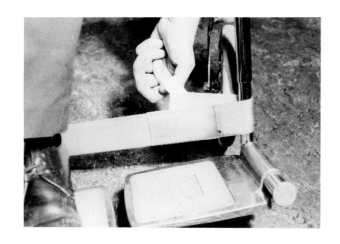

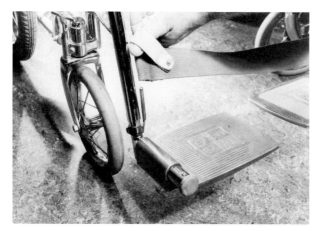

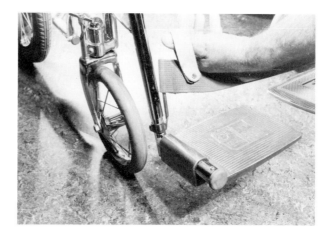

FIGURE 2-7A

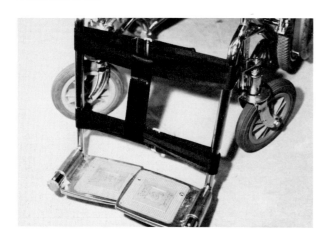

FIGURE 2-7B

22

A patient, learning to lower his legs, may drop a foot onto them and cause trauma. In addition, the straps must be pushed forward before the foot rests can be folded up.

BACKS

Back Height

When assessing back height, the cushion required must be included. A standard wheelchair back measures 16 inches (40.64 cm) from the seat rail to the top. Some wheelchairs have a modular back which comes in 8–1/2 inch (21.59 cm), 11 inch (27.94 cm), 13–1/2 inch (34.29 cm), and 16–1/2 (41.91 cm) heights. A modular back may be useful for assessing the height required by a quadriplegic patient and it will be useful for the patient who requires a high back at first, for balance, but who will progress to a lower back. If a modular or sectional back is not obtainable, a standard wheelchair back may be temporarily extended (Fig. 2-8) by adding aluminum tubing split down its length for about 4 inches (10.16 cm). The top of the cut is contoured to fit the curve of the pushing handle, thereby forming a continuation of the wheelchair back upright. An envelope of leather or other material is sewn to fit over these uprights and overlap the wheelchair back; the extension may be machine screwed, or held in place with hose clamps.

A high back may push a patient forward too far so that he tends to fall, and a lower back will often correct this problem (Fig. 2-9). It may also be a problem for a patient to fling his arm over the pushing handle of a high-backed wheelchair. The lower back will be an advantage to the patient to allow his shoulder blades to

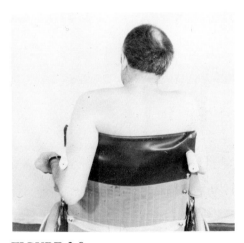

FIGURE 2-8

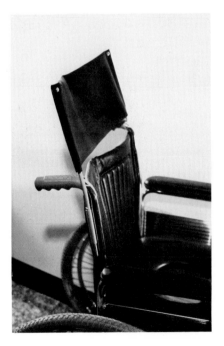

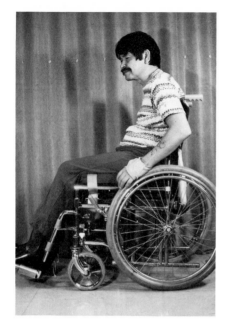
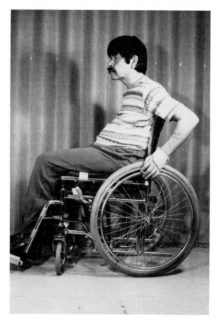

FIGURE 2-9   Back Too High   Correct Back Height For This Patient

move freely, permitting him to thrust hard on the wheel rims and increase the length of his stroke. The patient in a wheelchair with a back that is too low may fall backwards and be levered right out of the wheelchair.

Recliner Back

A recliner wheelchair will have both a high back and may also require a headrest. A nonpowered recliner wheelchair is hard to maneuver, and should not be ordered unless absolutely necessary.

Slightly Reclined Back

For the patient whose trunk is inclined to fall forward, the wheelchair back may be slightly reclined by using graduated spacers and longer screws to fasten the upholstery to the back upright. The top spacer can be up to 1 inch (2.54 cm) long. If the spacers are too long, the weight of the patient against the upholstery will tend to bend the screws, and the uprights may interfere with the patient's arms (Fig. 2-10).

Lateral Supports

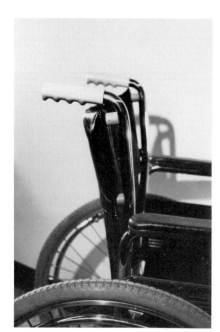

FIGURE 2-10

The patient who has a tendency to develop a "C" curve of the spine due to spasticity or muscle imbalance, may require padded lateral supports. Generally one such support is inadequate, and two- or usually three-point contact is required to correct the problem (Fig. 2-11).

24

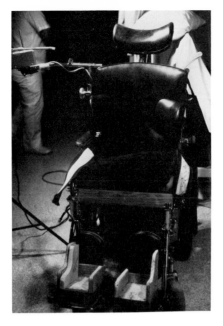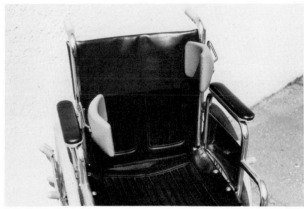

FIGURE 2-11

These lateral supports may be obtained commercially, either fixed or swing away. They are an obstacle to the independent patient, and to the attendant of the dependent patient. Supports therefore require careful fitting and good judgment of the patient's needs.

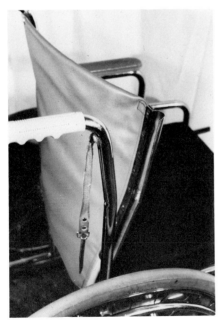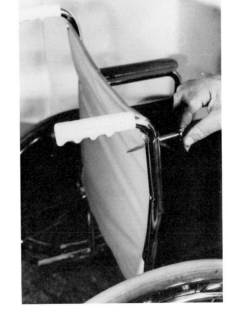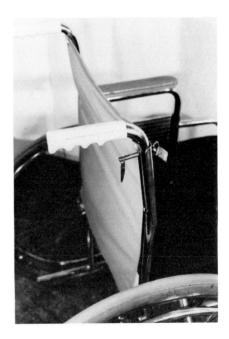

FIGURE 2-12

Semi-Detachable Backs

If a dependent patient needs to transfer through the back of the wheelchair, he may use a commercially available zipper back. The independent patient will find the zipper very difficult to manage. It is more practical to have a back that is removable on one side and fastened by a full-length contoured metal clip, which fits onto the front of the back upright and is secured by a small pin (Fig. 2-12).

Swivel Backs

Swivel backs will sometimes enable the patient to change position more easily in the wheelchair (Fig. 2-13). The position of the swivel on the uprights must be carefully adjusted to allow the patient to lean back in a controlled fashion so the seat will lever his buttocks forward.

Pressure Relief

The emaciated patient may have a tendency to have pressure areas caused by the back of the wheelchair rubbing on his spinous processes. If this occurs, the problem may be alleviated by making a detachable back which has two 3-inch (7.62 cm) wide pads of 1-inch (2.54 cm) foam rubber, glued down its length approximately 2 inches (5.08 cm) apart, which are then covered with soft leather. This back may be secured by two loops slipped over the pushing handles (Fig. 2-14).

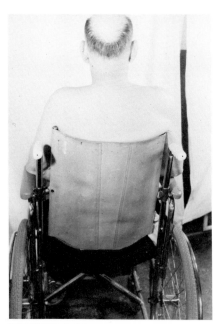 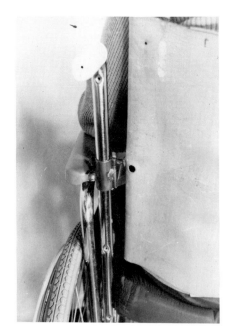

FIGURE 2-13

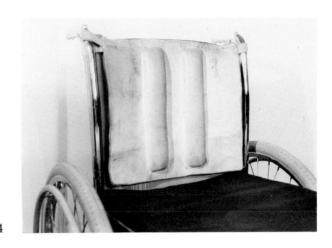

FIGURE 2-14

Arm Rests

Removable desk arms allow close approach to a desk or table. They are available as a standard or as a wrap-around arm. The wheelchair with a wrap-around arm is 1–1/2 inches (3.81 cm) narrower than a standard wheelchair. A person with restricted arm range may have difficulty in fitting the arm rest into the back sleeve, which is hidden behind the wheelchair back upright.

Many arm rests have a simple lever-action pin lock which can be managed without adaptions by most quadriplegics who are capable of removing the arm rests.

The high lesion level quadriplegic patient will probably require adjustable height desk or full-length arm rests with detachable arm troughs. These will aid in positioning and balance, protection of the shoulder joint, and in hand and wrist positioning (Fig. 2-15).

The sports model sloping arm rests are lighter, but do not afford as many pushing or gripping areas for transfers or weight shifts as the standard desk arm. They lack the skirt guard, leaving a possible hazard of scraping a hip on the wheel,

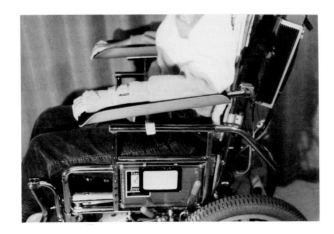

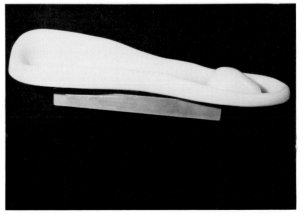

FIGURE 2-15

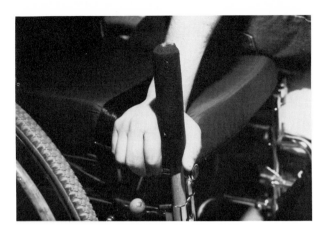

FIGURE 2-16

and also eliminating a useful storage area. If padded arm rests are required, they must be specially ordered for the sports arm rest.

Some patients may eventually wish to discard arm rests because it may be easier to push the wheelchair without the arm restriction, and there is more freedom of movement. A removable post which fits into the front arm rest sleeve, and which is padded on top is often more useful than the arm rest upright for positioning and transfer (Fig. 2-16).

WHEELS

Wheels and brakes are discussed on page 38. See Propelling the Wheelchair.

Tires

Tires can be obtained as solid, semi-pneumatic, pneumatic, or as a solid tire which resembles a pneumatic tire but which is filled with a porous material that is not affected by a puncture. Tires may also be obtained smooth or treaded and widths may vary. If a tire is hard, it rolls more easily than a soft tire, but the ride may not be as comfortable. The balance between ease of wheeling and comfort must be decided on an individual basis.

A smooth tire rolls easily and tracks less dirt, but a treaded tire may be required to provide friction for the person who pushes on the tire, or who requires it for traction on rough ground.

A narrow tire is easy to move on a hard surface, but a wider one is required for pushing over soft or rough ground; this is especially important for front tires.

Hub Types and Positions

Many wheelchairs have multi-axle positions (Fig. 2-17). The position of the wheel is important for efficient propulsion. If the hub is mounted forward, more weight is placed on the rear wheels, and less on the front castors. This makes the wheelchair easier to wheel, and often places the wheel in a more appropriate

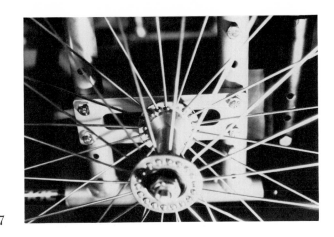

FIGURE 2-17

position for the patient's arm thrust. The wheelchair is less stable in this position, and the learner may require anti-tipping levers.

Mounting the hub higher or lower alters the tilt of the wheelchair. This tilt back may correct a tendency for the patient's trunk to fall forward and may prevent a person from sliding forward.

Precision bearings contribute greatly to easier wheeling.

Cambering (Fig. 2-18)

Cambering of the rear wheels contributes to stability and makes turning easier. If the camber is extreme, the wheelchair may be too wide at the base to go through narrow doorways, the top of the wheel may scrape the patient's hips, and the wheels may be so close at the top that the patient's wheeling becomes inefficient. In addition, the back upholstery sags and may require adjustment. The seat guide posts on some standard wheelchairs may lift right out of the chair frame when folding the chair unless longer posts are substituted.

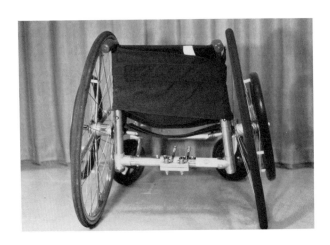

FIGURE 2-18

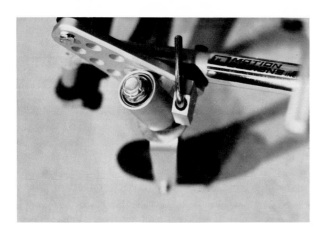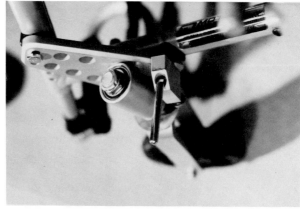

FIGURE 2-19
Off On

CASTORS AND CASTOR LOCKS

The greater the diameter of the castor, the easier it is to push the wheelchair on rough surfaces, but the smaller diameter castor permits easier turning on a hard surface. A major consideration is the stability of the wheelchair when the castor is turned forward, and the larger castor gives a longer wheelbase and therefore more stability. For these reasons most quadriplegic patients will choose an 8-inch (20.32 cm) castor. An extremely efficient moulded plastic castor has precision bearings on both spindle and axle and a pneumatic tire which gives a softer ride.

To ensure stability during transfer, castor locks on both sides may be used (Fig. 2-19). These should always be engaged with the castors in the forward position.

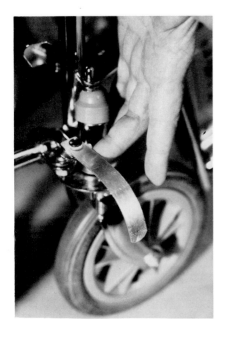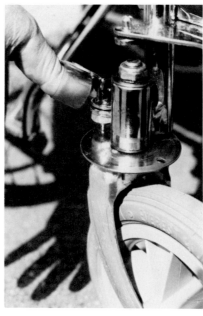

FIGURE 2-20   Extension Loop

30

The castor lock lever may be adapted with a loop or an extension for easier manipulation (Fig. 2-20).

RETAINER STRAPS

Chest Strap

A chest strap may be required for safety by the high lesion patient, especially early in treatment, or when wearing a Halo-thoracic type brace (Fig. 2-21).

Safety Belt

A safety belt of 2-inch (5.08 cm) webbing may be attached to the second retainer screw up on both sides of the back between the upholstery and the back upright. It may be fastened in front with a car safety belt buckle (Fig. 2-22), or a velcro D-ring fastening. Thumb loops may be sewn to the straps to make fastening

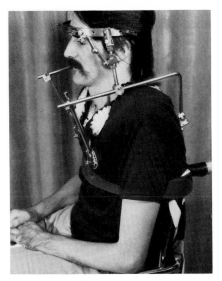

FIGURE 2-21

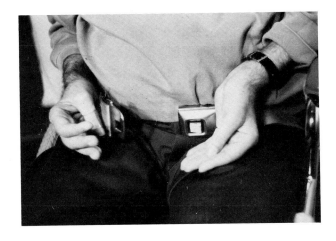

FIGURE 2-22

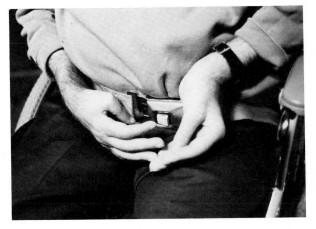

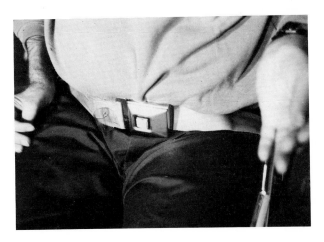

31

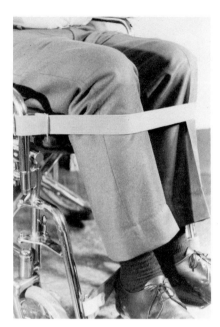

FIGURE 2-23

possible, and a knob may be glued to the release button on the car safety belt buckle to make release easier (Fig. 2-22).

It is desirable to do without a safety belt, so that weight reliefs can be done more conveniently.

Knee Strap

Occasionally a knee strap may be required to restrain the patient with gross extensor spasms who can slide under a waist safety strap. A strap passing across the shins, just below the knees is attached to the front uprights of the wheelchair (Fig. 2-23).

Ankle Strap

If extensor spasms are of the legs only, the strap can be attached to the frame of the leg rests (Fig. 2-24). Skin checks must be made regularly and the strap may have to be padded.

Toe Loops

Toe loops are seldom necessary and can cause leg injuries in a fall. They can also be inconvenient for an independent person. The toe loop illustrated (see Fig. 2-5) is being used in conjunction with a modified shoe to help to correct a deformity of extreme inversion of the foot.

CUSHIONS (FIG. 2-25)

The cushion which suits everyone has yet to be invented. Consideration must be given to patients with different builds, different types of skin, allergies, perspiration problems, flaccidity or spasticity, and different degrees of independence. Patients who are careful with their skin inspection, skin care, weight shifts, nutrition, and transfers, will encounter fewer skin problems. Some patients live in

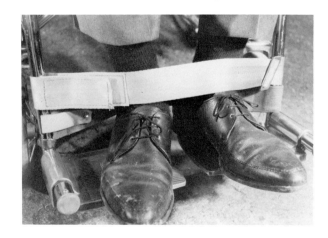

FIGURE 2-24

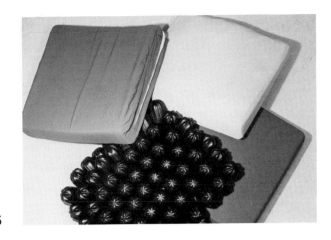

FIGURE 2-25

extreme climates or work in hot or cold environments. These are all factors in cushion selection.

A wheelchair cushion is usually a compromise between several differing needs. The patient learning independent transfers requires a firm cushion with a low friction surface. A person who sits for a long time requires a cushion which is soft or molded so that the weight of the patient on any portion of the cushion is evenly distributed, thus allowing good circulation. However, the patient may find it hard to maintain balance on the softer cushion, particularly on water or air filled types of cushion.

Moisture absorption is another important consideration in cushion selection for the incontinent patient or for the patient who perspires excessively. Ideally moisture should pass through the cushion without being absorbed, as in a closed-cell foam, a Roho, or Bye-Bye Decubiti cushion. If incontinence is a major problem, a cushion with a water barrier covering may be required. A material such as ensolite, which has a fatty texture, or a waterproof cloth which can breathe, such as "Gore-Tex" will protect the cushion. It is particularly necessary to protect a foam rubber cushion because washing destroys the chemicals and causes the cushion to lose density.

If the patient perspires excessively, the cushion and cover materials should allow circulation of air. Roho cushions and egg-crate type cushions meet this condition; the egg-crate type cushion must be frequently renewed as the convolutions flatten and their effectiveness is lost. Some types of cushions are very warm to sit on and may promote perspiration. These cushions may however be very suitable for cold climates. Such cushions as foam rubber or ensolite may be excellent in a cold climate, whereas rubber-type cushions such as Roho or Bye-Bye Decubiti may be too cold unless other insulation such as sheepskin is added. Temper foam becomes hard and brittle in cold climates, and "flows" in a hot climate.

The weight of the cushion is important for the independent person who must lift the cushion, as in car transfers. Water or gel-type cushions are generally heavy.

An extra firm density foam rubber cushion, 3 inches (7.62 cm) thick, is tolerated well by a majority of patients and is certainly the easiest to use while learning to transfer. Thinner cushions may be insufficient protection for the skin, and also leave the chair wheels higher and further forward, impeding transfers.

Relieving Pressure

Cushions may be adapted by layering different types of foam, or by placing different types of foam under the bony area. Foam cushions may be adapted by plucking or carving out areas which require pressure relief. This should preferably be done on the underside.

Excessive pressure areas may be located by feeling the pressure area with a flat hand between the buttocks and the cushion, or pressure gauges may be used. As it is difficult to seat a patient in exactly the same place each time he is transferred or shifted, any pressure relief cutouts must be made large enough to allow for this.

Wedge Cushions

Such adaptions as abduction wedges or wedge cushions may be required for posturing or balance, but these may interfere with transfers.

Knee abduction wedges (see Fig. 2-4) may be useful to reduce adduction and extensor spasticity. An abduction wedge may also be useful for the flaccid patient to position his legs to help prevent foot deformities, knee pressure areas, and to relieve pressure on the genitals or urinary apparatus.

The wedge cushion which is higher at the front than at the back may be required to prevent the patient from sliding forward, or it may help to prevent extensor spasticity. The foot rests must be raised to accommodate the increased height of the wedge.

Laterally-wedged cushions may be required in conjunction with lateral supports for the person with a scoliosis. It is very difficult to attempt a correction or accommodation of a scoliosis while maintaining normal pressure over the ischii. Often a compromise must be used and carefully monitored to maintain comfort, function, pressure relief, and position.

Cushion Covers

Some cushions may be used with no cover in order to provide direct skin contact. This is sometimes desirable when treating pressure areas. For general use a cover will be required. A light soft canvas cover is in common use because it washes and wears well and absorbs perspiration. A nylon taffeta cover over the canvas cover will facilitate sliding. The direction of weave of the material can affect sliding. It is possible to select the smooth direction of the material by passing a thumb nail across the material in two directions and listening for the softer sound. This will be the smooth direction which should be from side to side to permit easier sideways transfer.

A two-way stretch material makes a most desirable cushion cover because it does not exert a shear force on the skin. However, this type of material is not as easy to move on as nylon taffeta.

"Gore-Tex" is a material which breathes and is waterproof, has a two-way stretch and is fairly slippery. If this material stands up to wear, it or similar material should be very useful.

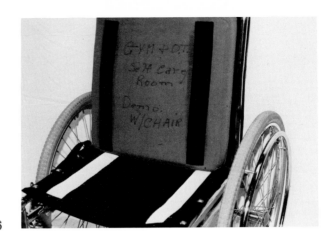

FIGURE 2-26

Anchoring Cushions

It is especially important for the person who does a sliding transfer to have the cushion anchored. Cushions can be anchored by sewing two strips of hook velcro to the wheelchair seat and two opposing strips on the underside of the cushion cover (Fig. 2-26). Alternately, a material such as dycem, thin foam rubber, or other sticky material may be placed between the wheelchair seat and the cushion.

If the cushion does not need to be lifted from the wheelchair, a wide nylon webbing belt may be placed over the front part of the cushion and seat rails to fasten underneath the seat. This not only holds the cushion down, but can also be used to hook a thumb under for purchase during transfers (Fig. 2-27).

If the patient must slide out of the back or the front of the wheelchair, a nylon flap may be sewn to the top edge of the cushion with a fluffy velcro strip sewn to the free end. An opposing strip of velcro is sewn to the underside of the wheelchair seat. This prevents the cushion from rolling up during transfer (Fig. 2-28).

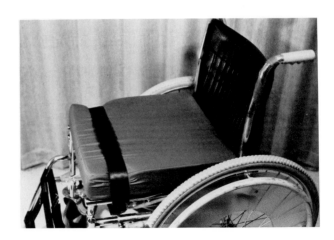

FIGURE 2-27

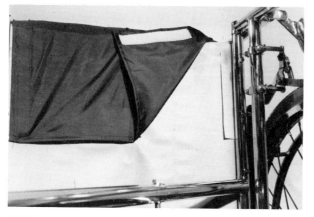

FIGURE 2-28

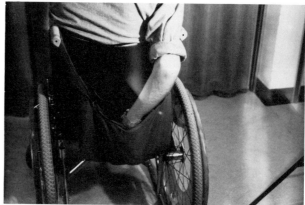

FIGURE 2-29

ACCESSORIES

Wheelchair Bags

Most patients will find a bag hung from the pushing handles very useful, particularly if no wheelchair arms are used. The bag must be hung low for the convenience of the patient who can reach in (Fig. 2-29).

Wheelchair Trays

A wheelchair tray is of use to the majority of quadriplegics. The advantages of the tray shown in Figure 2-30 are simple attachment, stability, and appearance. Two ³/₈ inch (.95 cm) holes are drilled in desk arm rests just in front of the pad and on the curve to accommodate the rods. The rods consist of ³/₈ inch (.95 cm) cold rolled steel 16 inches (40.64 cm) long, flattened at one end and bent at 90°, 5

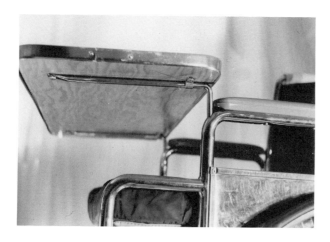

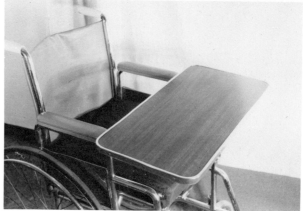

FIGURE 2-30

inches (12.70 cm) from the other end. The flattened end is drilled and bolted to the tray to line up with the chair arms. The rods are then placed in the holes in the chair arms to ensure a good fit before bolting them permanently into position under the tray using electrical cable straps. The tray is made of ¹/₂ inch (1.27 cm) plywood covered with Arborite or Formica, finished with aluminum edging to form a small lip around the tray.

The tray may be made to fold (Fig. 2-31A).

A transparent plastic tray allows the patient to see where she is going and also allows her to check her foot position and her clothing (Fig. 2-31B).

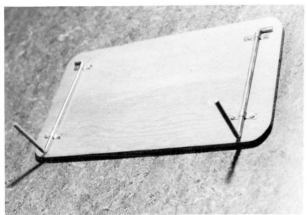

FIGURE 2-31A

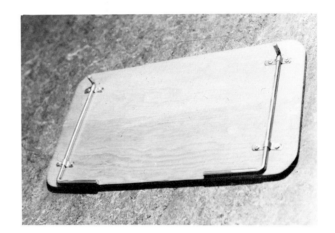

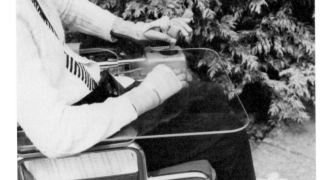

FIGURE 2-31B

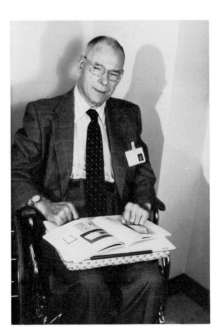

FIGURE 2-31C

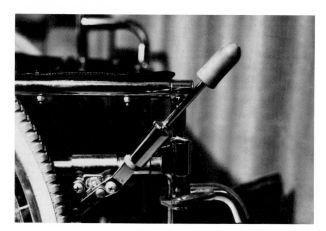

FIGURE 2-32

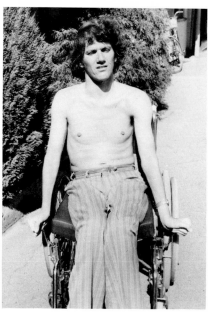

FIGURE 2-33

A "bean bag" or foam chip cushion with a tray attached on top may be easily transported. It can be placed so that it is angled for reading or writing, and flat for beverages or meals (Fig. 2-31C).

BRAKES

Brakes are essential to provide stability for transfers and for many other activities such as for working at a table or eating.

Brake Extensions

A removable brake extension gives more leverage but requires greater arm range (Fig. 2-32).

BRAKING

Applying

Pushing forward is the preferred movement for locking brakes because balance can be maintained more easily.

Many patients apply their brakes simultaneously, using the same movement as in wheeling-flexion of the shoulder with adduction and external rotation (Fig. 2-33).

To maintain balance some patients apply a brake with one hand using the other arm as a counterbalance (Fig. 2-34).

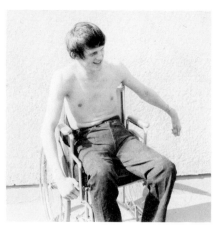

FIGURE 2-34

38

A patient may hook one elbow over the pushing handle and use it as an anchor point to develop more momentum to push against the brake (Fig. 2-35).

The hand position is determined by the degree of external rotation required and the presence or absence of wrist extensors. Wrist extension and/or external rotation can be used to flick the brakes on (Fig. 2-36).

The heel of the hand or the fingers push against the brake when elbow flexion and external rotation of the shoulder are used to apply the brakes (Fig. 2-37).

Releasing

The same methods of maintaining balance while applying the brakes are used for release, except that the maintenance of balance is made more difficult by the pulling action.

The brakes may be released simultaneously, usually using adduction and internal rotation of the shoulders (Fig. 2-38).

The brakes may also be released using a chopping action, hitting the side of the hand against the brake handle (Fig. 2-39).

PROPELLING THE MANUAL WHEELCHAIR

The patient must be correctly positioned in the wheelchair before he is ready to learn the techniques of propelling the chair.

Wheeling Forward

The patient places the heels of both hands on the drive rims as far back as possible. His shoulders are internally rotated and his elbows slightly flexed initially. A pushing action is developed by adduction and external rotation of the shoulders (Fig. 2-40). The upper trunk is extended to maintain balance as the hands move forward. Patients are inclined to move their hands only a short distance until they have learned to synchronize these movements. Greater speed and balance will be developed with practice.

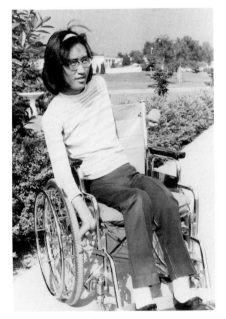

FIGURE 2-35

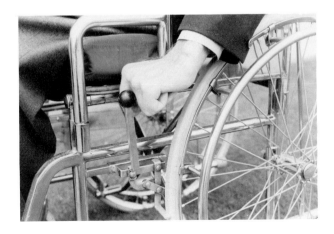

FIGURE 2-36

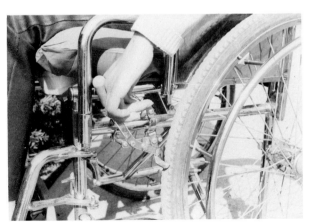

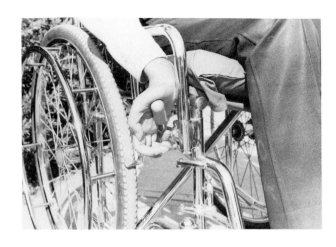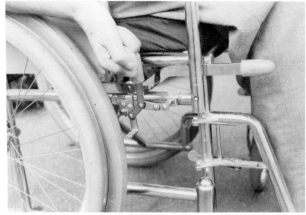

FIGURE 2-37

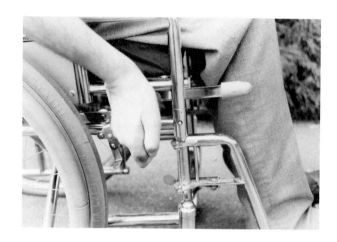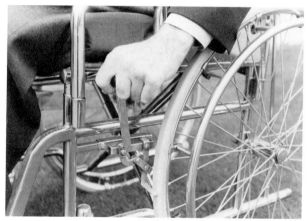

FIGURE 2-38

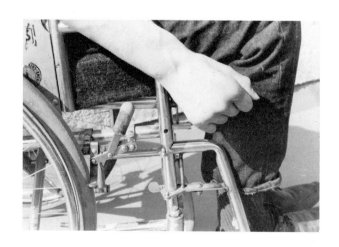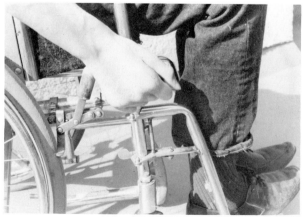

FIGURE 2-39

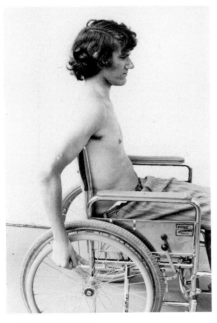 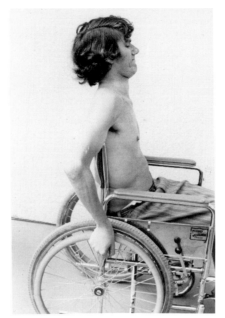 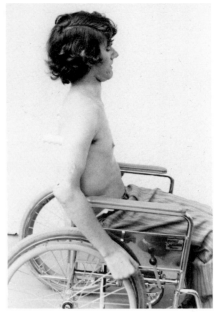

FIGURE 2-40

In some cases a patient is unable to maintain balance in the chair when wheeling and cannot tolerate a safety belt across the chest. In such instances he may wheel while placing one or both arms behind the pushing handles (Fig. 2-41). However, this restricts his shoulder flexion and causes him to lose a considerable amount of his driving power.

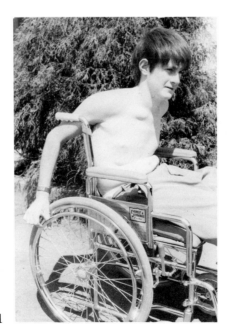 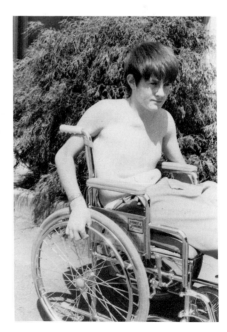

FIGURE 2-41

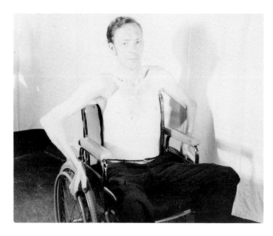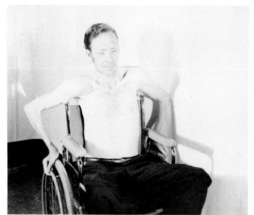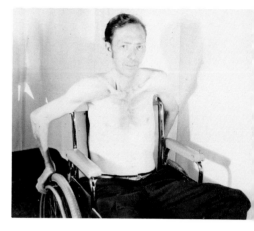

FIGURE 2-42

Wheeling Backward

The patient who uses drive rims will back up by placing his hands as far forward as he can reach, with elbows slightly flexed. With his back resting against the back of the wheelchair, he adducts and internally rotates his shoulders while he elevates and retracts his shoulder girdle (Fig. 2-42). This develops a pulling action that will not cause him to fall forward.

Some patients who use this technique also extend the upper trunk to gain additional pull and maintain balance (Fig. 2-43).

The patient who is unable to maintain balance while wheeling backward must place one or both arms over the back of the wheelchair. She places the heel of her hand against the inside of the tire and pushes by depressing her shoulder (Fig. 2-44).

Hand Positions and Adaptations

Covered Rims. If the patient's hands slip on the drive rims, the drive rims may be taped temporarily. This may indicate the need for commercially available

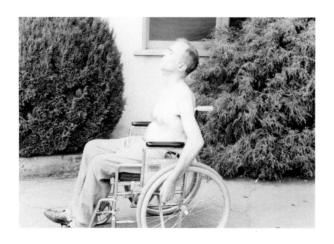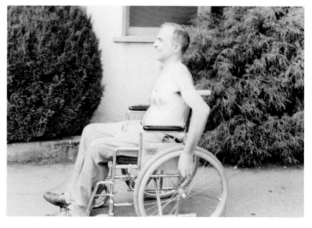

FIGURE 2-43

plastic-covered rims or rubber-covered rims. Note the hand position change as the shoulders rotate externally (Fig. 2-45).

To cover the rims with rubber, the drive rims are removed from the hangars and cut through. One inch surgical tubing is slipped onto the rim, and pulled back from the cut, which is then silver soldered. Sufficient tubing is used to ensure a tight butt fit when it is released. The rims are now remounted.

Pushing on Tires—Pusher Mitts. The patient who is unable to obtain sufficient purchase on the drive rims may push directly on pneumatic tires (Fig. 2-46). In this case he will probably require pusher mitts to protect his hands and gain friction. The spacers between the drive rims and the wheels are removed, and the drive rims bolted directly to the hangars. The drive rims are retained to prevent the fingers from becoming caught in the spokes.

Plastic Spoke Guards. Plastic spoke guards may also be used for this purpose (Fig. 2-47). A well maintained spoked wheel is lighter and easier to propel, but a molded plastic wheel is easier to maintain, and there is less hazard of catching fingers.

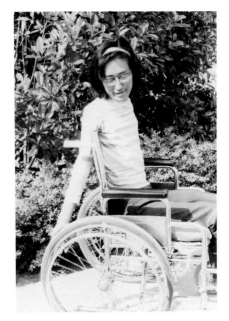

FIGURE 2-44

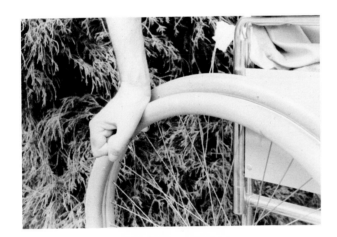

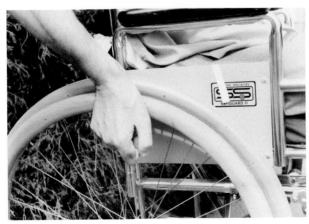

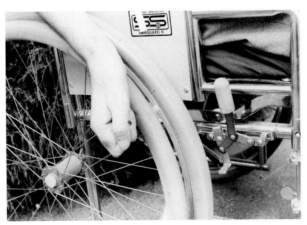

FIGURE 2-45   A, Forward

43

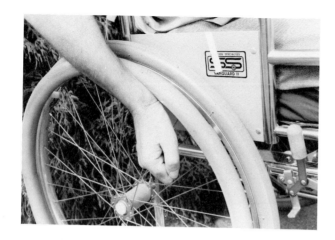

FIGURE 2-45   B, Backward

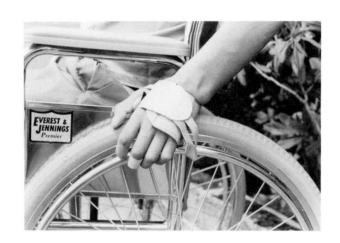

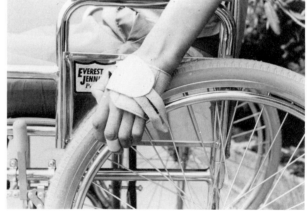

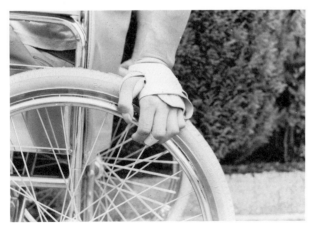

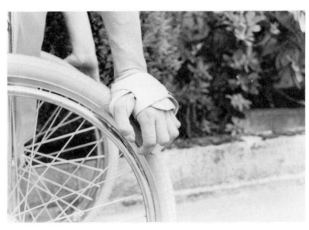

FIGURE 2-46

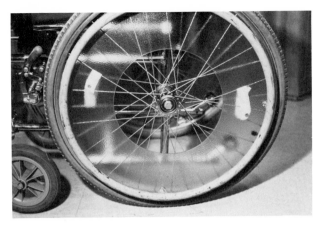 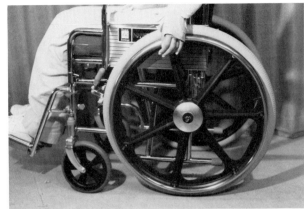

FIGURE 2-47

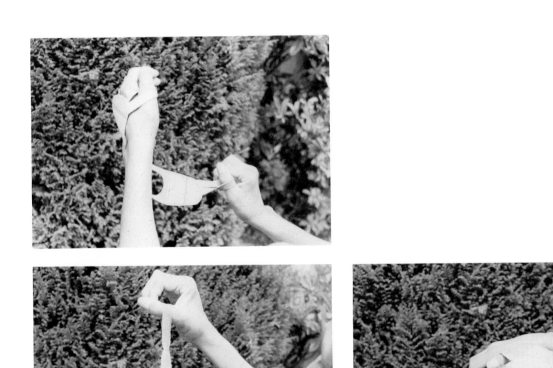

FIGURE 2-48

45

Putting on a Pusher Mitt. One type of pusher mitt (Fig. 2-48) may be made of cowhide with a velcro fastening and a hook velcro or rubber pushing surface (see Appendix). There is a thumb loop at either end with a hole to fit over the thumb at about a third of the distance from the end. The first loop is slipped over the thumb so that the pusher mitt lies over the back of the hand. It is then brought up over the palm of the hand, the thumb is inserted into the hole, and the mitt is fastened.

Wide Spacers. The patient who is unable to gain friction on the tire or rim may push on wide spacers. The patient places his thumb webs on the drive rims with his thumbs against the spacers (Fig. 2-49). It is possible to propel the chair using this method even though the shoulder adductors may be weak. To adapt the wheelchair, replace the four ³/₄ inch (1.91 cm) spacers with eight 1¹/₂ inch (3.81 cm) spacers.

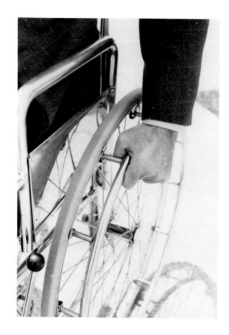

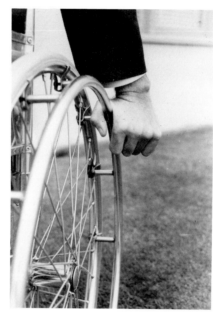

FIGURE 2-49   A, Forward B, Backward

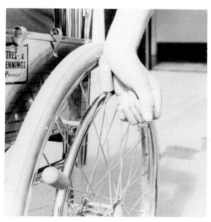

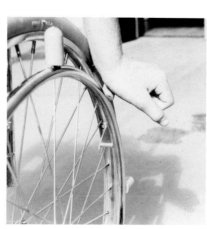

FIGURE 2-50   A, Forward B, Backward

46

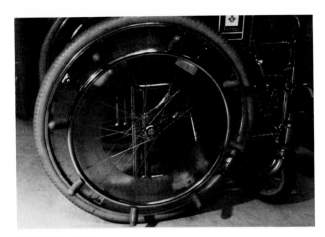

FIGURE 2-51

Vertical Lugs. Vertical lugs may be added if the patient is unable to position his hand to utilize spacers (Fig. 2-50). Eight to twelve lugs will be necessary. They should be covered with rubber brake handle tips. Horizontal lugs are not recommended as they are hazardous and widen the chair.

Angled Lugs. Angled lugs also widen the chair, but may be required by some patients (Fig. 2-51).

Pushing Splints. A molded splint, extending from behind the metacarpophalangeal (MP) joints to half way up the forearm, will stabilize a flail wrist. Pushing hooks, appropriately positioned and bent for the individual patient, may be attached to the molded splint (Fig. 2-52). The patient can push against spacers, wide spacers, or against vertical lugs inside or outside the drive rim.

Grade Aids. Many quadriplegic patients require grade aids to allow them to push up a hill. The grade aids hold the chair still until the hands can be repositioned (Fig. 2-53). They may also be useful for a helper when pushing a chair up a steep slope.

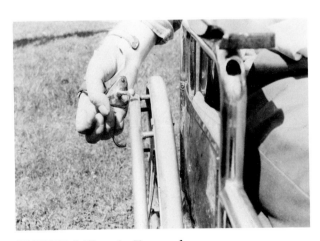 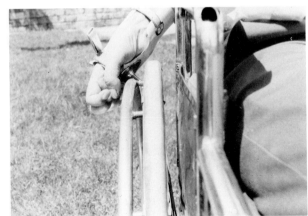

FIGURE 2-52   A, Forward

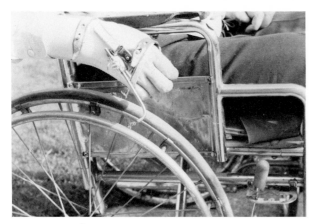
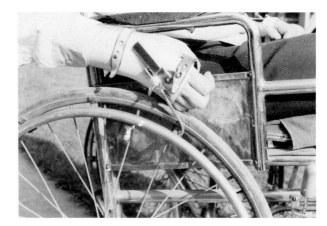

FIGURE 2-52   B, Backward

Jumping or Balancing the Chair

Some quadriplegics are able to jump the front castors over small obstacles such as carpet edges or weather strips. The chair must be rolled back slightly before pushing sharply forward to lift the front wheels (Fig. 2-54), but the castors must remain in the trailing position.

The patient with a low lesion and with good strength and balance may learn to balance his chair on two wheels, a great advantage in clearing obstacles and managing rough ground (Fig. 2-55). To balance the chair the patient must sit well back. He maintains the chair in the balanced position by slight counteracting wheel movements, pushing forward if the wheels drop, and back if they should lift too high.

When learning this skill the patient is tipped back into the balanced position and the helper keeps both hands just under the pushing handles of the chair so that he is in position to catch them when the patient tips too far. Once the patient has

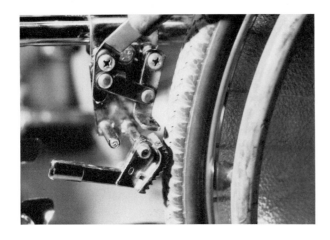

FIGURE 2-53

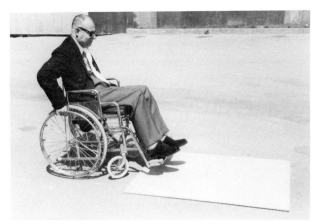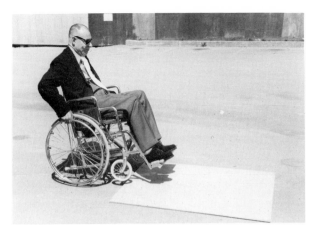

FIGURE 2-54

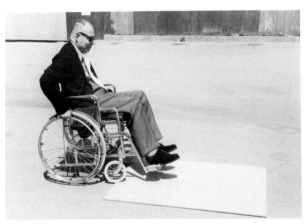

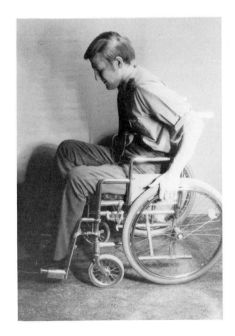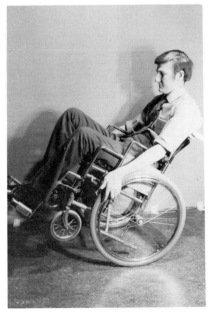

FIGURE 2-55

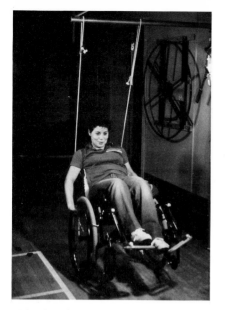

FIGURE 2-56

learned the feel of balance he can start to learn the more difficult maneuver of flicking the chair into the balanced position.

A patient may safely practice balancing alone (Fig. 2-56) using training ropes. These ropes may be suspended from a horizontal bar or doorway. The loops tighten around the pushing handles, and the ropes may be made adjustable for various patients.

GETTING IN AND OUT OF THE CHAIR TO THE FLOOR

When moving from the chair to the floor (Fig. 2-57), the patient wheels forward to turn the castors back and applies the brakes. He turns one armrest so that it projects forward of the chair. He puts his feet ahead of the footrests and drops a cushion onto the footrests. He slides to the edge of his chair until the chair tips forward and lowers himself the remaining short distance.

Getting back into the chair (Fig. 2-58), the patient lifts himself onto the cushion previously placed on the footrests. He grasps the projecting wheelchair arm and places the other hand against the inside of the other wheelchair arm. Strength, skill, and balance are required for the lift back into the wheelchair.

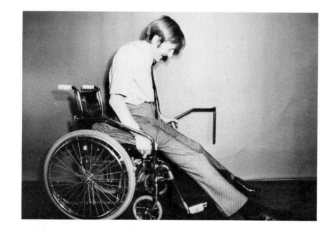

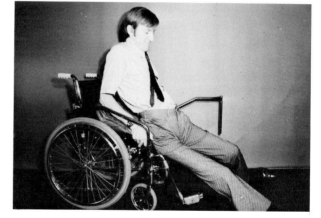

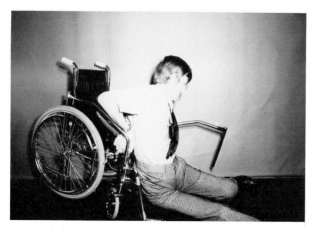

FIGURE 2-57

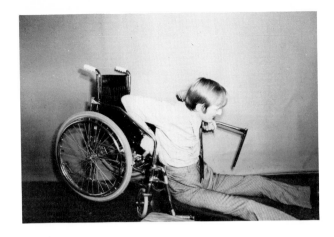
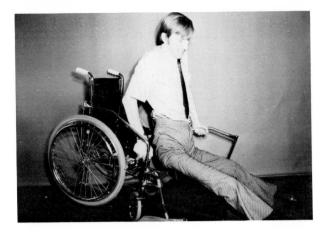
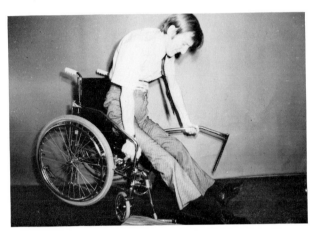
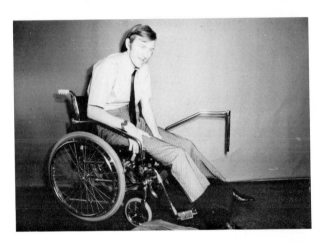

FIGURE 2-58

Replacing the Cushion

To replace the cushion (Fig. 2-59), the patient puts his foot on a high leg retainer strap and pushes the cushion well under his raised knee. When he does a pushup the cushion springs partially under him; he can square the cushion by doing a pushup and actually place the cushion with his buttocks.

To replace a foam cushion, the cushion is folded in half and wedged between the arm of the chair and the hip. A pushup on the folded cushion and the opposite armrest will flip the cushion under him. It is squared into position again by using the buttocks.

The patient illustrated has just completed a transfer from the floor to the chair and has left his front castors turned back because he does not need to lean forward while replacing the cushion.

ELECTRICALLY POWERED WHEELCHAIRS

A patient who can propel a manual wheelchair may use an electrically powered wheelchair as his second wheelchair for traveling distances encountered

51

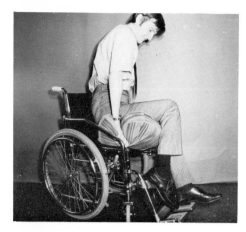 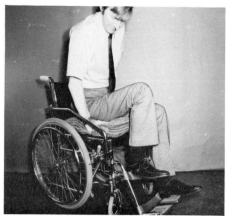

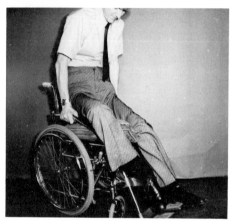

FIGURE 2-59

when shopping, going to school, and social activities. It must be remembered that it is very difficult to take a powered wheelchair up stairs or curbs, and it is generally not easily transported in a family car, and may require the family to purchase a van with a lift.

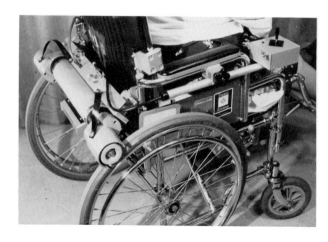

FIGURE 2-60

52

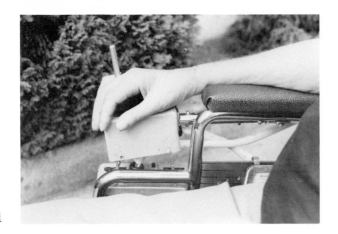 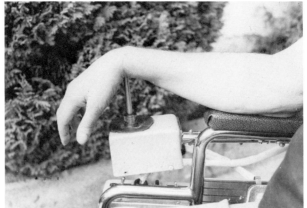

FIGURE 2-61

Many quadriplegic patients who use an electric wheelchair as a primary wheelchair may still want a manual wheelchair for greater mobility on outings where architectural barriers are likely to be encountered, and also because they may enjoy the exercise from wheeling.

Detachable Power Unit

Alternatively, a detachable power unit on a manual wheelchair will make transport in a family car practical, and can be used part-time if desired (Fig. 2-60).

Joystick Control

The normal method of control of an electrically powered wheelchair is by use of a small joystick, which may be placed on the right or the left chair arm (Fig. 2-61).

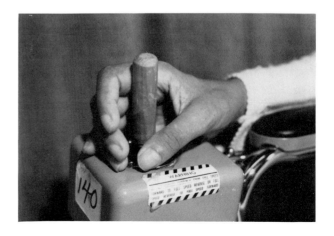

FIGURE 2-62

Adapted Joystick

A thicker or longer removable plastic, wood, or metal dowel may be added. The bottom end of the dowel must be bevelled so that the range of the joystick is not restricted (Fig. 2-62).

"T"-Bar

A "T"-bar, usually with stops on either end, may be added, which can also be offset to let gravity assist the patient on the longer side of the "T" (Fig. 2-63).

"J" Shaped Handle

"J" shaped handles may be tilted at angles from vertical to horizontal depending on the patient's ability to place a hand on the joystick, the amount of supination the patient can control, and his range of pronation and supination (Fig. 2-64).

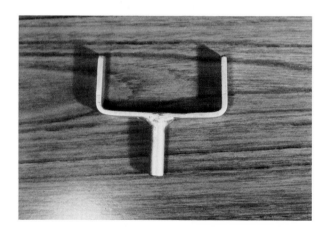

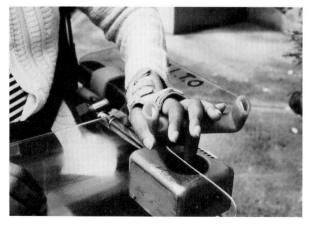

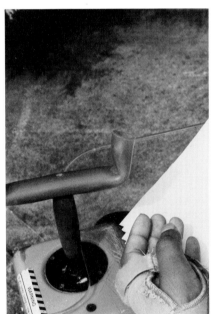

FIGURE 2-63

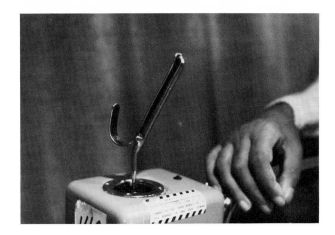

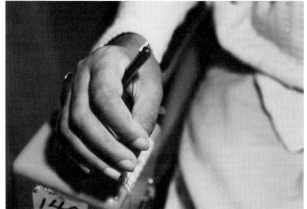

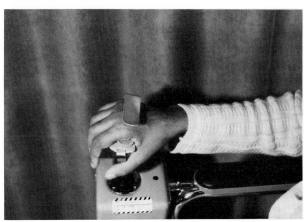

FIGURE 2-64

Palmar Pocket Strap

Hand splints or hand and wrist splints may be used to keep the hand on the controls. These splints may consist of a simple velcro D-ring pocket splint with a removable joystick attached (Fig. 2-65).

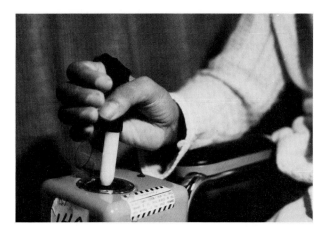

FIGURE 2-65

55

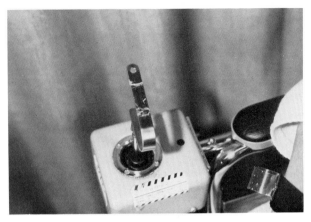
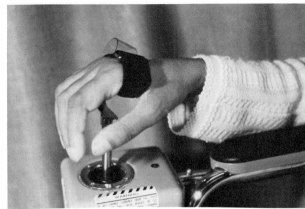

FIGURE 2-66

Horizontal Bar

If the patient has more control with the hand in pronation, a pocket splint may be slipped over a horizontal bar (Fig. 2-66).

Elastic Assist

A light elastic band may also be used to assist in one direction, but care must be taken that the elastic cannot force the joystick into contact on its own (Fig. 2-67).

Wrist Support With Pocket

A patient who requires wrist support may use a wrist support splint with a pocket in the palm. This pocket may be a simple webbing pocket, or a metal sleeve which can accept a joystick. This joystick has a limited movement universal joint which allows a straight-forward movement of the arm to be transformed to the rocker movement required to guide the joystick (Fig. 2-68).

Arm Supports and Restraints

An elbow stop attached to the armrest may be required to prevent the elbow from slipping outwards, losing power required for the hand control (Fig. 2-69).

The trough illustrated can be slipped onto an armrest and used as an arm positioner (Fig. 2-70). A hole may be cut through the support to accommodate a joystick. These armrests are made of polypropylene, which has low friction and is also easily cleaned.

Mobile Arm Support

A mobile arm support may be required, which must be carefully fitted and balanced (Fig. 2-71). Rocker arm supports can be used as a basis for this. The type

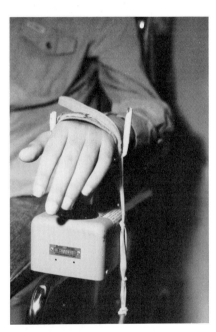

FIGURE 2-67

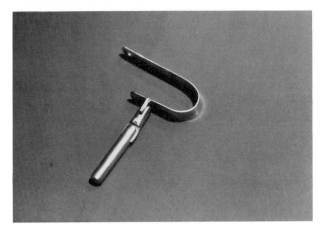
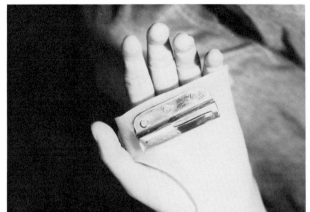

FIGURE 2-68

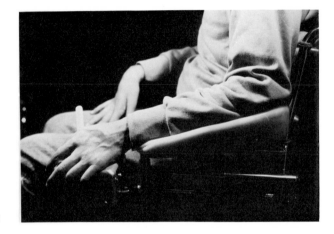
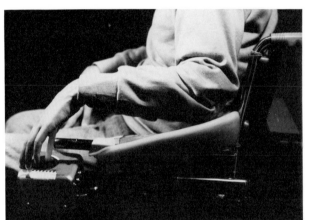

FIGURE 2-69

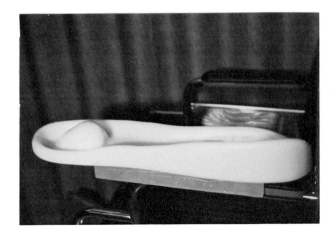
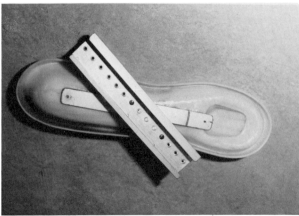

FIGURE 2-70

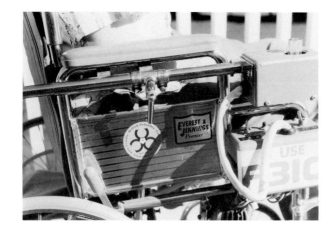
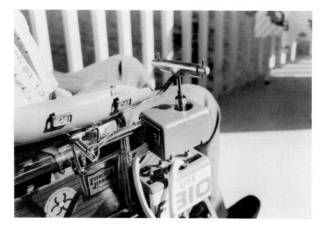
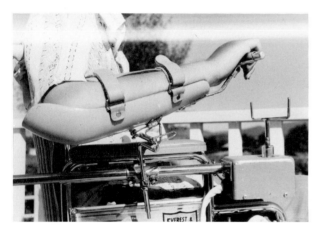
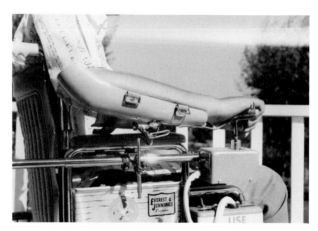

FIGURE 2-71

with proximal and distal ballbearing arms should be shortened so that no large protrusions are left to impede passage through doorways.

Overhead Sling

An overhead sling suspension may be used to support the arm and eliminate gravity (Fig. 2-72). It allows great freedom of movement within its arc, and when balanced may be used as a permanent method of control. The sling suspension may also be used for assessment or for training. Extensor spasticity of the arm may preclude the use of ballbearing arms or sling suspensions. However, if the patient is able to control a safety switch, he may be able to learn in time not to trigger extensor spasms, in the meantime operating the chair safely.

Control Box Adaption for Hand Use

The effort required to move the joystick may be reduced by reducing the spring tension within the box.

Control Positions

The position of the box may be adjusted forwards or backwards, and can also be moved from outside the armrest to the inside (Fig. 2-73). If the box must be moved closer to the center of the wheelchair, more extensive adaption will be required. In this case a swing away arm will be necessary to allow the patient to get out of the wheelchair.

The box may be tilted so that gravity assists the patient to move the joystick in one direction.

Switching Adaptions for Hand Use

The switch control may be adapted by lengthening the switch lever. A finger loop may be attached to the switch lever, or to the lengthened switch lever. A length of cord may be fastened to a fixed point and to the lever so that any pressure on the cord moves the switch in one direction. This may be used as a temporary measure.

A pressure or heat-sensitive switch may be available on some electric wheelchairs. If the wheelchair does not have this type of switch, it can be adapted by a qualified person. The switch can be located so that it can be operated by elbow, shoulder or head movement (Fig. 2-74).

Some patients who use the arm trough type of support for steering may have sufficient power to lift their hand. In this case a padded "dead man" type of switch can be used so that the wheelchair operates only when the hand rests in the trough, on the switch.

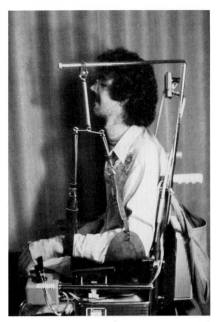

FIGURE 2-72

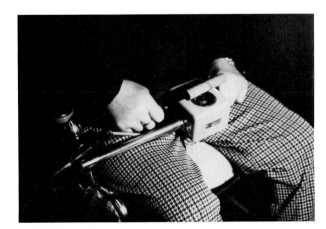

FIGURE 2-73

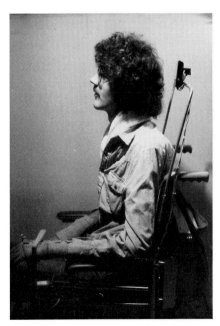

FIGURE 2-74

59

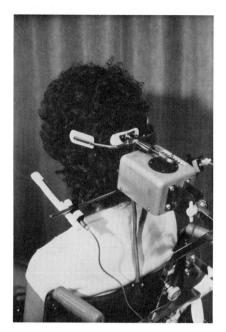

FIGURE 2-75

A patient who has occasional extensor spasms while operating an electric wheelchair will be in danger unless he has an on/off control switch which he can operate even while he is in spasm.

Alternate Controls

Instead of hand controls, head, chin, breath (sip and puff), moisture, heat sensitive, myoelectric, voice or optical head pointer controls may be used. All of these controls are interfaces to microswitches, except the head and chin controls, which are themselves direct proportional controls, and therefore require no interface. If proportional controls can be used, they provide finer maneuverability for the wheelchair; however, the head control cannot be used with a recliner wheelchair because of the need for a headrest in the recliner position. Head, breath, and chin controls require exact positioning of the patient, especially in the early days of learning.

Head Control. The patient who does not require a recliner wheelchair may find the head control very acceptable because it is unobtrusive (Fig. 2-75). All of the proportional controls require on/off switches, which are usually controlled with a shoulder shrug to operate a lever arm. This switch may alternatively be positioned so that it can be operated by pressing the lever with the cheek.

There are two methods of control for use with a microswitch. A switch is turned on and operated continuously until it is turned off. This is called a "latching" type of switch. The alternate method is a "momentary" or a "dead man" switch in which pressure or contact must be maintained for the switch to operate. As soon as pressure is released, the switch is off.

The latching mode, where a switch is turned on and continues to operate until another switch is made, can be dangerous because the moving chair will not stop if the patient drops the interface or loses control of the switching mechanism. The momentary or dead man mode may be tiring for the patient because the switch pressure must be maintained to move the wheelchair. It is, however, safe.

Sip and Puff Control. The patient must be able to move her head enough to reach forward for the tubing if a sip and puff interface is used (Fig. 2-76). Most

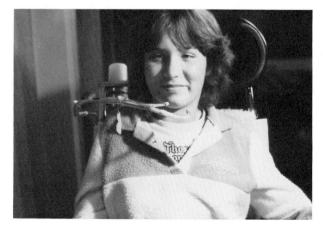
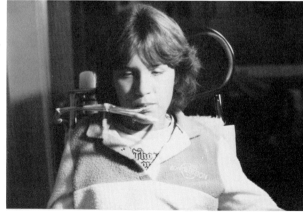

FIGURE 2-76

modes, that is, forward, or backward are latching switches, and are usually operated by hard or soft puffs or sips, singly or doubled. Some modes, such as for turning, may be momentary, for instance, a continuous soft puff may be required to turn right.

Short Throw Control. Dependent on head control, this short throw system can be mounted in a variety of fixed or movable positions (Fig. 2-77). The short

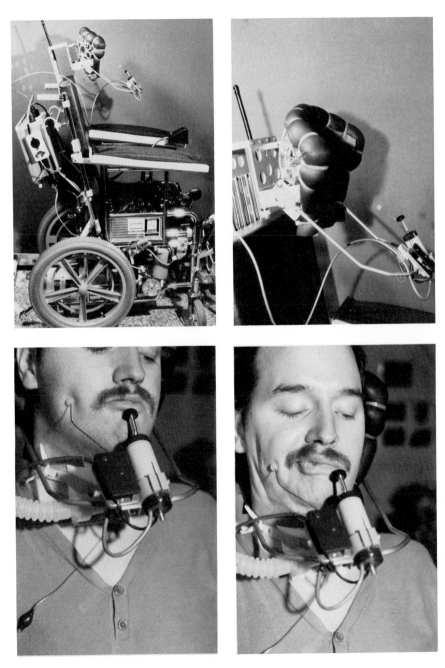

FIGURE 2-77

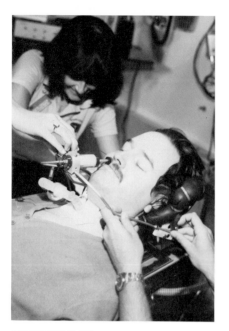

FIGURE 2-78

throw control is a proportional mechanism which can operate the chair or can be switched to operate environmental controls. The system is appropriate for a patient with weak or absent neck musculature. In Figure 2-77 the individual is unable to move his head forward to reach the controls, so they must be positioned within easy facial access. As well, the head piece is molded so that it fits the patient, and the controls can be placed accurately each time.

Control Placement. Before attempting to place controls, the patient must be well positioned; and careful note, or a photograph, may be taken of the position so that it can be reproduced.

The controls must be carefully placed for comfort and for ease of operation (Fig. 2-78). It should be remembered that the patient may fatigue quickly at first, and also his abilities may vary slightly from day to day in the earlier stages, and he may therefore become frustrated.

Power Reclining Wheelchairs (Fig. 2-79)

These wheelchairs may be required for weight relief, for people who cannot tolerate sitting for long periods, for people with persisting dizziness, and for those who require frequent rests. To avoid a shear force on the skin of the buttocks, a seat that moves back as the legs are lifted and the back is reclined is ideal. If this is not available, a cushion with a lower shear factor, such as a Roho cushion may be used. The switches may be pressure, toggle, or heat sensitive, operated by shoulder, head, or tongue, or they may be breath, voice, or myoelectric switches. When respirators are required they are attached to the wheelchair. A separate battery is mandatory for the safe operation of the respirator. The wheelchair battery must never be used to operate the respirator.

Progression

While the patient is learning to operate the controls, his positioning may be critical, and he may become frustrated by the variation in his ability caused by small changes in his position. As his ability improves, his positioning becomes less critical. Frequently a patient who has only just been able to operate the control at

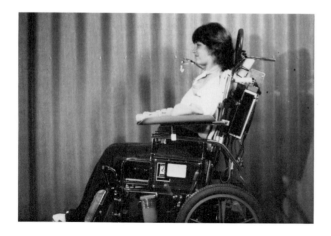

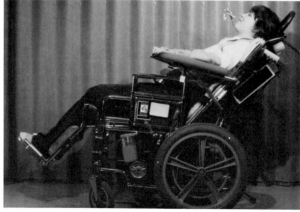

FIGURE 2-79

one time may progress to a different type of control. The therapist must remain alert to these possible changes, which may take place over several years.

It is very important for the quadriplegic person to learn to move in the chair so that he can position himself for comfort and posture, adjust his clothing, position his cushion and pre-position himself for transfers.

Moving Backward and Sitting Up in the Wheelchair

When moving back in the chair, the patient leans forward and transfers part of his weight from his buttocks to his feet. Some of the body weight is placed forward of the knees, which act as a fulcrum. The mechanical advantage gained by this position will enable the buttocks to be levered up and pushed back with the help of shoulder flexion.

Method 1. (Fig. 2-80) In this method the patient places the palms of his

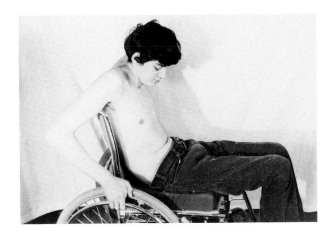
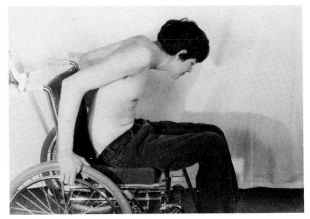
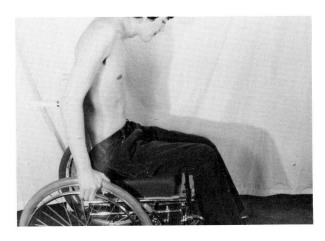
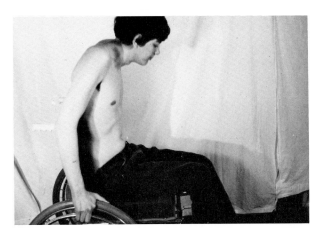

FIGURE 2-80

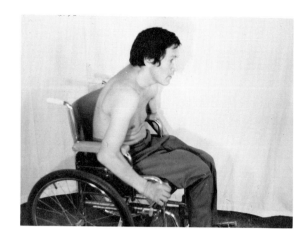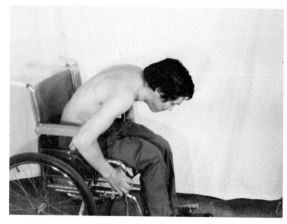
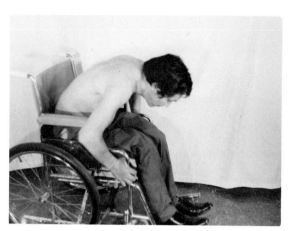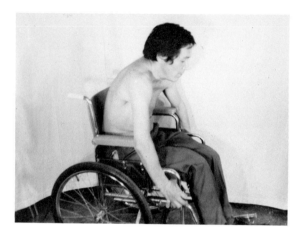

FIGURE 2-81

hands on his wheels and leans forward, so that by depressing his shoulder girdle and flexing his shoulders, he will take the weight off his buttocks and move them back.

Method 2. (Fig. 2-81)   With this technique, the patient places his arms outside the armrests, positioning his thumbs against the inside of the front of the armrests. By flexing his elbows, he pulls his trunk forward; then, flexing his shoulders, he pushes his buttocks back into the chair. A continuation of shoulder flexion will push him to the upright position.

Method 3. (Fig. 2-82)   The patient puts his arms inside the chair arms and places his thumbs against the inside of the front of the armrests. He moves back in the wheelchair, using the same technique as in Method 2. To sit up, he places his elbows on the armrests and works his elbows toward himself as far as possible, using adduction of the shoulders initially and protraction of the shoulders as he progresses to the upright position. He extends his neck quickly to gain momentum as he nears the upright, throwing him past his point of balance against the back of the chair.

64

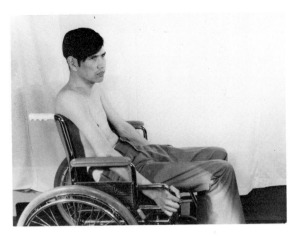

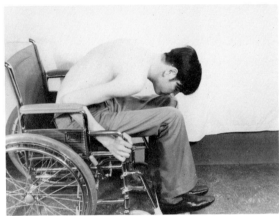

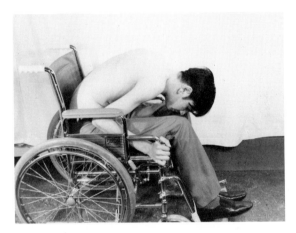

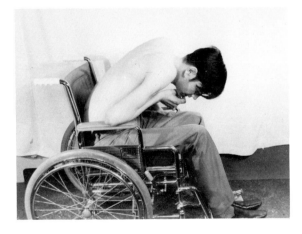

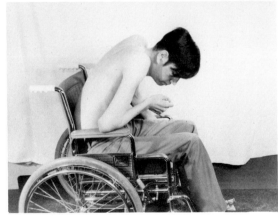

FIGURE 2-82

65

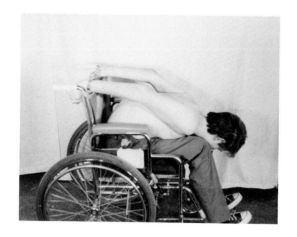
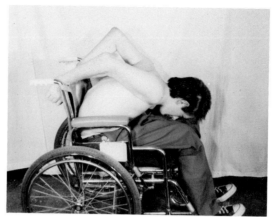
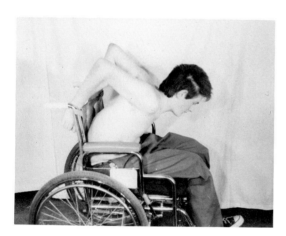
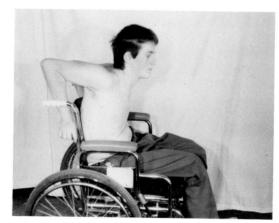

FIGURE 2-83

Method 4. (Fig. 2-83)   Placing both extended wrists over the back of the chair, the patient flexes his trunk forward as far as possible and flexes his elbows both to pull himself back into the chair and to sit himself up. Mechanical advantage is increased by the patient's sliding his hands down the back of the chair as he comes to a sitting position.

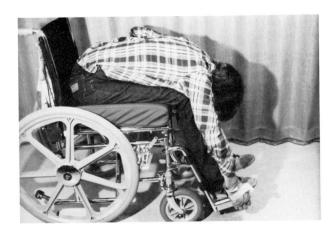
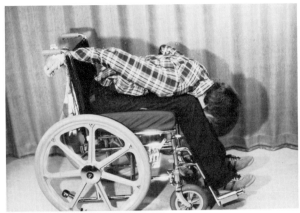
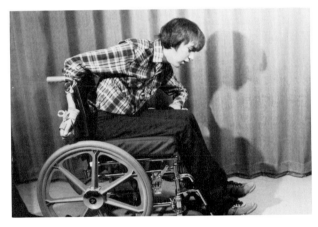
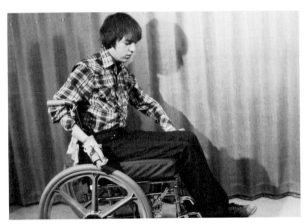

FIGURE 2-84

Method 5. (Fig. 2-84)   After moving back in the wheelchair, the patient swings one hand back to hook over the back of the wheelchair. This may be easier if the patient pushes himself over towards the swinging arm to increase the momentum and to shorten the distance that the arm must swing to hook over the wheelchair back. The patient now leans away from the hooked arm by pushing against his knee with the other hand and his trunk swings around and up in a circle away from the holding arm. As soon as possible he slides his holding arm down the back of the wheelchair to gain height.

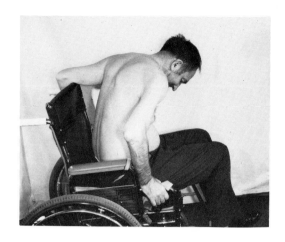

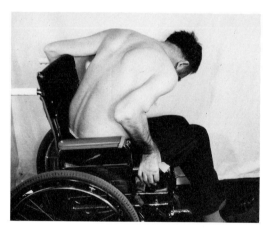

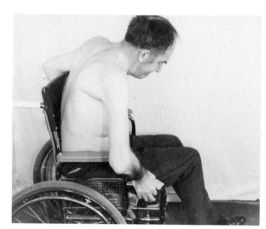

FIGURE 2-85

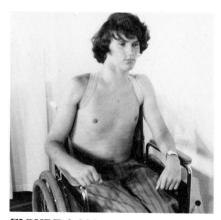

FIGURE 2-86A

Method 6. (Fig. 2-85)   The patient places one arm over the back of the chair and positions his wrist under his knee or chair arm to flex his trunk forward. The arm over the chair back is flexed at the elbow to move himself back in the chair. The other arm is used simultaneously to push against the armrest. Since there is some tendency to twist to one side using this method, the patient may have to repeat the action using the opposite arm over the chair back.

An aid which is very useful in training the quadriplegic in trunk mobility and the development of confidence, is made in the following manner. Two loops of light elastic are fixed to the first screw from the top of the wheelchair back on each side. The loops are placed around the shoulders of the patient, the left loop around the right shoulder and vice versa (Fig. 2-86A). These act as spring assists in lateral and forward trunk movements and eliminate the danger of falling (Fig. 2-86B). The tension can be decreased by elongating the loops as the patient becomes more adept.

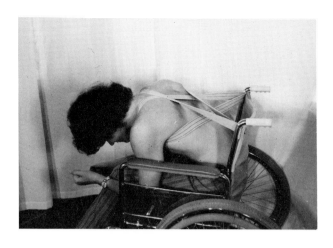

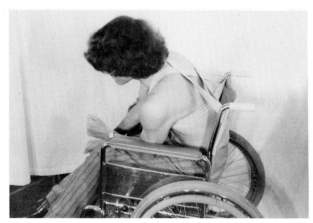

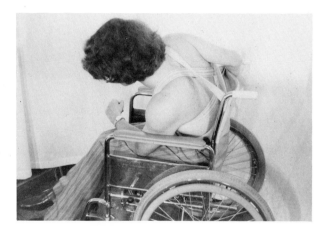

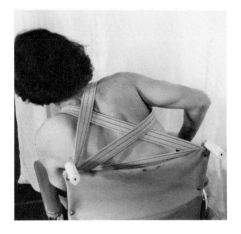

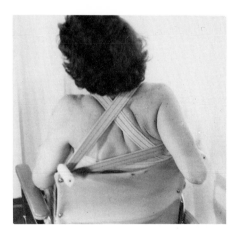

FIGURE 2-86B

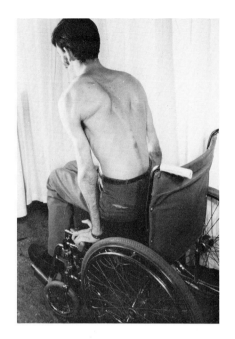

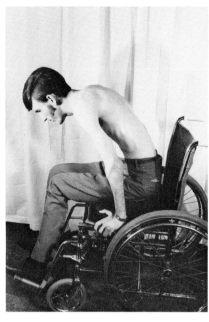

FIGURE 2-87

Moving Forward

   Method 1. (Fig. 2-87)   In this method the patient places both palms on the wheels and locks his elbows. By depressing his shoulder girdle and extending his neck and shoulders sharply he throws his buttocks forward in the chair.
   Method 2. (Fig. 2-88)   The patient puts his thumbs in his pants pockets or

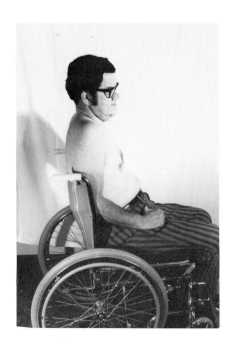

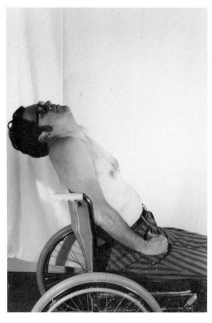

FIGURE 2-88

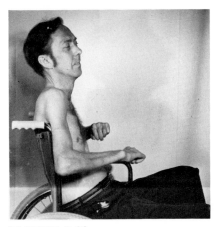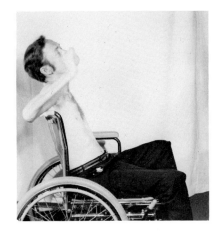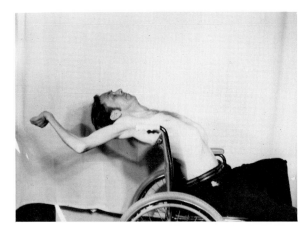

FIGURE 2-89

belt tabs and places his elbows against the chair back as close to his body as possible. He pushes his buttocks forward in the chair by extending his wrists, upper trunk and neck.

Method 3. (Fig. 2-89)   Simultaneously the patient extends his neck and throws both arms up and over his head. This gives sufficient momentum to slide his buttocks forward on the chair seat.

Method 4. (Fig. 2-90)   One arm is hooked around the pushing handle of the chair; the patient flexes this shoulder to pull the trunk over and into rotation and extension. This action relieves the weight from the opposite buttock and tends to move it forward. This forward movement may be enhanced by either swinging the free arm forward vigorously, or by pushing against the arm or wheel of the chair. The action is repeated using opposite arms and alternated until the desired position is reached.

Method 5. (Fig. 2-91)   The patient swings both arms behind the pushing handles of the chair. When he flexes his shoulders vigorously he will extend his

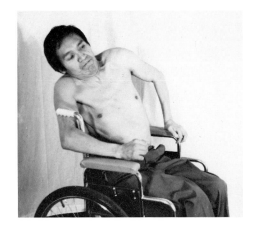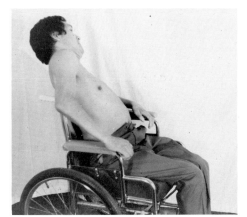

FIGURE 2-90

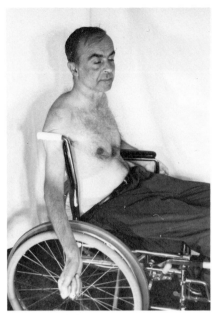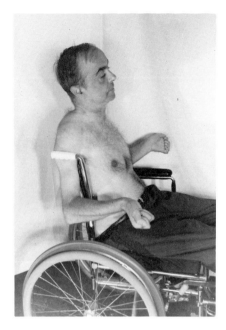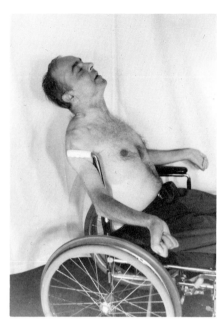

FIGURE 2-91

trunk over the back of the wheelchair, making it into a fulcrum and levering his buttocks forward.

Method 6. (Fig. 2-92)   Extension of neck and shoulders will rock the patient back, causing the bottom of the swivel back to swing forward. This relieves some weight from his buttocks and slides him forward. A stop should be placed so that the patient who cannot adequately control the movement will not slide forward

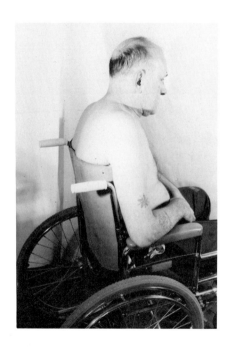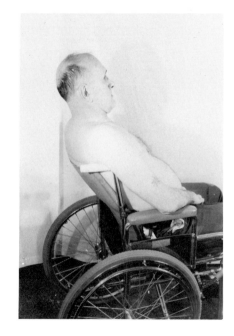

FIGURE 2-92

too far. The stop may be a length of leather running between the two back uprights and behind the swivel back uprights, near the top.

Moving Across the Chair Seat

Method 1. (Fig. 2-93)   Some patients can do a straight-arm pushup on the wheels of the chair. In this situation the patient leans forward until he reaches his

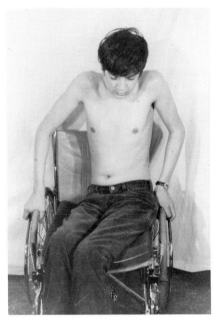
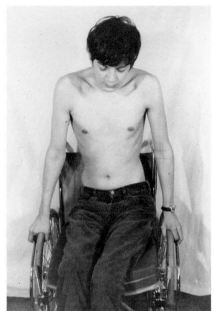
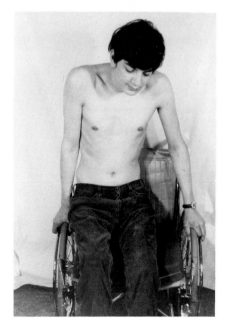
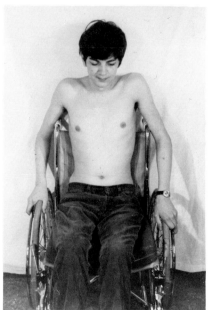

FIGURE 2-93

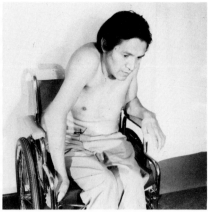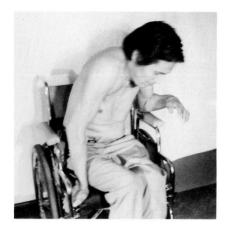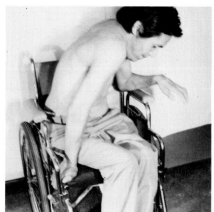

FIGURE 2-94

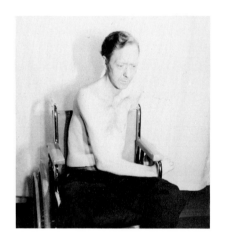

point of balance. He does his pushup using his shoulder depressors, thus enabling him to swing his buttocks laterally. When he is learning this movement he starts by swinging his trunk from side to side in pendulum fashion. This enables him to move further because of the developed momentum.

Method 2. (Fig. 2-94) The patient places a forearm on the inner side of the armrest and leans over this arm. He puts the other hand on the wheelchair cushion at midthigh level and locks the elbow. By depressing both shoulders and flexing his trunk forward and over the armrest, some of the pressure is relieved from the buttocks and they are levered sideways and back.

Method 3. (Fig. 2-95) Placing one arm over the chair back, the patient hooks his elbow under the pushing handle. The other arm is positioned across his body with the thumb web hooked into the chair front upright. This causes him to twist and lean over the armrest with his forearm resting on his thighs. By throwing his trunk forward and flexing both shoulders, his buttocks will move back and towards the opposite side of the chair.

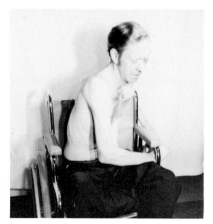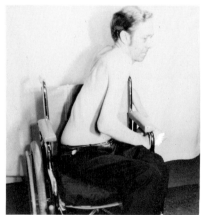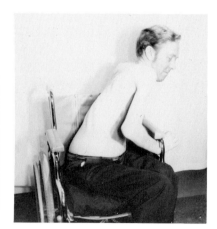

FIGURE 2-95

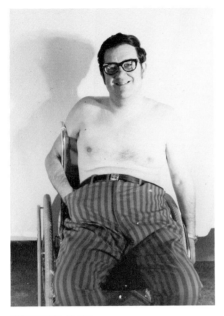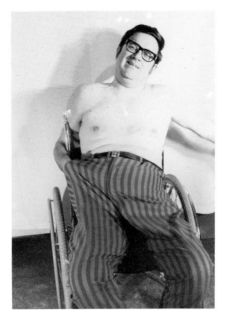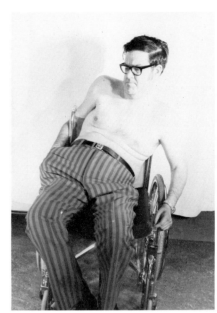

FIGURE 2-96

Method 4. (Fig. 2-96)   This is a particularly useful method for a patient who is wearing a splint on one hand. The patient places one arm over the chair back, hooks his elbow around the pushing handle, and puts his hand into his pants pocket. By throwing his weight over the chair back and simultaneously rotating his shoulder externally he will lever his buttocks over. This also ensures that the pants are wrinkle-free beneath the buttocks.

WEIGHT RELIEF

A seated person who has anesthesia of the buttocks must have relief of pressure, particularly from the bony areas such as the ischial tuberosities and the sacral

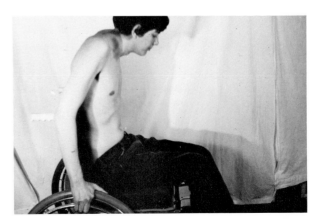

FIGURE 2-97

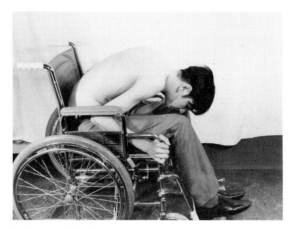

FIGURE 2-98

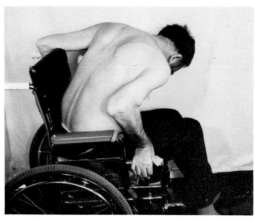

FIGURE 2-99

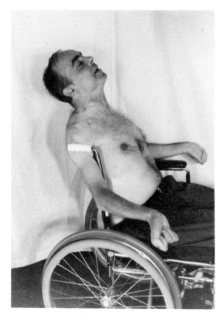

FIGURE 2-100

area. In early rehabilitation, weight relief will have been done at least every quarter of an hour, but with frequent skin inspections individual tolerance can be assessed and increased. Skin condition, patient weight and type of seating required (see Cushions) will vary tremendously and tolerance must be built up carefully.

Weight Relief Methods

Pushing Up. A push up on the wheels is a most effective method of relieving weight from the buttocks (Fig. 2-97).

Leaning Forwards. The person can lean forward and rest his trunk on his knees or on a table surface to take some weight off the buttocks (Fig. 2-98).

Leaning Sideways. The person can lean his trunk sideways over the arm of the chair to relieve weight, leaning first to one side and then to the other (Fig. 2-99).

The wheelchair may be placed parallel to the bed with the brakes on and the armrest removed. Pillows may be positioned on the bed and over the chair wheel so that the patient can be reclined sideways comfortably. He should not be left in this position for long, as while weight is relieved on one side of his buttocks, it is increased on the other. The chair is reversed to allow him to recline on the other side. This method is often used in early days when a patient cannot tolerate leaning forwards onto his chest.

Leaning Backwards. The person can relieve weight by leaning back over the chair back (Fig. 2-100).

The chair may be tipped back to relieve the weight from the patient's buttocks (Fig. 2-101). This position may also be very useful for the patient who is becoming used to the upright position but who has dizzy spells (postural hypotension) and who must be reclined to prevent a black-out. This blackout is caused because patients who are brought to the upright position in the early stages may experience a rapid fall in blood pressure due to the inability of the vasoconstrictors to act, thus allowing pooling of the blood in the lower extremities.

If the person must be reclined for more lengthy periods, the chair may be

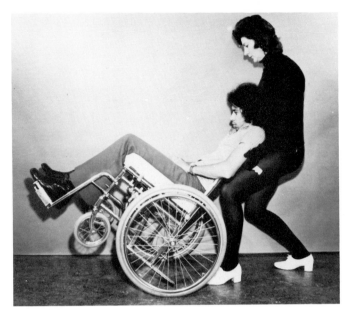

FIGURE 2-101

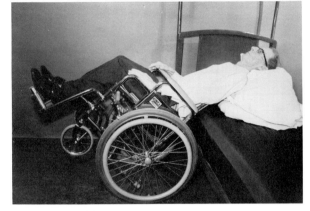

FIGURE 2-102

tipped back and the pushing handles rested on a bed. If a pillow is placed under the head and shoulders, this position can be very comfortable and save transfers to the bed (Fig. 2-102).

The person who uses a reclining chair may recline the back to change position and to take weight from the buttocks (Fig. 2-103).

Tolerance. Weight can be relieved by having only short periods in the chair, increasing tolerance by degrees. Bedrest may be used in the early stages to alternate with the chair, but later, and particularly if areas of skin redness begin to develop, a stretcher or prone board may be used to allow continued mobility (Fig. 2-104 and 2-105).

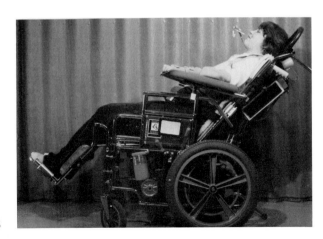

FIGURE 2-103

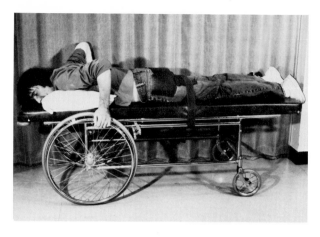

FIGURE 2-104

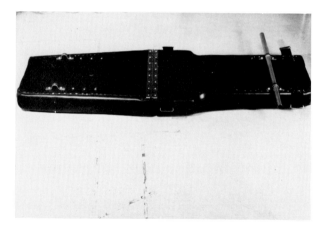
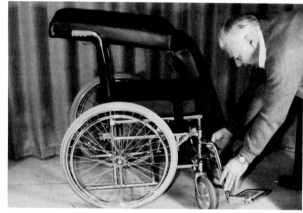

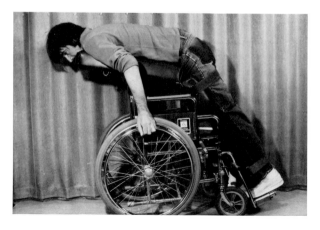
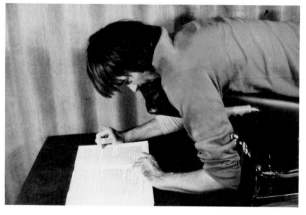

FIGURE 2-105

Stretchers and Prone Boards

A patient who is unable to sit because of incipient or developed decubitus ulcers may use a stretcher for mobility (see Fig. 2-104).

A stretcher is useful in an institution, but in a home it is very clumsy and hard to maneuver. The person at home may find a prone board, which fits onto a wheelchair, very practical and comfortable (see Fig. 2-105). The prone board is made of two pieces of 3/4 inch (1.91 cm) plywood, hinged together. The lower section is attached to the wheelchair by an adjustable bar designed to slip through the swing-away footrest supports. This is the only fastening that is required since the prone board rests against the front of the wheelchair seat and the top of the wheelchair back. If the patient is heavy, or will use the prone board a great deal, a belt across the pushing handles will preserve the back upholstery. The prone board is upholstered with 4 inches (10.16 cm) of covered foam. Many people find this very comfortable and can work or read for hours resting the chin on the edge of the padded board.

Some patients cannot use the prone board because of flexor spasticity of the legs, causing great difficulty in getting the patient onto the board, and once he is on, in keeping his feet positioned. Some patients have trouble breathing well in this position and cannot tolerate it.

If a person has a decubitus ulcer, he should be lifted onto the prone board from the prone position in bed. If he can sit for short periods, he may sit facing the prone board on the edge of the bed with his feet on the foot rests of the wheelchair; the ankle strap is then fastened. If the patient is tall, the wheelchair may be tipped forward so that the foot rests are on the floor. A shorter person may require a block under the foot rests. The castors are turned back and blocked with a foot while the patient is pulled forward and levered up onto the prone board by a person on either side. The wheelchair is lowered to its normal position, the thigh strap is then fastened, and the patient can become mobile. Care must be taken that the feet are close together so that the castors do not touch the toes during a turn. In some cases longer footrests may be required for the person who is very flaccid or has large feet.

MAINTENANCE

The necessity of weekly maintenance should not be overlooked, since the wheelchair is the equivalent of legs to a quadriplegic. The following should be done once weekly:

The tubing should be cleaned with a type of cleaner that leaves a wax finish, and which when polished provides a protective coating.

Lint should be removed from around the axles with a bottle brush.

Vinyl cleaner will both clean and preserve the upholstry.

The wheels should be checked for loose spokes and worn bearings. Pneumatic tires should be tested for correct pressure.

A few drops of light oil should be applied to the bearings at the hubs. Care must be taken not to apply too much oil because it will drip and gather lint.

The patient himself may do as many of these tasks as he can, depending on the severity of his disability. He will be more efficient if he can work from a firm padded surface on the floor. Regular maintenance will reduce the number of costly repairs and the possibility of being without a wheelchair.

USEFUL REFERENCES AND AIDS

BROWN, JC, ET AL: Late spinal deformities in quadriplegic children and adolescents. Journal of Pediatric Orthopedics. 4 (4): 456-61. Aug. 1984. (Discusses prevention of spinal deformity in the paralyzed growing person. Shows why seating should be an important concern.)

GARBER, SL, ET AL: A system for clinically evaluating wheelchair pressure-relief cushions. The American Journal of Occupational Therapy. Vol. 32, No. 9. Oct. 1978.

GARBER, SL: A classification of wheelchair seating. The American Journal of Occupational Therapy. Vol. 33, No. 10. Oct. 1979.

GARBER, SL, Krouskop, TA: Body build and its relationship to pressure distribution in the seated wheelchair patient. Archives of Physical Medicine and Rehabilitation, Vol. 63, Jan. 1982.

GARBER, SL: Wheelchair cushions for spinal cord injured individuals. The American Journal of Occupational Therapy. Vol. 39, No. 11. Nov. 1985.

GARBER, SL and KROUSKOP, TA: Wheelchair cushion modification and its effect on pressure. Archives of Physical Medicine and Rehabilitation, Vol. 65, Oct. 1984.

McCLAY, I: Electric wheelchair propulsion using a hand control in C4 quadriplegia. Physical Therapy, Vol. 63, No. 2. Feb. 1983. (Describes the progression in ability which often occurs, and which makes an early decision on the type of interface required for the wheelchair so difficult.)

3

Bed Mobility and Transfers

BED TYPES	Mattresses
Three Quarter Bed	Additional Equipment
Double Bed	Overhead Equipment
Bed With Head Gatch	Self-Positioning In the Bed
Adjustable Height Bed	Sitting Up In Bed
"Sitting Bed"	Transferring
Turning Bed	

BED TYPES

The bed should have a sturdy metal frame if equipment is to be attached. These beds are obtainable as a single bed from hospital suppliers. The deck of the bed should be 13–1/2 inches (34.29 cm) from the floor if a 6-inch (15.24 cm) spring filled mattress is used. This will bring the top of the mattress to the same height as the top of the 3-inch (7.62 cm) foam cushion on the standard wheelchair with the seat rails 19–1/2 inches (49.53 cm) from the floor when both cushion and mattress are compressed equally. There must be adequate room under the bed frame for the footrests to allow a close and angled approach of the wheelchair for transfers.

THREE QUARTER BED

The width of the bed may be increased by adding a 3/4 inch (1.91 cm) thick plywood deck to extend beyond the sides. The weight of most patients will not be sufficient to tip a single bed if the width is increased to three quarter size. This size may facilitate independent turning. The dependent patient is more easily managed in a single bed so that the attendant does not have to reach so far.

Double Bed

Couples who wish to use a double bed may find that two single beds pushed together is more practical. This allows easy bedding changes in case of accidents, and also allows one partner to have a waterproof mattress, or a gatch head if required.

Bed With Head Gatch

A head gatch, either manually or electrically operated, may be extremely useful for the management of the dependent patient. Sitting in bed with the head portion elevated for long periods should be avoided, as the mattress folds and wrinkles under the buttocks. The electric head gatch may be useful for the independent patient during dressing and for assisting him to sit up in bed.

Adjustable Height Bed

An adjustable height bed is useful for the nursing care of the dependent patient. The patient who is learning to become independent may also find this bed useful, so that the bed can be lowered when he is transferring into bed, and raised when he transfers to the wheelchair.

"Sitting" Bed

A commercially made bed for general public use which positions a person so that he sits with bent knees, may be useful for a quadriplegic to relieve the pressure on his heels so that clothing may be put on more easily over his feet (Fig. 3-1). It also assists him to sit up in bed.

Turning Bed

A bed which turns the patient from side to side, either by time switch, or microswitch, can be a major contribution to allowing a patient to remain with his

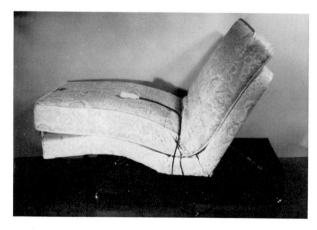

FIGURE 3-1

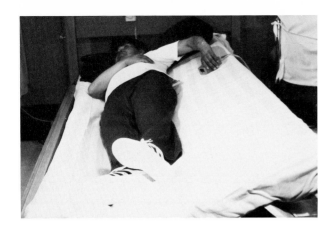

FIGURE 3-2

family (Fig. 3-2). Many quadriplegic patients must turn or be turned every two hours during the night, and this may be an unacceptable drain on the patient or on the family.

All of the beds described should have rubber tipped legs to prevent any sliding. Wheels or castors, even with the brakes applied, are less secure.

MATTRESSES

Spring-Filled Mattress

A firm, spring-filled mattress facilitates movement on the bed and is commonly used by an independent patient. This type of mattress does not bend easily, therefore a firm foam mattress is required if a gatch bed is used. These mattresses must be covered with waterproof ticking in case of accidents. The ticking must be smooth and free of buttons.

Alternating Pressure Pads, Water, Gel, or Air Mattresses

A person prone to pressure sores may use an alternating pressure pad. This pad will allow longer periods between position changes. Water, gel, or air mattresses are alternatives that may suit some individuals. None of the flotation mattresses are easy to move on independently, as the patient's hands and buttocks sink into them. If any mattress, such as a waterbed, requires a containing wall, the top of the wall must be well padded to prevent trauma during transfer.

Sheepskin Covering

Any of these mattresses may be covered in addition to the normal bedding, by sheepskin or a synthetic substitute. The latter is easier to wash and dry. The independent patient may require the sheepskin to be anchored like a drawsheet.

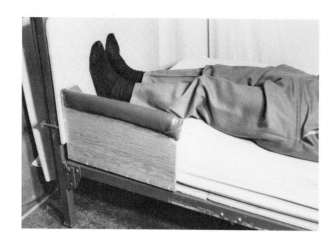

FIGURE 3-3

Footboard

A footboard will take the weight of the covers from the feet, which will facilitate movement in bed.

Leg Retainer Board

A leg retainer board will provide leverage and prevent the legs from falling off the bed during transfer (Fig. 3-3). The top and inside should be padded with 1-inch (2.54 cm) foam rubber, and upholstered.

Slippery Surfaces

A nylon contour sheet will be an advantage to patients who must move by sliding. The sheet should be a tight fit to prevent wrinkling and should have a conventional sheet beneath it to absorb moisture. The contour sheet is useful if a patient requires a sliding surface everywhere on the bed, but a nylon draw sheet will allow the buttocks to move while preserving a nonskid surface for the patient's hands on the linen sheet near the head of the bed.

There are two methods shown for fastening drawsheets. Figure 3-4A shows a thin walled conduit tube, sleeved through a hem on the nylon sheet with hooks and elastic to hold the sheet taut to the bedframe. Hooks and elastics are not commercially available, but are easily constructed.

Figure 3-4B shows a draw sheet on a gatch bed where a tube attachment cannot be used. A heavy canvas is placed under the mattress, and the draw sheet is fastened to it with velcro. The heavy canvas is required to prevent the sheet from ruckling.

Stabilizing

Generally, castor locks on the wheelchair will be sufficient to prevent the front of the wheelchair from moving sideways (Fig. 3-5). Occasionally, bed hooks

84

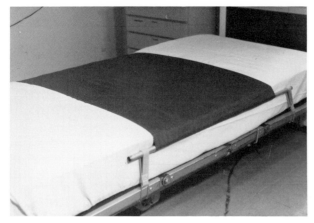

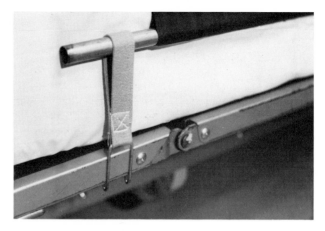

FIGURE 3-4 A

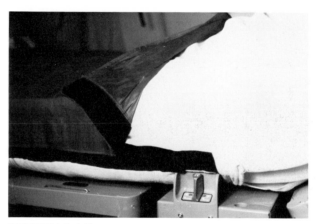

FIGURE 3-4 B

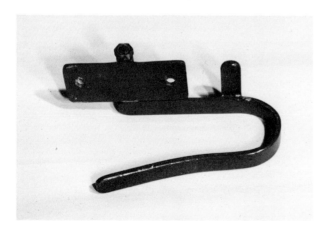

FIGURE 3-5

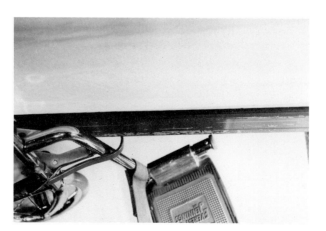

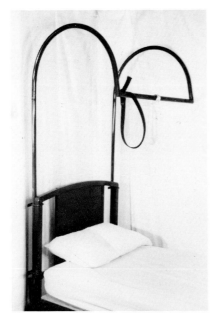

FIGURE 3-6

may also be required to prevent either front or rear wheels from sliding away from the bed during transfers. If these are to be permanently installed they should fold away, for safety (See Appendix II).

For front approach transfers, hooks with an automatic spring lock can be used. (See Appendix II).

OVERHEAD EQUIPMENT

Overhead Bar

If an overhead bar is required it must be strongly constructed, and may be attached either to the bed frame or the wall behind the bed (Fig. 3-6). The bar should run the full width of the bed and be approximately above the elbows of the patient when his arms are by his side. The minimum height of the bar should be just beyond arms reach when the patient is sitting. Final adjustments must be made to suit the individual patient.

Overhead Bar With Projections

A projection from the center of the bar may be added, which runs horizontally toward the foot of the bed for no more than half the length of the bed (Fig. 3-7). A longer projection requires attachment at the foot of the bed (Fig. 3-8).

Double Bars

Two bars, one on either side and eight inches in from the edge of the bed, may be attached to overhead bars at the head and foot of the bed (Fig. 3-9).

Outrigger

An outrigger is a continuation of the overhead bar that projects out over the wheelchair (Fig. 3-10). The end of the projection must be padded to protect people who may inadvertently walk into it.

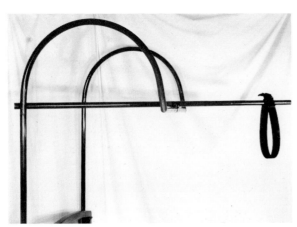

FIGURE 3-7

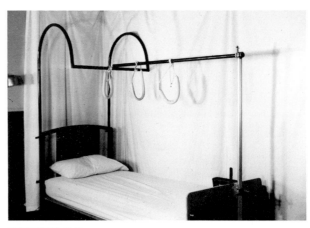

FIGURE 3-8

86

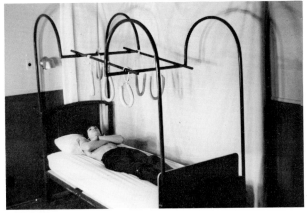

FIGURE 3-9

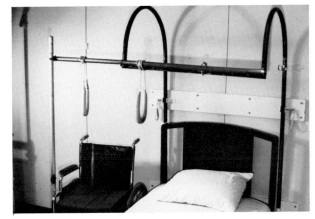

FIGURE 3-10

Fastening Method For Bars

These may be fastened temporarily by interlocking two hose clamps fastened around the bars.

Acceptable Décor

Once final positioning of overhead straps is established and the patient has been able to discard equipment required only during training, overhead bars, if required, can be built to the individual's needs and tastes. Overhead bars can be camouflaged as part of a four poster bed, or as part of the décor of the room (Fig. 3-11).

Overhead Straps

Floating straps are placed around the overhead bars and left free to slide along the bar. The buckle must be firmly fastened with no projections (Fig. 3-12).

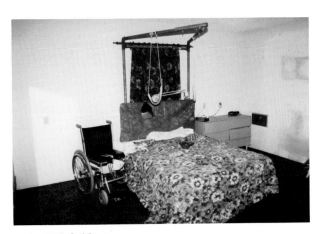

FIGURE 3-11

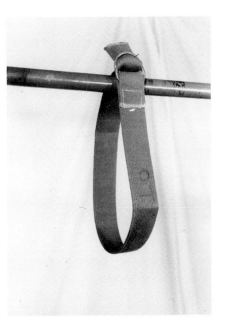

FIGURE 3-12

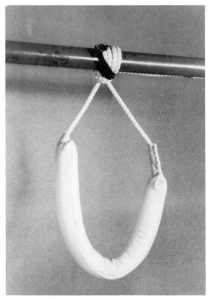

FIGURE 3-13

Fixed straps are placed around the bar and taped or bolted into position (Fig. 3-13).

Turning in Bed

Supine to Prone. (Methods of turning can be learned most easily on a gymnastic mat).

Method 1. (Fig. 3-14)   The patient tucks one arm under his body palm up, then flings his other arm and shoulder violently across his body. He turns his head sharply in the direction of his arm to add momentum. This twists his upper trunk, and the rest of his body follows until he is prone.

Method 2. (Fig. 3-15)   The patient sits up, works one extended arm behind him close to his body, pivots on it, and throws himself over the arm onto his face. This can be accomplished more easily if his legs can be crossed first. This is often done by leaning forward and inserting an arm under one leg and over the other. Lifting the elbow will lever the leg over.

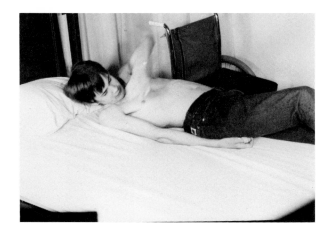

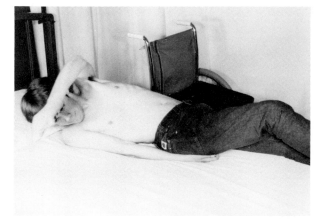

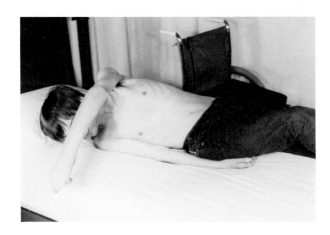

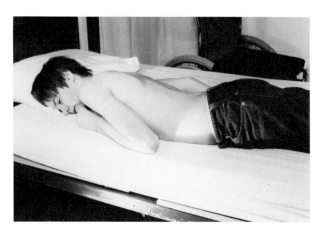

FIGURE 3-14

88

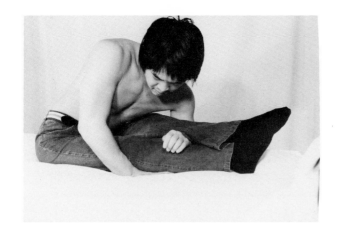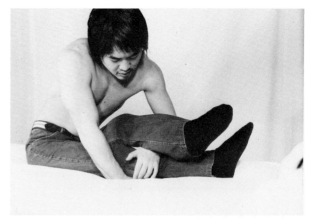

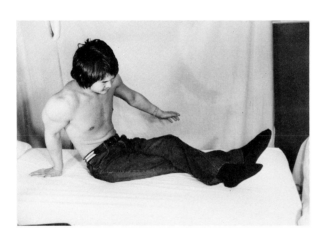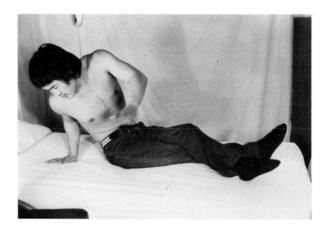

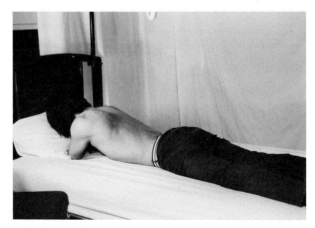

FIGURE 3-15

89

Method 3. (Fig. 3-16)   The patient inserts her wrist into an overhead strap and pulls up, enabling her to work her elbow underneath her upper trunk. She takes her arm out of the strap and throws her trunk over the elbow. She

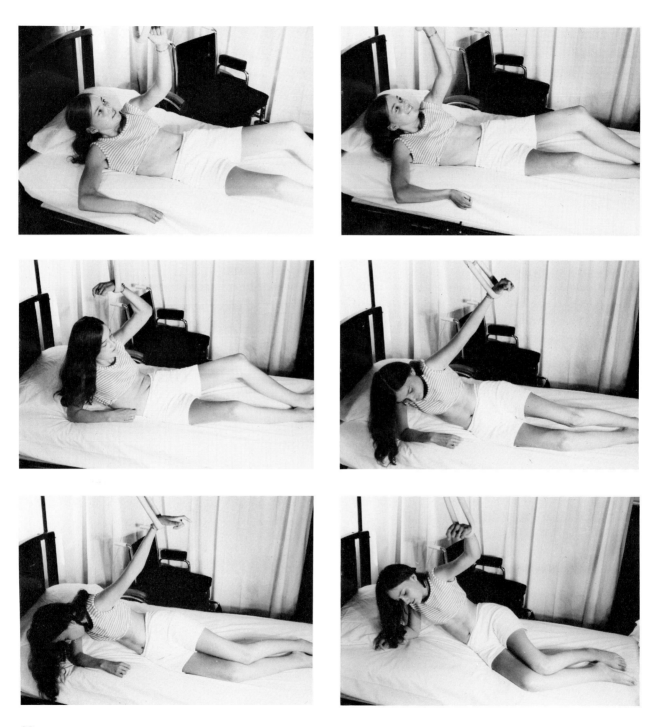

FIGURE 3-16

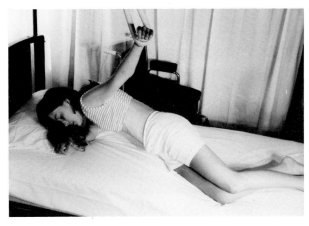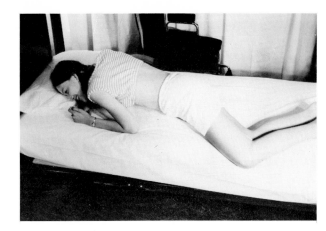

FIGURE 3-16   Continued

may have to reach over and hook her wrists through a strap at the side of the bed or use the edge of the mattress to pull herself completely over.

Method 4. (Fig. 3-17)   The patient flexes his trunk to one side, using his head and elbows to lever himself over, or by pulling on the edge of the bed. The arm on the extended side is swung in behind the back of his head. He reaches vigorously over his trunk with the other arm, thus gaining momentum to roll partially onto his side. He places his free hand on the bed, and turns by using the friction of this hand on the bed to pull himself over the flexed arm.

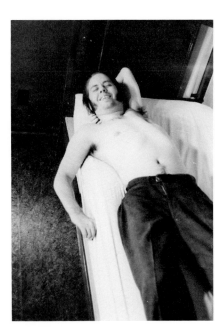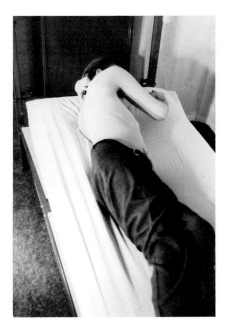

FIGURE 3-17

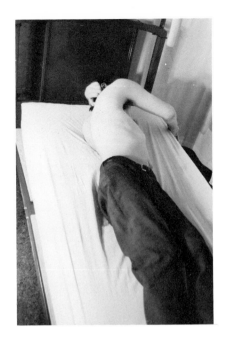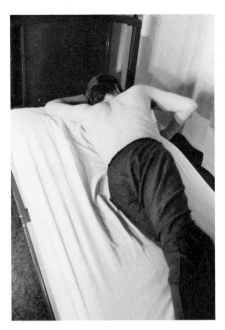

FIGURE 3-17   Continued

Method 5. (Fig. 3-18)   A patient may turn independently using an electric hydraulic turning bed. This can be activated by a manual switch operated by the patient, or he can program the control to turn from side to side at regular intervals. Many patients will not awaken during the turning process, once they are used to it.

Prone to Supine, Right to Left (Fig. 3-19). The patient flexes his trunk to the right. He places his right hand on the bed level with his shoulder, his elbow flexed at 90° above his hand. The left arm is placed under his head. As he pushes with the right hand on the bed, the left arm is worked further under his head until the left elbow points towards the right shoulder. In this position, he can maintain balance. By pushing with the left elbow and flinging the right arm backwards, he

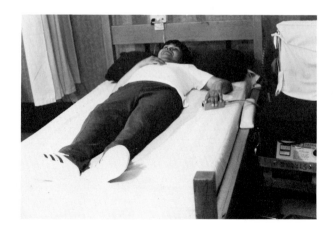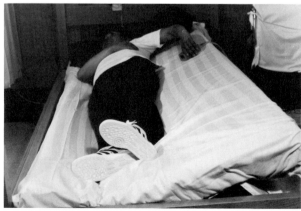

FIGURE 3-18

will roll over to his left. The patient may, when balanced on the elbow, reach with the right hand for the overhead strap to give additional leverage.

Basically, all quadriplegics use this method to turn from prone to supine, although slight variation of hand, arm and head positions might be noted.

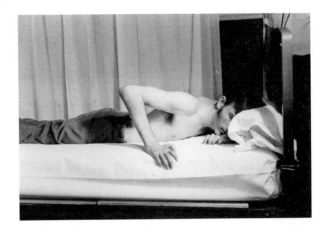

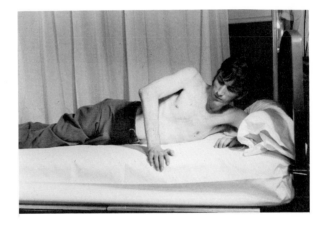

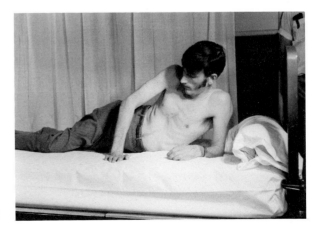

FIGURE 3-19

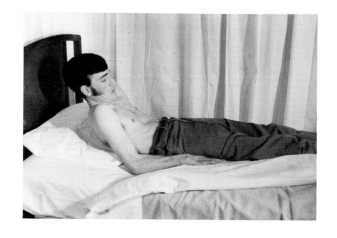
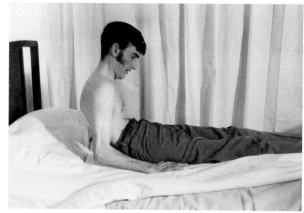
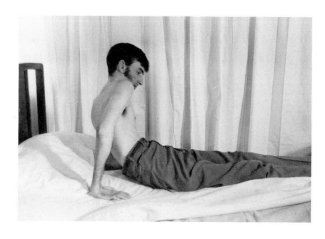
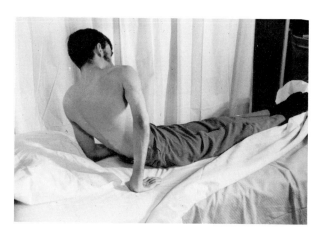
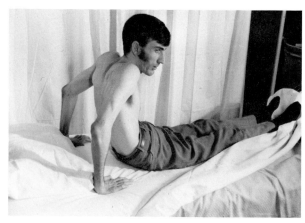

FIGURE 3-20

94

Sitting Up In Bed

Method 1. (Fig. 3-20) The patient slides his hands palm down under his buttocks and uses his wrist extensors, elbow flexors, and shoulder adductors and flexors to pull himself up onto his elbows. He now leans over one elbow and balances on it while flinging the other arm behind his buttocks and locking the elbow. He balances on the locked arm while flinging the other arm behind and locking it also.

Method 2. (Fig. 3-21) The patient rolls to one side. He places his wrist in an overhead strap, which is just within his reach, and he pulls his head and shoulders

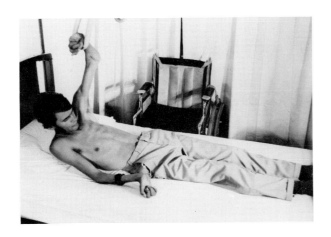
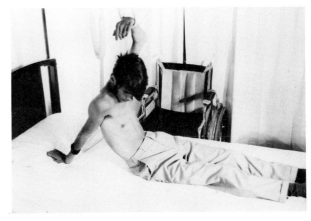

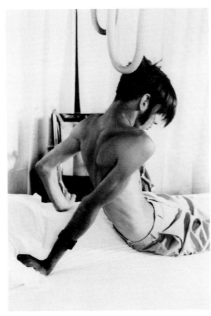
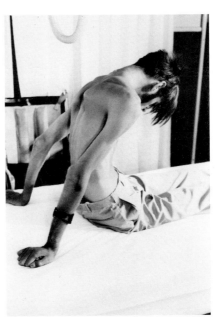

FIGURE 3-21

off the bed. This allows him to throw his disengaged arm behind him and to lock the elbow. He now removes his arm from the sling and, balancing on the locked arm, he throws his other arm behind him and locks the elbow. By flexing his head and shoulders sharply, a bouncing motion is produced, giving him the opportunity to slide his hands forward on the bed until sitting balance is reached.

Method 3. (Fig. 3-22)   The patient rolls to one side and up onto his elbow. He uses his legs as an anchor point for his arm to hook around to pull himself around and up to sitting; the other arm helps by pushing against the wheelchair.

Method 4. (Fig. 3-23)   The patient may use an overhead strap to lift himself up so that he can work his way around using his other elbow on the bed. The patient must check the skin on his elbow frequently if he uses this method because of the friction of the sheet.

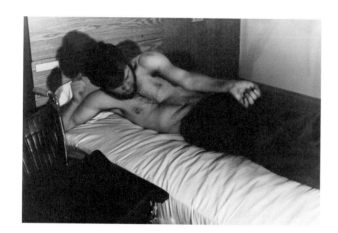
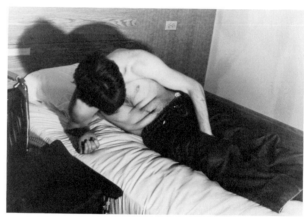
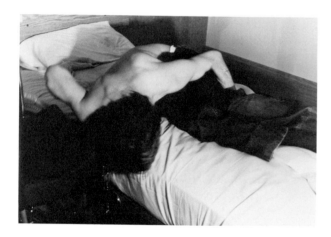
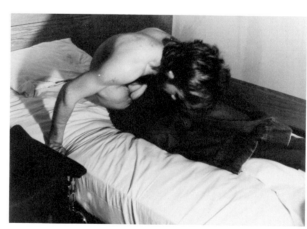

FIGURE 3-22

96

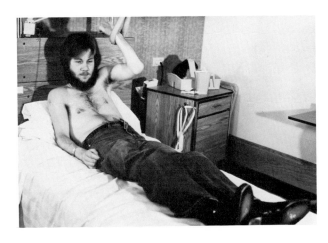
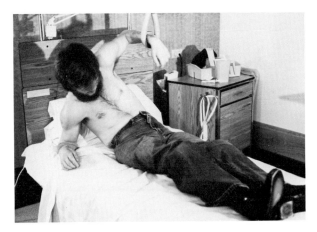
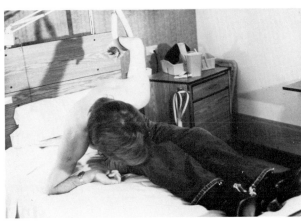
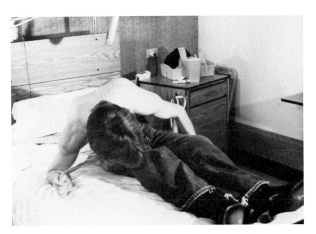
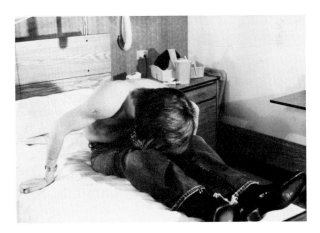

FIGURE 3-23

97

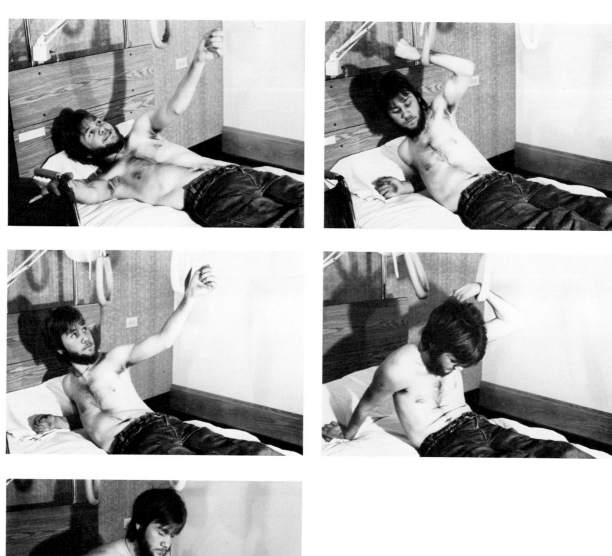

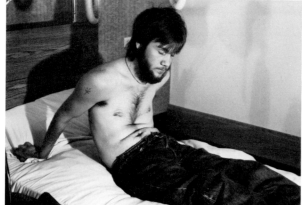

FIGURE 3-24

Method 5. (Fig. 3-24)   In this method, it is important that the patient pull high enough on the first strap to move his elbow well underneath his trunk to balance on the elbow before reaching for the second overhead strap, so that he does not fall back. Once he has pulled up on the second overhead strap he should be sitting high enough to fling an arm behind himself and lock the elbow. This hand must also be well behind him to enable him to balance and release his other hand from the strap.

Method 6. (Fig. 3-25) The patient rolls to one side. He places his wrist in an overhead strap, which is just within his reach, and he pulls his head and shoulders

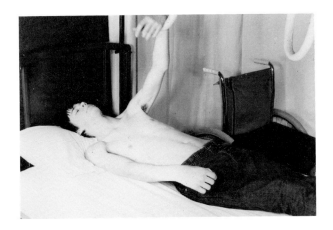 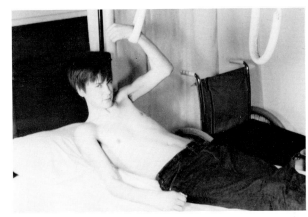

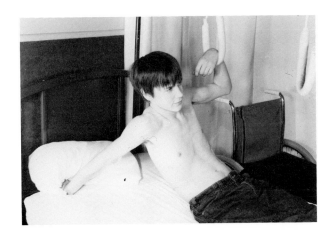 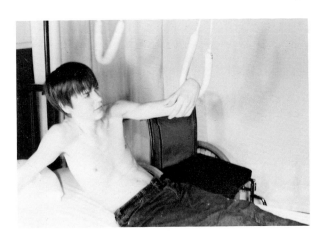

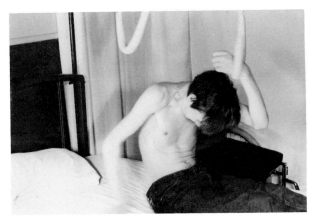

FIGURE 3-25

off the bed. This allows him to throw his disengaged arm behind him and to lock the elbow. He now removes his arm from the sling and, balancing on the locked arm, he reaches for a fixed sling that had been placed in a more forward position. He now pulls himself to the upright position. He slides his locked arm forwards towards his buttock until he can remove his other arm from the sling.

Method 7. Two overhead bars are fixed, one at the head and one at the foot of the bed. A rope ladder is attached to the corners of these bars, thus giving maximum stability. The ladder is allowed to hang loosely so that the patient can just reach it (Fig. 3-26A). The smoothly padded rungs should be spaced as far

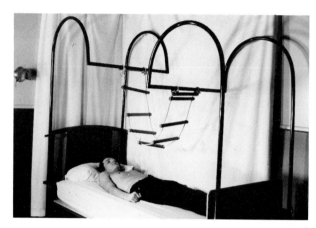

FIGURE 3-26 A

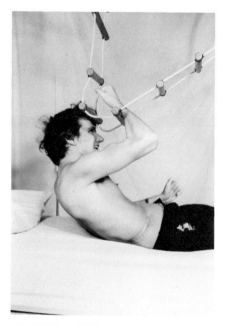
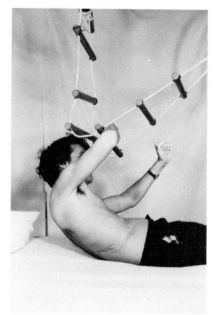

FIGURE 3-26 B

100

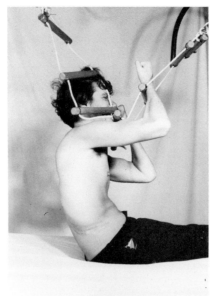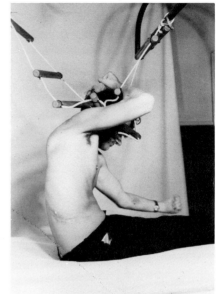

FIGURE 3-26 B   Continued

apart as possible within the patient's reach. He reaches forward and hooks his wrist up behind the first rung (Fig. 3-26B), and pulls himself up as far as possible before reaching for the next rung with his other wrist. He repeats this until he reaches sitting balance.

A more permanent arrangement can be made with two balkan beams placed about 8 inches (20.32 cm) in from the edges of the bed. Fixed and floating straps can be attached to these in the positions predetermined by the rope ladder (Fig. 3-27). This equipment is more stable than the ladder.

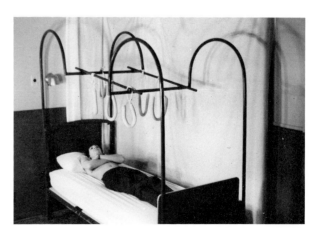

FIGURE 3-27

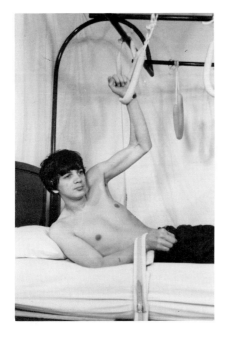

FIGURE 3-28

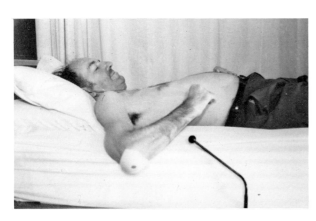

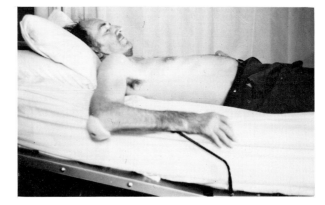

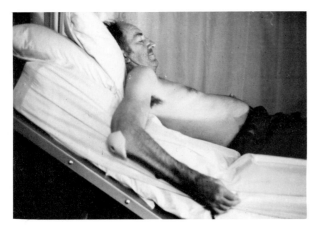

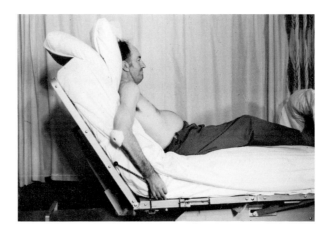

FIGURE 3-29

Method 8. A strap may be fixed to the bed frame for insertion of the wrist, giving initial leverage so that an overhead sling may be reached (Fig. 3-28).

Method 9. A bed with an electrically operated gatch may be required. The lever or micro-switch should be operable by the patient if possible (Fig. 3-29).

Sitting To Lying

Method 1. (Fig. 3-30) The patient is in long sitting position with his hands on the bed at midthigh level and his elbows locked. He pushes his trunk back to just beyond the point of balance. He quickly extends his shoulders and flexes his elbows so that as he drops back, he rests his weight on his elbows. He lowers himself the remaining distance by abducting his shoulders.

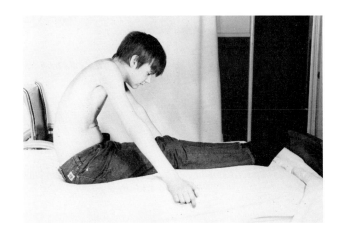 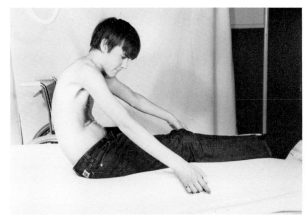

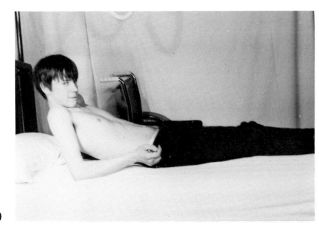 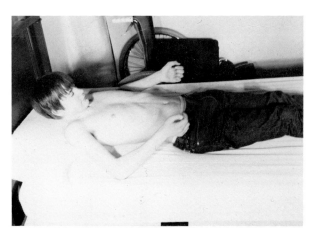

FIGURE 3-30

Method 2. (Fig. 3-31)　The same technique is used as in Method 1, but rather than drop back onto his elbows he throws his arms back into the locked position, thus giving him more control of his rate of fall. He drops onto an elbow by internally rotating the shoulder, thus releasing the elbow lock. He drops onto the other elbow and continues as in Method 1.

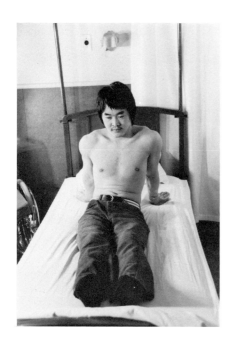
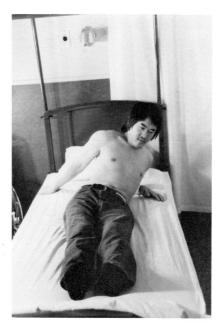
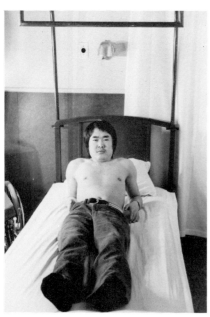
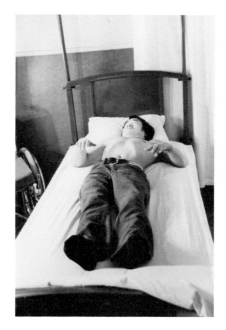

FIGURE 3-31

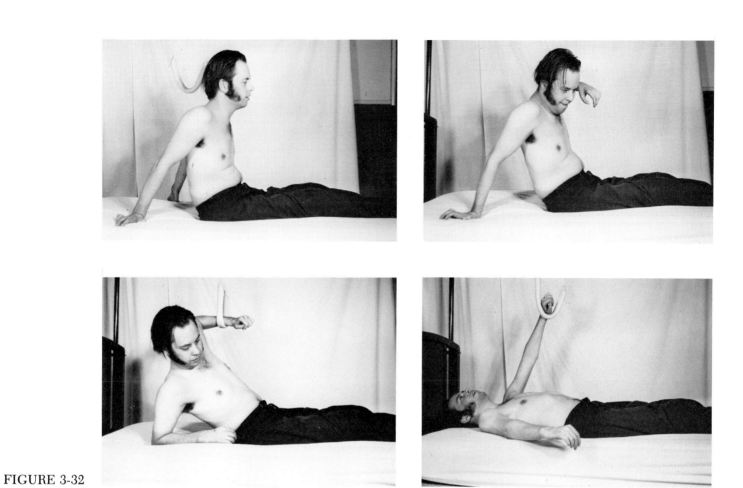

FIGURE 3-32

Method 3. In this method the patient places his wrists in suitably placed overhead straps and lowers himself to the bed (Fig. 3-32).

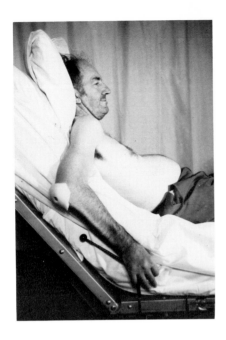 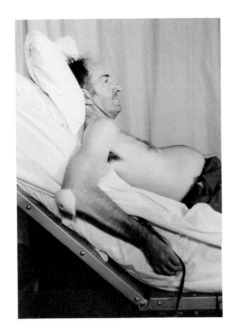 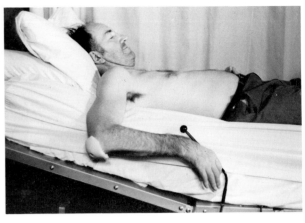

FIGURE 3-33

Method 4.   When a patient is able to raise an electrically operated head gatch himself, the control must be located so that he can also lower it independently (Fig. 3-33).

Moving Up The Bed

Method 1. (Fig. 3-34)   The patient sits with his arms locked and his hands on the bed at about midthigh level. As he flexes his head and shoulders sharply, his buttocks are lifted from the bed and moved back.

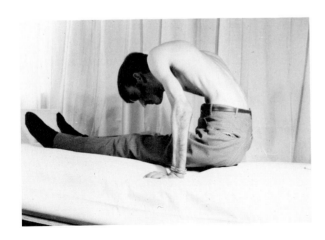

FIGURE 3-34

Method 2. (Fig. 3-35)   The patient sits with his arms locked, hands on the bed well behind his buttocks. He moves up the bed by extending his upper trunk over his arms and adducting his shoulders, stopping just before he reaches a point where he would lose his balance.

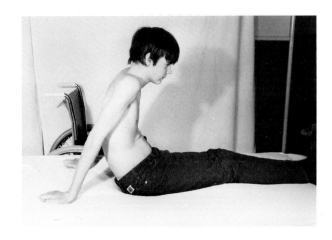

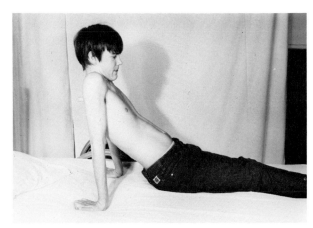

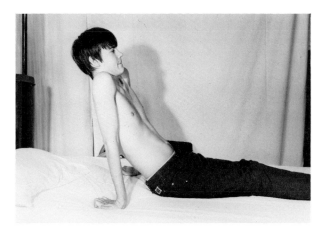

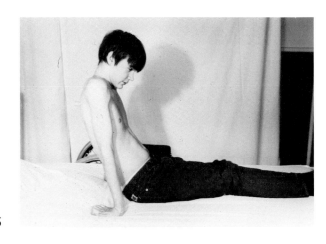

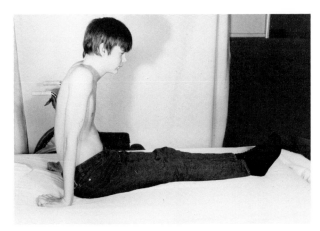

FIGURE 3-35

107

Method 3. For the patient who sits, but requires an overhead strap for balance, a twisting method is used (Fig. 3-36). A wrist is placed in the strap, and the other hand is placed on the bed with the elbow locked. The patient leans over the locked arm, twisting his buttocks back and to one side. As he alternates the arm positions and repeats the action, his buttocks move further back and to the middle of the bed again.

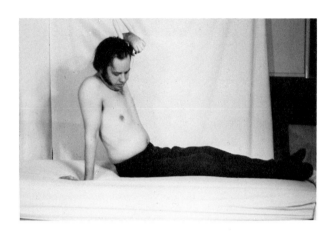
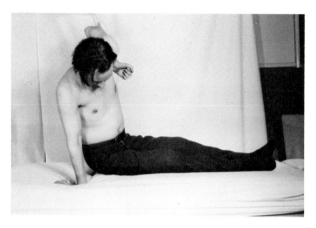
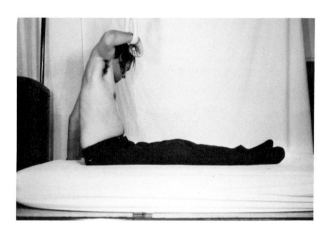
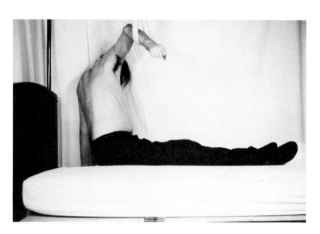

FIGURE 3-36

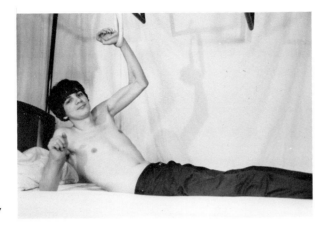
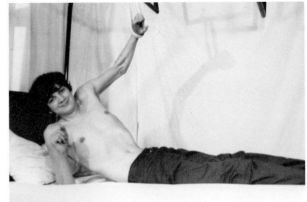

FIGURE 3-37

Method 4. (Fig. 3-37) The patient with tight hamstrings or interfering spasms will have difficulty sitting up in bed. This patient hooks an arm into an overhead strap to pull himself up onto the opposite elbow. He works this elbow towards the head of the bed, then quickly flexes and adducts the shoulder, pulling himself up in bed. It may be necessary to change arm positions and repeat the maneuver in order to centralize the buttocks on the bed.

Method 5. When the patient is lying within reach of the head of the bed, he can hook his wrists from the outside around the head panel of the bed and, by pulling, move up the bed (Fig. 3-38).

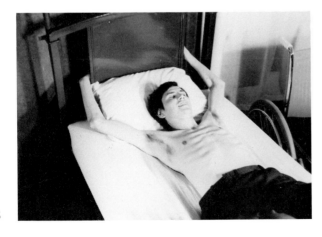
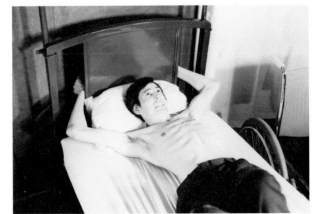

FIGURE 3-38

Method 6. Cribsides or ladders can be used on either or both sides of the bed. After hooking the wrists around the rungs from the outside as far up the bed as possible, the patient will pull himself up the bed (Fig. 3-39). Extremely weak quadriplegics can learn this method.

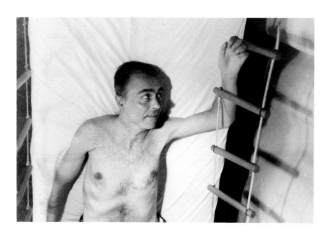
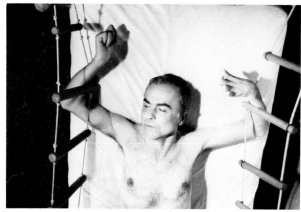
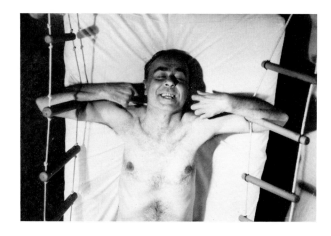

FIGURE 3-39

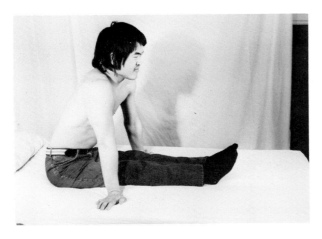

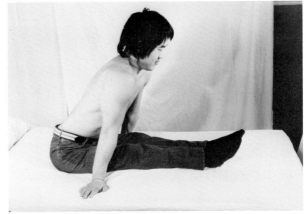

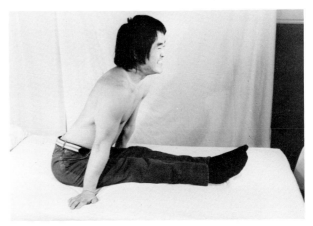

FIGURE 3-40

Moving Down The Bed

Method 1. (Fig. 3-40)   The patient sits with elbows locked and his hands on the bed at midthigh level. He flexes his trunk forward as far as possible and he briskly extends his upper trunk and neck while remaining in the forward position. The resulting bouncing action raises his buttocks and moves him forward.

111

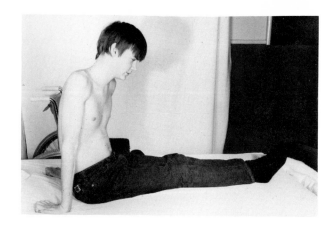

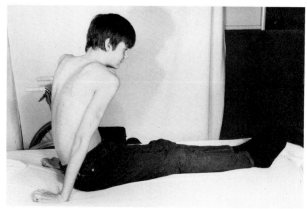

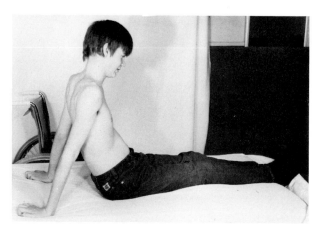

FIGURE 3-41

Method 2. (Fig. 3-41)   The patient sits with his arms locked, hands on the bed slightly behind his buttocks. A wriggling motion is produced by extending his upper trunk over his arms and extending his shoulders alternately. Along with this motion the patient leans first on one arm, then the other, thus taking the weight off the buttocks alternately. This will result in the patient sliding down the bed.

Method 3. For the patient who can sit, but requires an overhead strap for balance, a twisting method may be used (Fig. 3-42). With one wrist in a strap, placed as far forward as possible, he puts the other hand on the bed close to his buttock and locks the elbow. Pulling himself up by the strap, he relieves some of the weight from his buttocks. He depresses and externally rotates the shoulder of the locked arm, producing a pushing motion. The combination of this push on the bed and pull on the strap will move him down the bed.

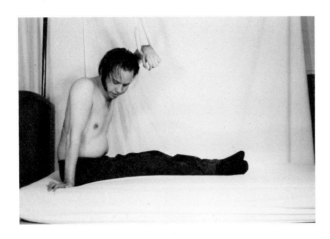
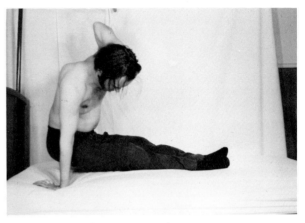
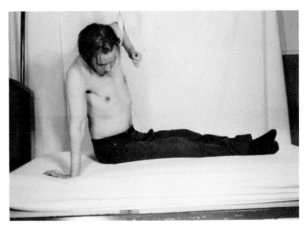

FIGURE 3-42

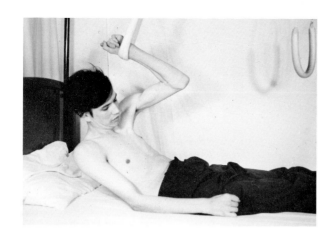
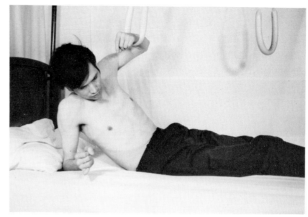

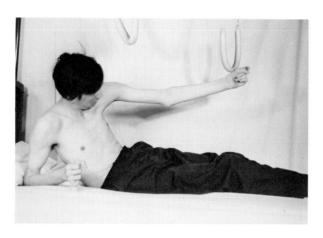
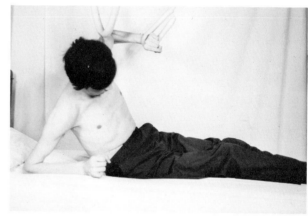

FIGURE 3-43

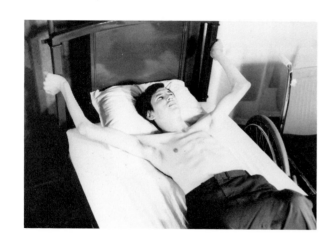
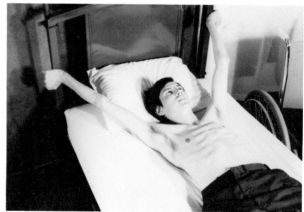

FIGURE 3-44

114

Method 4. (Fig. 3-43)   The patient with tight hamstrings or interfering spasms may not be able to sit up in bed. This patient hooks his arm into an overhead strap, pulling himself onto the opposite elbow. While balancing on the elbow, he reaches for another overhead strap further forward. He moves his elbow as far forward as possible keeping it close to his body. He slides down the bed by pulling with the arm in the strap and extending the other shoulder.

Method 5.   When the patient is lying within reach of the head of the bed, he can place the palms of his hands against the head panel in line with his shoulders, and push to slide down the bed (Fig. 3-44). This is a functional push developed through the shoulder girdle, not by active extension of the elbow.

Method 6.   The patient with restricted hip flexion may use an overhead rope ladder (Fig. 3-45). When the patient pulls on the ladder, he only partially raises his trunk. Therefore, further pulling will slide him down the bed.

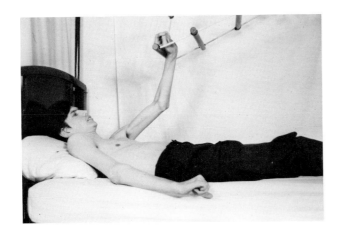
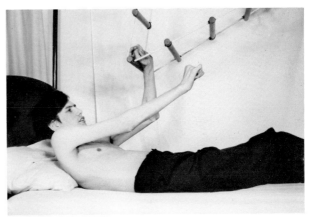
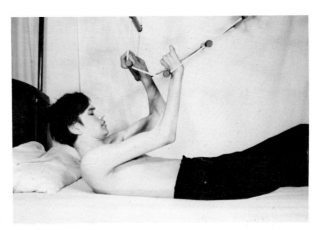

FIGURE 3-45

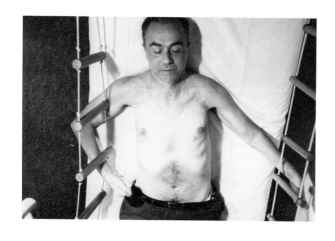
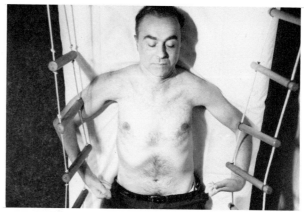
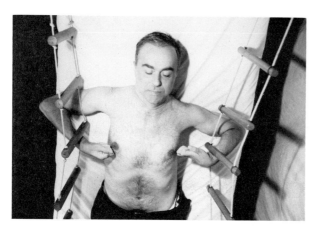
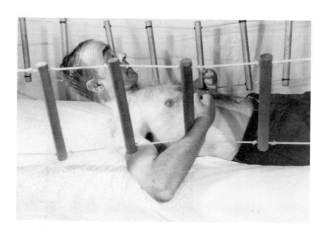

FIGURE 3-46

Method 7. Cribsides or rope ladders may be used by a very weak patient. The ladders provide a better angle of pull because they move close to the patient's trunk as he flexes his elbows (Fig. 3-46).

116

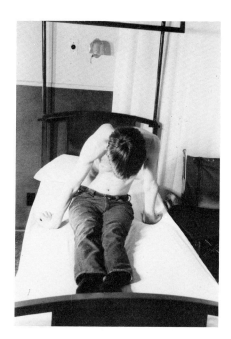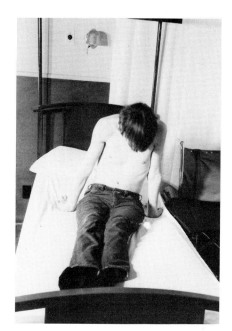

FIGURE 3-47

Moving Across The Bed

Method 1. The patient who moves up or down the bed by using locked arms, hands on the bed, will use the same method for moving across the bed (Fig. 3-47). One hand is placed about a foot away from the body and the patient leans over this arm, permitting his other hand to be placed on the bed under the buttock. The patient then does a push up and his body swings from the near to the far arm. He must now move his feet across and, if necessary, repeat the whole action.

Method 2. (Fig. 3-48)   Instead of swinging between his locked arms, the patient may twist his trunk and place both hands on the bed on one side. Throwing his weight over his locked arms, he will push his buttocks away.

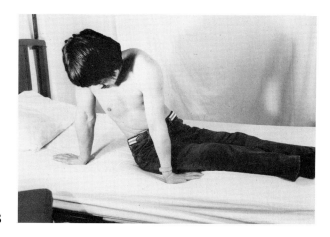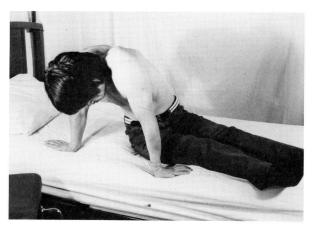

FIGURE 3-48

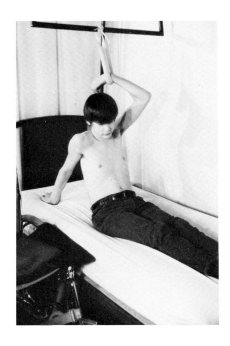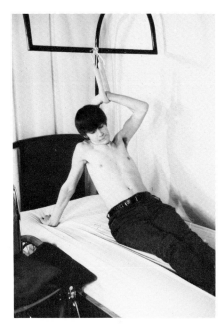

FIGURE 3-49

Method 3. (Fig. 3-49)   The patient places a wrist in an overhead strap, slightly forward of and in line with the opposite shoulder. The other elbow is locked with a hand on the bed close to the buttock. A pull on the strap, together with a push on the bed, will move the buttocks over.

Method 4. (Fig. 3-50)   The patient who is unable to sit up, lies on his side and pulls himself onto an elbow using an overhead strap. By pushing away with the elbow and pulling on the strap, he moves his buttocks over and down the bed. The amount of flexion of his trunk determines his direction of travel. The greatest sideways travel occurs when the patient is most flexed.

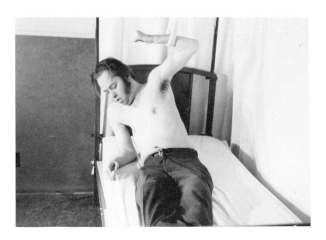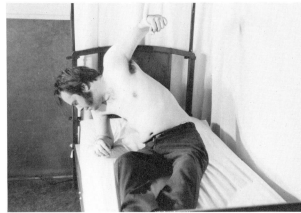

FIGURE 3-50

Bridgeboards

Bridgeboards, (also called sliding boards or transfer boards), are usually necessary to facilitate transfer from chair to bed, toilet, shower, bath, or car. Whatever design is used, it should be suitable for as many transfer situations as possible except transfer to car. A different design is usually required for the latter. An unpadded board may be used only by patients with good skin tone and muscle bulk. A ³/₁₆ inch (0.48 cm) tempered hardboard is strong and develops a highly polished surface when rubbed with talcum powder. The corners must be rounded, bevelled, and well sanded. Patients who are prone to skin breakdowns should be provided with boards which are padded and nylon covered (See Appendix II).

Placing the Bridgeboard in Position

Method 1. (Fig. 3-51)   The patient slides forward in the chair and removes the chair arm. He places the board on the bed and pulls it under the buttock as far as possible using his wrist over the far side of the board. He then hooks the arm furthest from the bed over the chair arm, and raises the buttock by pulling his trunk away from the bed. He may now pull the board further under him.

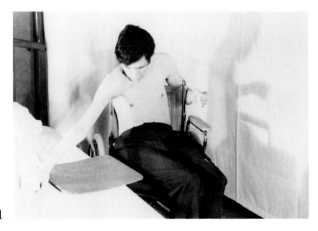 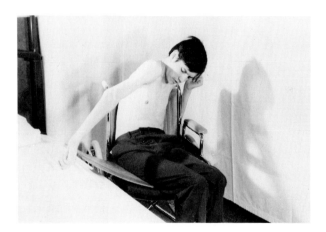

FIGURE 3-51

Method 2. (Fig. 3-52) The patient rests one end of the board on the bed and the other end just on his thigh. By pulling his trunk away from the bed using both arms over the outer chair arm, the board will fall into place as his buttock is raised. Methods 1 and 2 can be used with legs up or down.

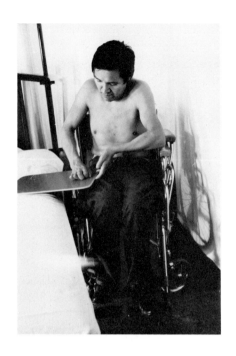 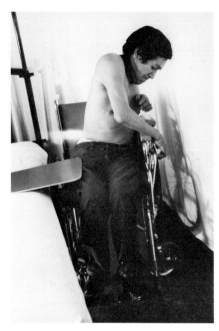 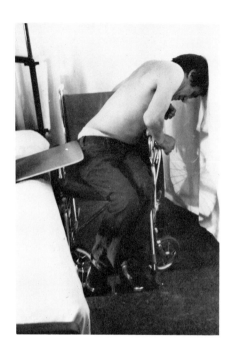

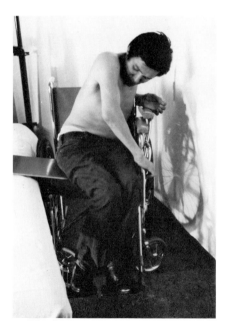 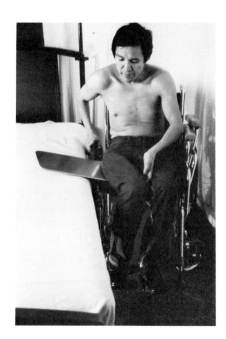

FIGURE 3-52

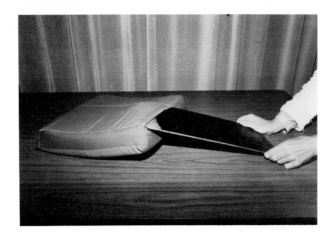
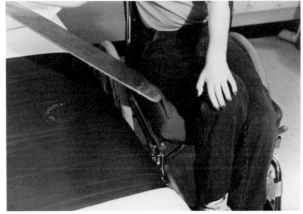

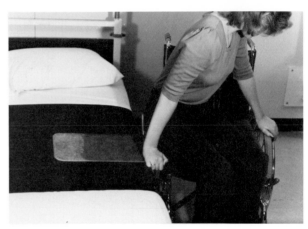

FIGURE 3-53

Method 3. (Fig. 3-53)   Sometimes it is difficult to insert a bridgeboard because it catches on clothing. To solve this problem an open-ended pocket may be
sewn into the cushion top, and the bridgeboard may be inserted into this.

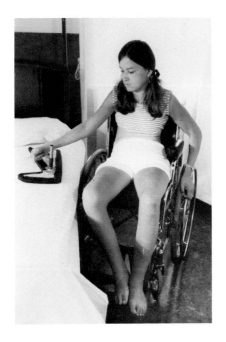
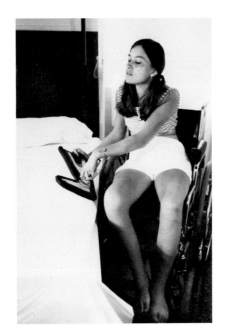
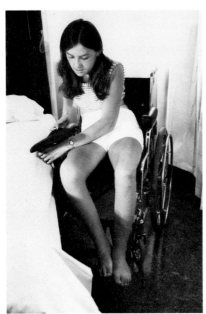
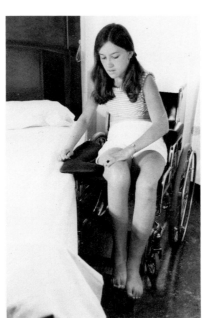

FIGURE 3-54

Method 4. (Fig. 3-54)   The padded board must be placed in position before the legs are lifted onto the bed either before or after sliding forward in the chair. The post on the underside of the board is placed in the arm rest socket and the wheel recess is placed over the wheel. This board leaves no gap between bed and chair and increases the size of the sliding area. (See Appendix for construction and plans.)

122

Lifting Legs Onto the Bed

The quadriplegic person commonly approaches the bed from the side. The chair faces the foot of the bed and the front is turned in at a 30° angle. This angle puts the seat closer to the bed and positions the patient so that his legs are easier to lift onto the bed.

The patient wheels back and puts on the castor locks before wheeling forward again into position. This is an easy way to turn the castors forward to ensure stability of the wheelchair.

The patient locks the brakes and removes the arm of the chair nearest the bed. He then shifts his buttocks forward in the chair. There are two reasons for the maneuver: first, so that the buttocks will clear the wheel and second, so that the patient has room to rock his trunk back, giving added leverage as he lifts his legs onto the bed. The padded bridgeboard must be in position before lifting the legs onto the bed. In some cases a leg retainer board will also be required, to prevent the feet from slipping off and to add leverage. The feet are lifted onto the bed one at a time.

Method 1. (Fig. 3-55)   The patient places the arm furthest from the bed over the back of the chair and under the pushing handle. This enables him to lean forward safely. The other wrist is inserted from the lateral side under the knee nearest the bed. By flexing the shoulder of the arm over the back of the chair and the elbow of the arm under the knee, the foot is raised to the level of the bed. The foot is levered onto the bed by external rotation of the shoulder and extension of the wrist against the calf. At this point the knee is flexed and the hip internally rotated; pressure on the knee will extend the knee and slide the foot further onto the bed. The other leg is raised in a similar manner except that the wrist is inserted from the medial side of the knee. When the foot is on the bed, the hip is externally rotated before pressure is applied to extend the knee so that the foot is 'steered' further onto the bed.

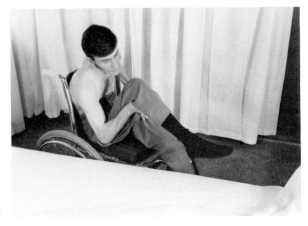 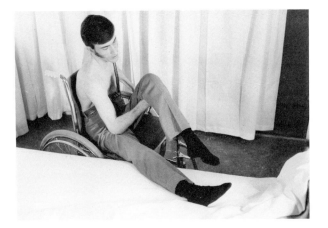

FIGURE 3-55

123

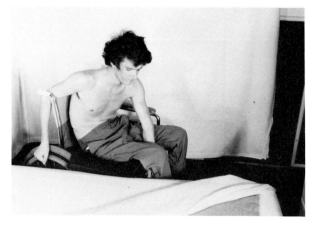 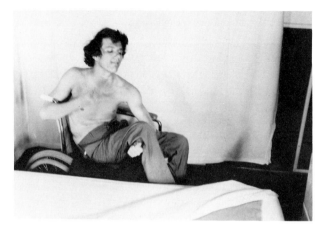

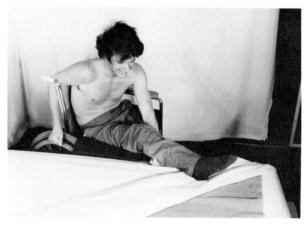 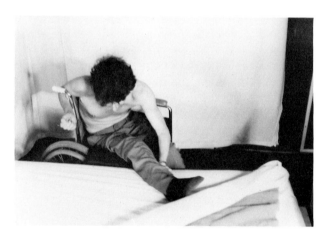

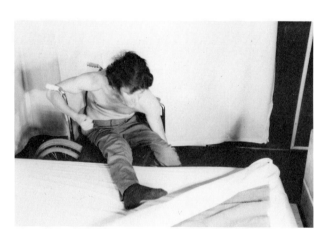

FIGURE 3-56

124

Method 2. (Fig. 3-56)   The patient with weak external rotators of the shoulders places the arm nearest the bed over the back of the chair and under the pushing handle. He inserts the wrist of the other hand under the knee nearest the bed from the medial side and flexes the elbow. Flexion of the shoulder over the back of the chair will rock the patient back, raise his leg, and rotate him in the chair, thus moving his leg towards the bed. Protraction and flexion of both shoulders in a hugging action will swing the foot onto the bed. The knee is straightened as in Method 1. The other leg is raised in a similar manner except that the wrist is inserted from the lateral side of the knee.

Method 3. (Fig. 3-57)   A patient who can lift the first leg onto the bed sometimes has difficulty with the second, because when the effort is made to lift the leg, the trunk rotates and the hips slide across the chair away from the bed. This also causes the trunk to fall towards the bed, so that all effort to lift the leg only pulls the patient more off balance.

Until the patient can learn to lean away from the bed while lifting the second leg, a small foam rubber cushion may be used as a block between the hip and the wheelchair arm to prevent the buttocks from sliding across the chair seat and to stabilize the patient so that her efforts can lift the leg (Fig. 3-58).

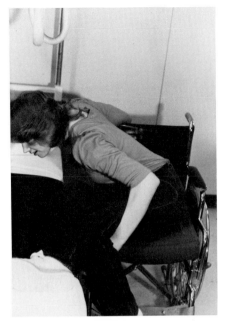

FIGURE 3-57

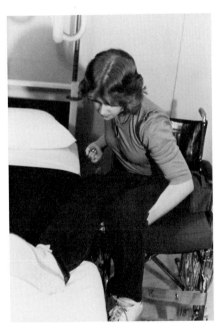

FIGURE 3-58

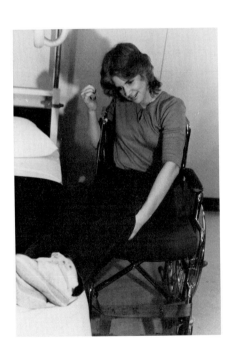

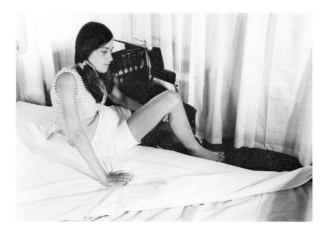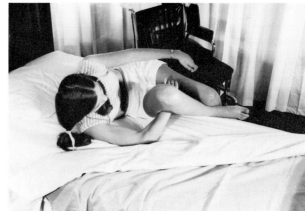

FIGURE 3-59

Method 4.   Most patients who transfer onto the bed before moving their feet from the footrests do so because they have tight hamstrings or spasm. Once seated on the bed, the patient inserts a wrist under the knee nearest the bed and rolls sideways onto the bed, pulling her leg up as she rolls (Fig. 3-59). In a patient with flexor spasm the other leg will frequently follow the first leg onto the bed; and the patient can be encouraged to control this spasm.

Method 5.   When spasm cannot be used to raise the second leg, the patient inserts one wrist in the overhead strap and the other under the knee nearest the bed. By rocking back and pulling on the strap the leg is pulled onto the bed (Fig. 3-60). The same procedure is used for the second leg. Some patients are able to insert a wrist under both knees, thereby pulling both legs onto the bed together.

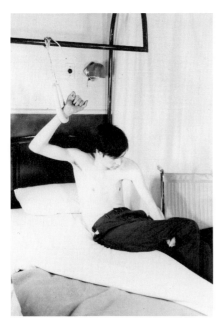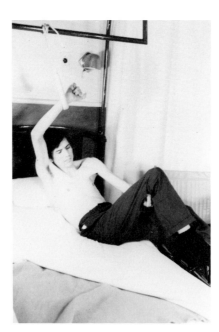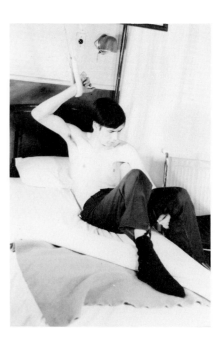

FIGURE 3-60

Method 6.   The patient may use a loop of rope or webbing to swing his legs to the bed (Fig. 3-61). In this case the foot is moved forward on the footrest so that the instep is free. This is done by raising the foot partially and swinging it forward by extending the wrist against the calf. The patient sits with the arm nearest the bed over the back of the chair and the elbow flexed around the pushing handle. He inserts his other wrist into the loop of webbing and flexes his trunk forward as far as possible to place the loop of the strap over his forefoot. The loop should be as short as possible to allow the greatest lift. The forearm rests on the thigh with the hand on the medial side of the leg so that leverage can be obtained by using the thigh as a fulcrum to extend the knee. The hip is internally rotated, permitting the foot to swing over onto the bed. Knee extension and hip rotation occur simultaneously as the patient rocks back using both shoulder flexors and protractors. (Leg position is determined by placing the hand on one or the other side of the knee.)

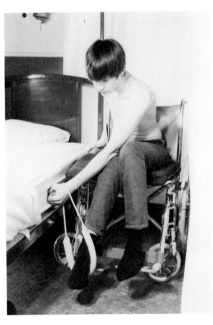 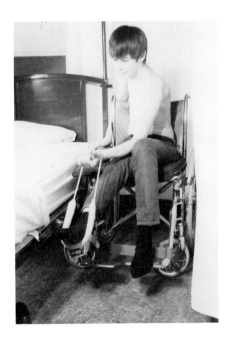 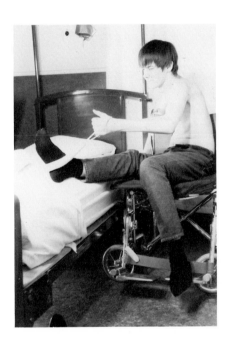

FIGURE 3-61

Method 7. (Fig. 3-62)   A figure 8 loop with a wire core may be used to lever the leg up. The crossover should be just below the kneecap, thus simulating the action of the quadriceps muscle to extend the knee. The assistant should try the action of the loop to ensure that the mechanics are correct before asking the patient to attempt the maneuver. Once the knee is straightened it is easier to lift the leg over to the bed.

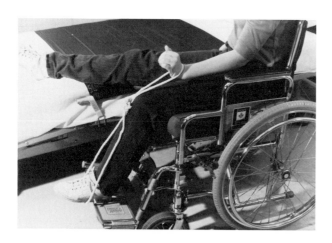
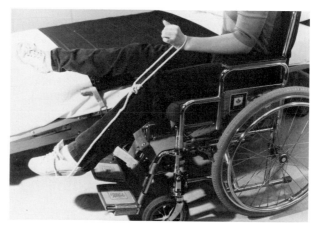
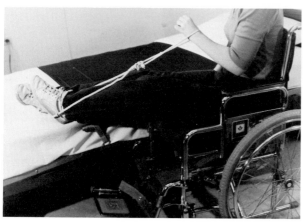

FIGURE 3-62

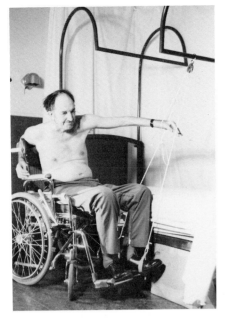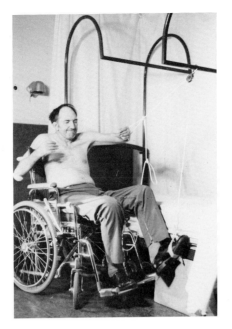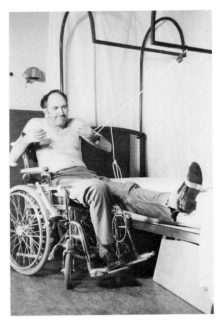

FIGURE 3-63

Method 8.   The patient may use a pulley that is attached to a balkan beam at the point above the bed where the foot is to be placed (Fig. 3-63). A rope is sheaved through the pulley and a loop formed at one end to pass over the forefoot. A loop, large enough to enable the patient to insert his wrist, is tied at the other end as close to the pulley as possible. As many other loops as are necessary are tied in this tail end of the rope. These merely enable the patient to pull the loop nearest the pulley within reach and so keep the rope taut. A strong pull should elevate the leg and carry it onto the bed.

Wheelchair to Bed Transfer

When it is stated in this section that a side approach is used, it indicates that the patient places his chair at a 30° angle to the bed, facing the foot of the bed with his shoulders just behind the level of the overhead bar. When it is stated that the patient prepares to transfer, it signifies these steps: he applies his brakes and castor locks, slides his buttocks forward in the wheelchair, removes the armrest on the exit side of the wheelchair, and places his bridgeboard if necessary. The necessity for complete stability of the wheelchair cannot be overemphasized.

It is desirable to push down to do a transfer where possible, avoiding the use of an overhead strap, as the shoulders are less protected in the pulling position. A "pulling" transfer may, however, be most useful, particularly if this is the method of maintaining balance, but care must be taken not to damage the weak shoulder.

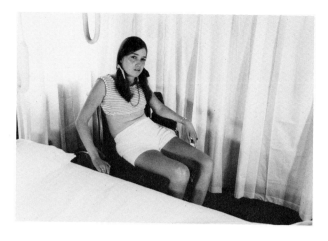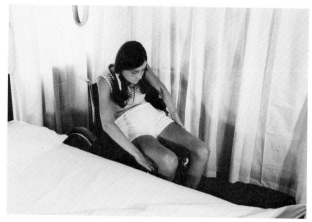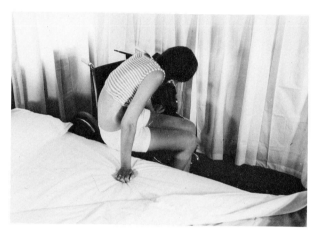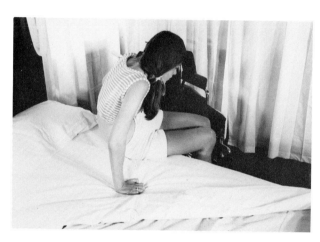

FIGURE 3-64

Method 1. The patient with a low cervical lesion and good balance should accomplish transfers without the use of overhead bars. She uses a side approach and prepares to transfer with her feet on the footrests (Fig. 3-64). She places one hand on the bed and the other close to her buttock, then locks both elbows. She leans forward until she reaches her point of balance, then depresses her shoulder girdle and flexes her shoulders. She swings her buttocks across by abducting and externally rotating the far shoulder while adducting and internally rotating the near shoulder. To gain added momentum and lift, she flexes her neck and turns her head away from the bed. At first she may move only a short distance, in which case a bridgeboard will be necessary. The bridgeboard may not be necessary as she improves her technique, so that one movement takes her over to the bed.

The more flaccid patient may place his legs on the bed first (Fig. 3-65).

Method 2. (Fig. 3-66) The patient moves himself well forward in the wheelchair and sits up by pushing on the wheel and using head and shoulder momentum. He places his hands, one close to his hip, and the other level with his hip, but further away, to allow room for movement. He pushes up with his arms and

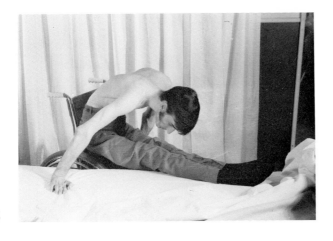 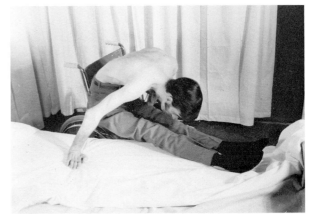

FIGURE 3-65

simultaneously bends his head and shoulders away from the direction of travel. This movement must be done vigorously. Repetitions may be required to move him further onto the bed.

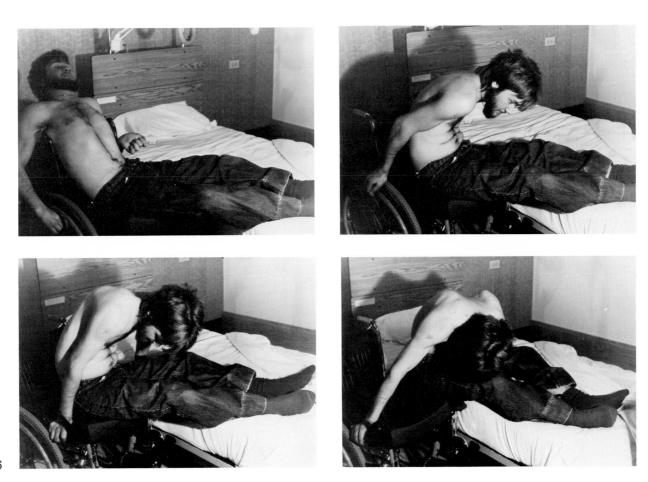

FIGURE 3-66

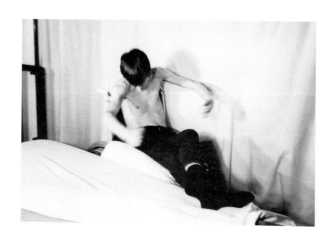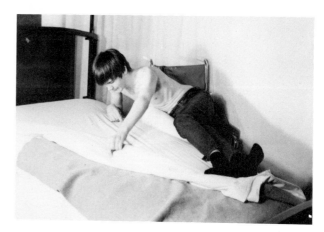

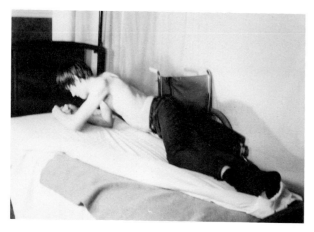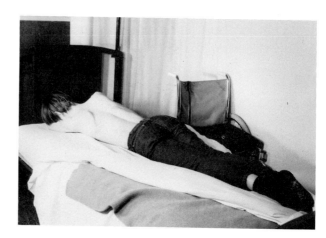

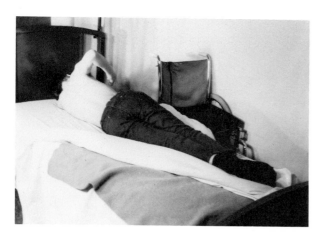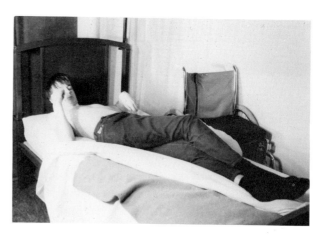

FIGURE 3-67

Method 3. (Fig. 3-67)   The patient prepares to transfer using the side approach, in this case from the left of the bed. He places a small cushion in the gap between wheelchair and bed and over the wheel. He now places his right leg on the bed. He picks up the left leg and places the heel over the knee of the right leg. When pressure is exerted on the left knee, it will straighten with the legs crossed. The patient now abducts the left arm and adducts the right arm across his chest at shoulder level. He then swings both arms rapidly across, turning his head, shoulders and upper trunk towards the head of the bed. As he rolls into bed he drops onto his right elbow. The left shoulder is flexed above his head so that his head rests on his forearm. He is now in position to roll over onto his back, using the momentum gained from rolling out of the chair.

This is a quick and useful transfer, but is not applicable in many other situations, and is therefore often learned as an alternative transfer.

Method 4.   The patient who can move on the bed in long sitting by locking his elbows and doing a pushup to shift his buttocks, can use the following method to transfer from wheelchair to bed (Fig. 3-68). He faces the middle of the bed and locks his chair about a foot away from the side of the bed. This leaves room for

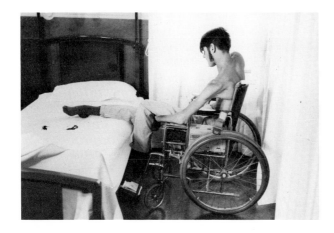
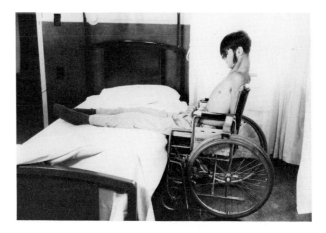
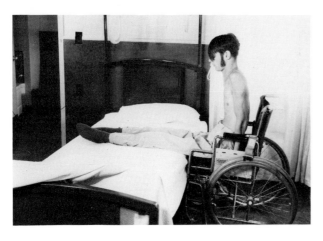
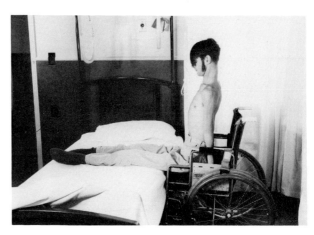

FIGURE 3-68

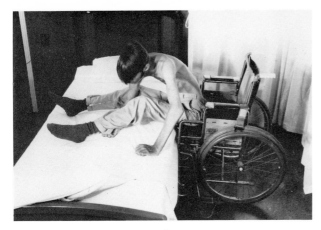 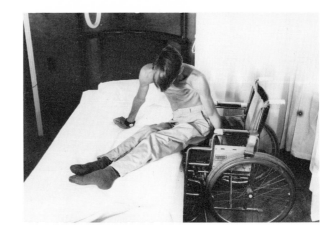

FIGURE 3-68   Continued

him to put his feet on the bed and swing his footrests away. He unlocks his brakes and wheels his chair forward until the chair seat is against the mattress. Automatic spring locks may be required to secure the wheelchair to the bed frame (see Appendix). He slides his buttocks forward in the wheelchair and then leans forward and locks his elbows. He shifts his buttocks forward until he is almost on the bed before levering his legs over towards the foot of the bed. He now shifts sideways to the center of the bed and levers his legs over again if necessary.

Method 5. (Fig. 3-69)   Using Method 3, but with overhead bars as described earlier in this chapter, the patient reaches the point where a pushup would be required. He reaches for a fixed strap on the near bar with the arm nearest the foot of the bed. He levers his feet towards the foot of the bed, using the free arm. He now reaches for a fixed strap on the far bar with his free arm, and pulls up with both arms, lifting his buttocks up and over onto the bed. These transfers do not allow mechanical advantages to be used, but may be required for people who have complications such as elbow contractures.

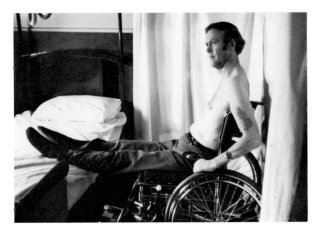

FIGURE 3-69

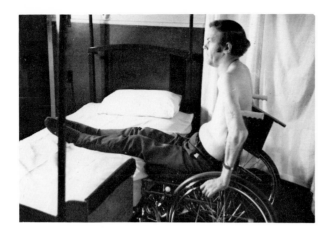
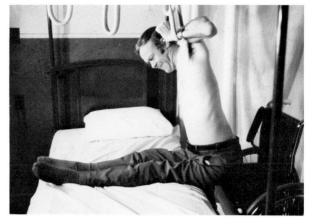
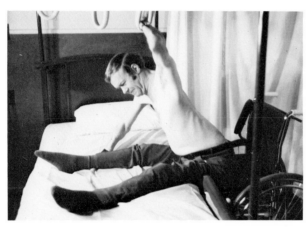
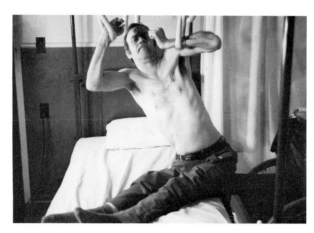
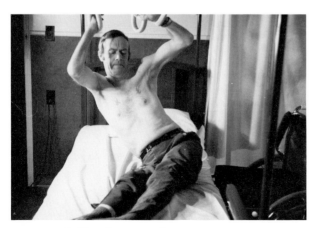
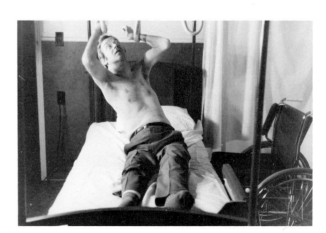

FIGURE 3-69　Continued

135

Method 6. (Fig. 3-70)   The patient prepares to transfer, using the side approach, and places his legs on the bed. He uses one overhead bar with one floating strap adjusted so that he can insert his wrist into it when sitting. He puts the arm nearest the bed through the strap. The other hand, wrist extended, can be placed against the far tire behind the chair back, or against the arm of the chair. The patient then leans his trunk away from the bed to gain the fullest mechanical advantage. By strongly contracting his elbow flexors and shoulder adductors bilaterally, he will develop a pushing action with his hand on the wheelchair and a pulling action with his arm in the strap. This will move him from the chair to the edge of the bed. At this stage, he must move the floating strap further away from himself along the bar. His other hand is moved to either the seat of the chair or the wheel nearest the bed. A repetition of the bilateral pull will place him well on the bed.

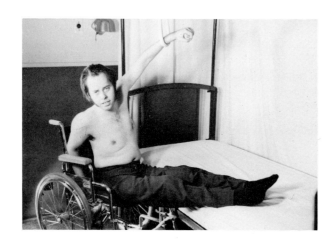
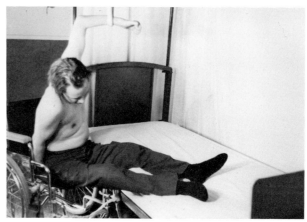
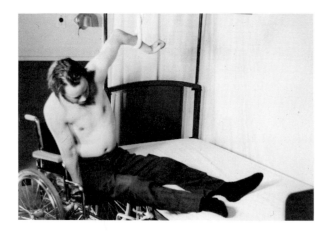
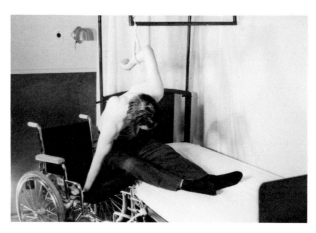

FIGURE 3-70

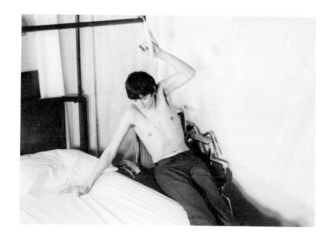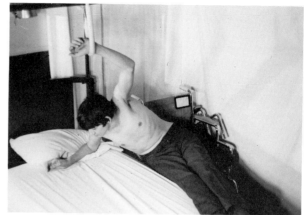

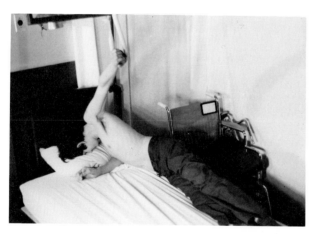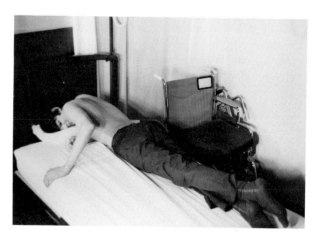

FIGURE 3-71

Method 7. (Fig. 3-71)   The patient uses the same equipment and the same method for initiating the move as in Method 6. He reaches the edge of the bed and places the arm furthest from the bed in the strap. He places the other hand on the bed with the wrist extended, while he moves the strap further over. He rolls himself by pulling on the strap, dropping onto his elbow, and twisting his body towards the bed. He is now on the bed in side lying and can remove his arm from the strap.

Method 8. The patient who uses a side approach and is unable to make use of trunk torsion because of flaccidity, may use an overhead bar with several fixed straps at intervals along the bar (Fig. 3-72). He prepares for transfer in the usual way and places his feet on the bed, but instead of leaning away from the bed, he leans towards it. He gains no mechanical advantage from this position and must rely solely upon muscle strength. He inserts the wrist nearest the bed into the second strap to pull his trunk over. This enables him to reach the first strap with the other arm. He pulls himself as far as possible towards the bed. He now moves his wrists into straps further along the bar to give him fresh purchase to pull and so continues until he is on the bed.

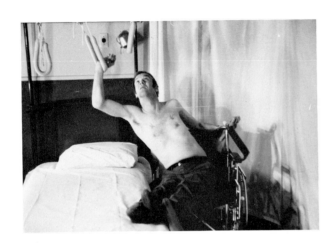
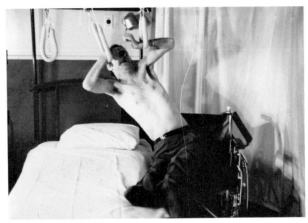
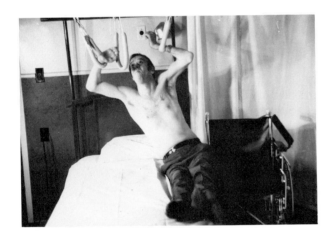
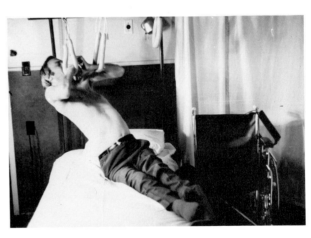

FIGURE 3-72

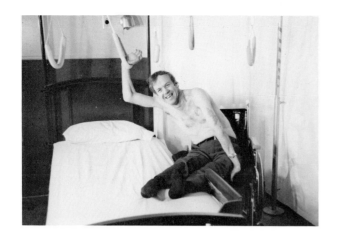
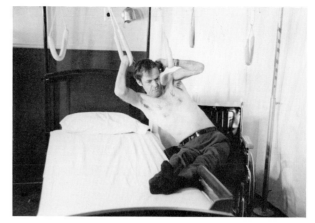
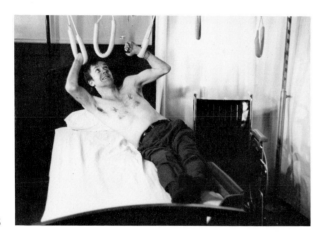
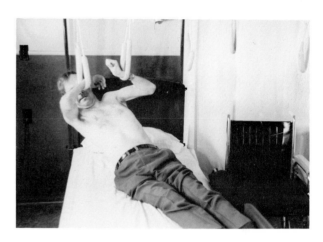

FIGURE 3-73

Such a patient may require the outrigger (described on page 86) during the learning process (Fig. 3-73).

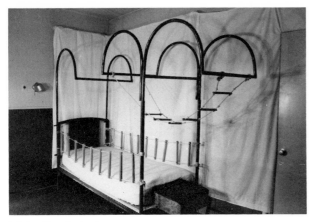

FIGURE 3-74 A

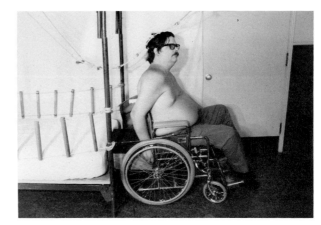

FIGURE 3-74 B

Method 9.   On rare occasions a practical and permanent method of transfer can be accomplished through the back of the chair with the chair positioned at the foot of the bed. This method is very useful as a demonstration to the patient of his ability to move independently. It is also useful as a strengthening exercise to enable the patient to use another transfer method utilizing less equipment at a later date. For this method of transfer three overhead bars are required (Fig. 3-74A), one at the head of the bed and two at the foot facing in opposite directions. In the place of the footboard, a special end is made to support the two overhead bars and permit entry. A box is made and padded with 1 inch (2.54 cm) foam rubber and is nylon covered. This fills the gap at the end of the mattress and projects to the seat of the chair (Fig. 3-74B). Two eye bolts are fastened to the uprights of the overhead bars at the level of the wheelchair arms. Hooks are made of a 3/16 inch (0.48 cm) welding rod. These hooks are hung from the eyebolts and are dropped into holes drilled in the top back of the wheelchair arms to lock the chair to the bed. The chair must be equipped with a detachable back. A horizontal rope ladder is fastened to the foot and head at each side of the bed. The bottom of these ladders should be about 4 inches (10 cm) above the mattress to permit the patient to place his wrists underneath. The rungs should be about 10 inches (25 cm) apart, although this distance may have to be modified. Another rope ladder is attached to the bar that projects over the chair. The other end is tied to the other bar at the foot and is looped downwards so that the patient can reach it when lying.

To transfer (Fig. 3-75), the patient first locks the chair in position and removes the back. He then lowers his trunk to the bed, usually using the rope ladder looped at the foot of the bed. The patient reaches up the bed to put a wrist under each ladder and behind a rung. By adducting his shoulders and flexing his elbows, he will move up the bed. This process is repeated until he reaches the desired position. When the patient is learning this process, he will be greatly assisted if his knees are extended for him.

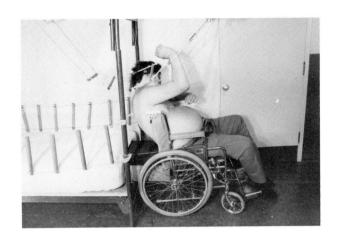 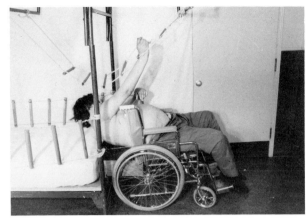

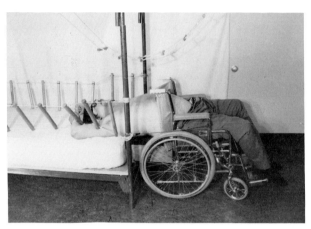 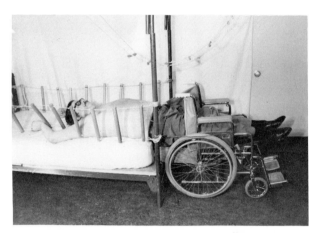

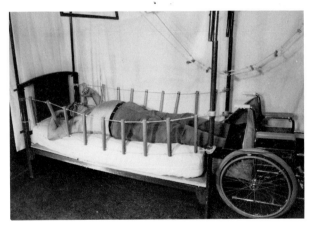

FIGURE 3-75

141

The patient reverses the process to get out of bed (Fig. 3-76), reaching down as far as possible and pulling on the ladder rungs. When his feet are on the footrests of the chair, he reaches for the overhead ladder and pulls himself to the sitting position. The chair back is fastened and the locks are removed.

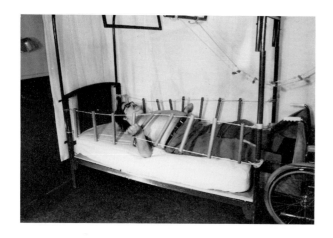 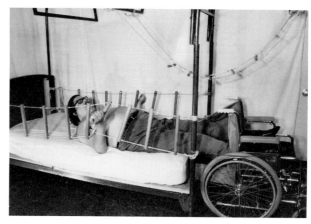

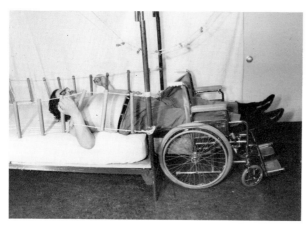 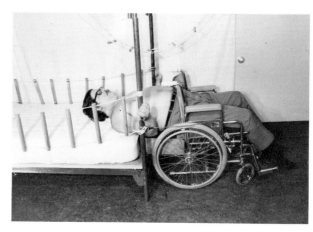

FIGURE 3-76

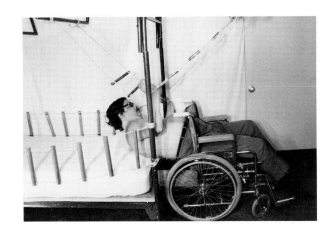
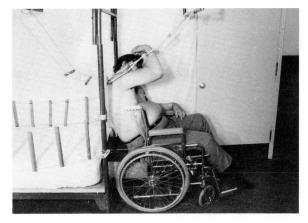
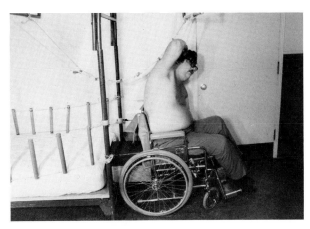
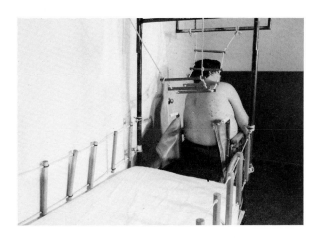

FIGURE 3-76   Continued

143

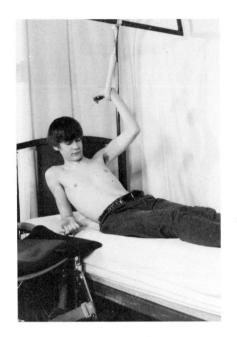

Lowering Feet to Footrests from the Bed

If a patient has tight hamstrings, he will have to put his legs down onto the footrests before transferring from bed to chair. Many patients without tight hamstrings manage better also with legs down. There are several methods of moving the legs from the bed. The patient must first learn the correct position of his body in relation to the chair, so that his feet will make contact with the footrests each time.

Method 1. (Fig. 3-77) The patient with flaccid lower extremities may sit up, and hook the wrist furthest from the chair into an overhead strap. He then leans forward, placing his wrist under the knee nearest the chair. He inserts the wrist from the lateral side of the leg. By pulling with both arms he will rock to the upright position, and bring the knee up to his chest. By outwardly rotating his shoulders, he can place his foot over the edge of the bed, and then lower it to the footrest. The other leg is lowered, using the same method except that his wrist is inserted from the medial side of his leg.

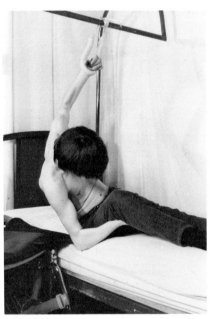
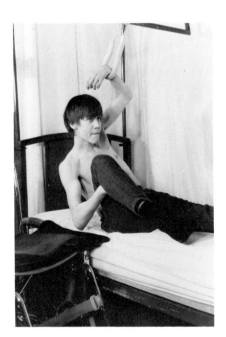
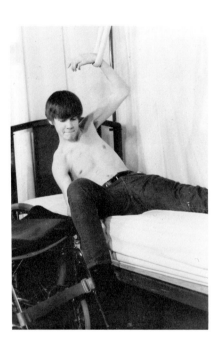

FIGURE 3-77

Method 2. (Fig. 3-78)   From the long sitting position, the patient leans forward. He maintains balance by using an overhead strap for one arm, by resting on one elbow, or by relying on the normal tension of his hip extensors to hold his position. By inserting a hand under a leg and raising his elbow, the lever action will move his leg over until the heel slides off the bed and to the footrest. Alternatively a bridge board may be slipped under the leg to be used as a lever.

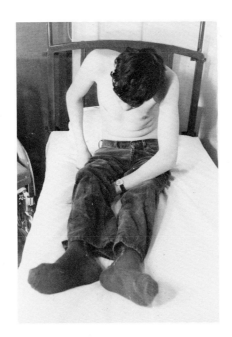
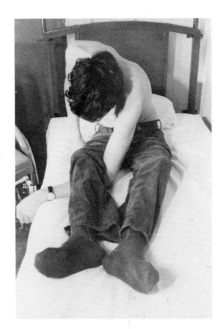
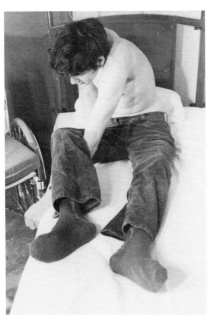
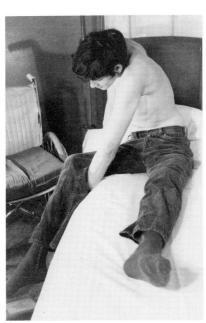

FIGURE 3-78

145

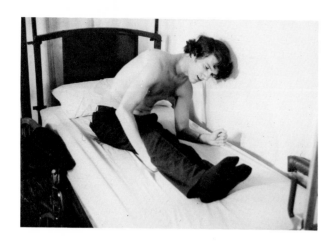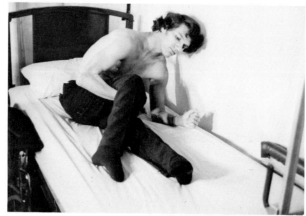

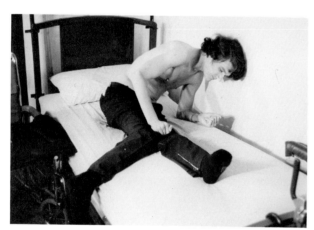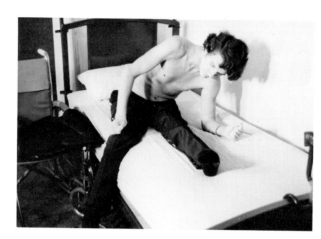

FIGURE 3-79

Method 3. (Fig. 3-79)   Sitting up and leaning away from the chair on one elbow, the patient reaches down and hooks his wrist behind his knee. He pulls his knee up as far as possible so that he will be able to pull his foot towards his buttocks. He then pushes on the knee, extending the leg. This may have to be repeated to move the leg over the edge of the bed. The other leg is managed similarly.

Method 4. (Fig. 3-80)   The patient with some rigidity of trunk and hip may side flex his trunk away from his chair so that his legs will swivel towards the footrests.

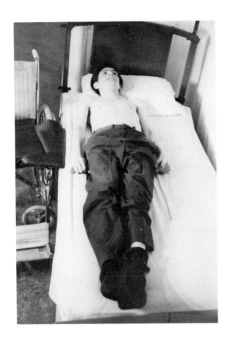
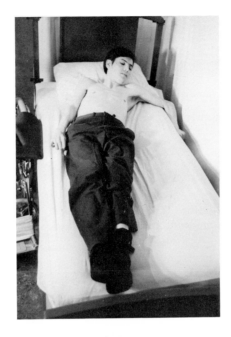
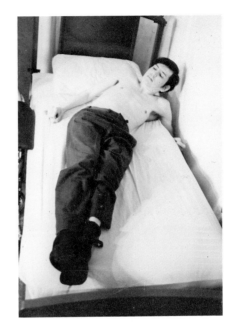

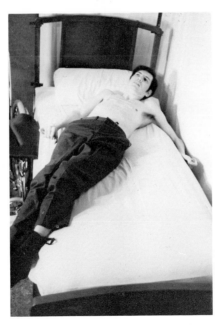
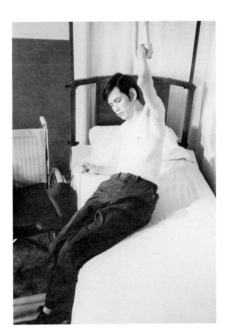

FIGURE 3-80

Bed to Chair Transfer

The patient starts in long sitting near the side of the bed, forward of the rear wheels of the chair. If a bridgeboard is used, it is positioned at this time. The patient may lower his feet to the footrests either during the transfer or when he is in the chair.

Method 1.   The patient who is able to transfer onto the bed without the use of an overhead bar will use the same pushup method to transfer back to the chair (Fig. 3-81). He may lower his feet to the footrests either before or after transferring. The hand nearest the chair may be placed on the chair seat or on the armrest. The patient leans forward until he reaches his point of balance; then he depresses his shoulder girdle to raise his buttocks from the bed. He flexes his neck sharply and turns his head away from the chair to give him extra momentum as he lifts himself over into the seat.

Method 2. (Fig. 3-82)   The patient sits up and places his hands, one near his hip, and the other level with his hip, but further away to allow room to move towards the wheelchair. He pushes up with both arms and simultaneously bends his head and shoulders sharply away from the direction of travel. These movements are repeated vigorously until his seat is partly on the wheelchair. In order to get back into the wheelchair he puts one hand on the front edge of the wheelchair, and one on the wheel; by ducking his head and shoulders and pulling with his biceps, he moves back.

The removable post in the arm rest socket may be most useful in this transfer to provide a purchase point for the hand on the wheelchair seat.

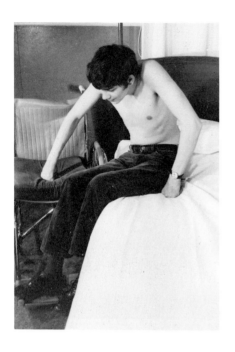

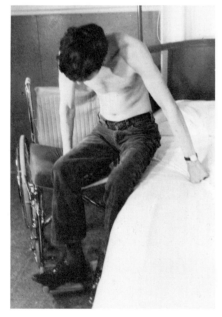

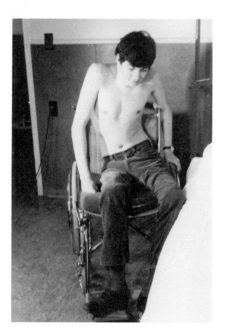

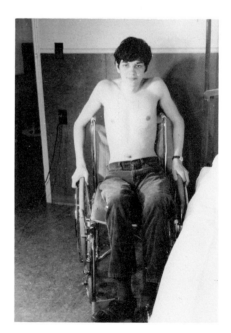

FIGURE 3-81

148

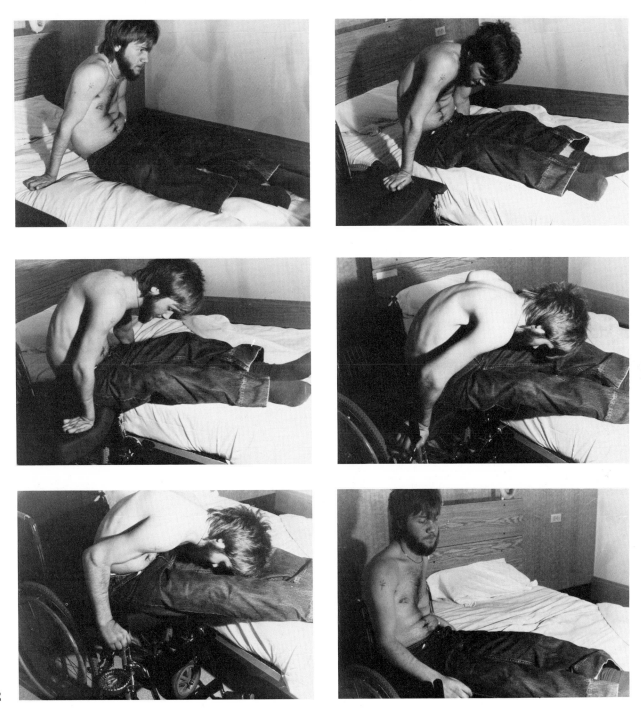

FIGURE 3-82

149

Method 3. (Fig. 3-83)   The patient places the wrist furthest from the wheelchair in an overhead floating strap. He places the other hand on the wheelchair seat and locks his elbow. He pulls up on the strap so that his buttocks are raised from the bed. Simultaneously, adduction and flexion of the other shoulder will pull him into the wheelchair seat. He remains leaning forward to move his buttocks back into the chair.

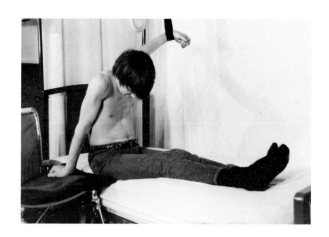
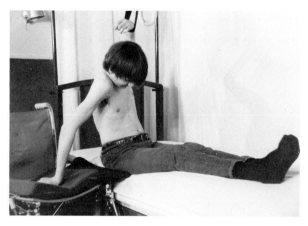
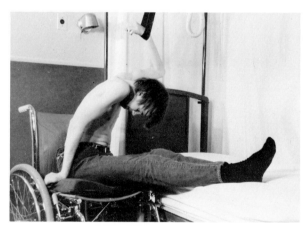

FIGURE 3-83

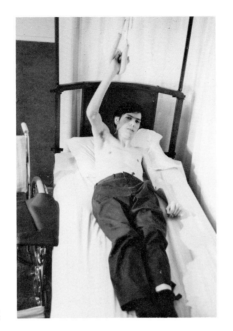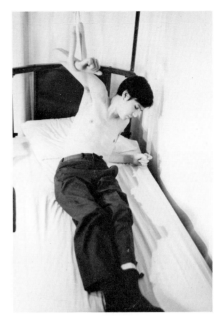

FIGURE 3-84

Method 4. (Fig. 3-84)   The patient sits up and puts the wrist nearest the chair into an overhead strap. The other hand is placed on the bed behind him with the elbow locked. (If unable to straighten his arm he can lean on his elbow.) The patient then leans forward over the locked arm. This, in conjunction with a pull on the strap, will move the buttocks towards the chair. It may be necessary to repeat this procedure to move onto the wheelchair seat. At this point, the patient must lean forward and move back into the chair.

This method may be very useful for a patient with spasticity, since he can maintain a flexed position and avoid triggering extensor spasm.

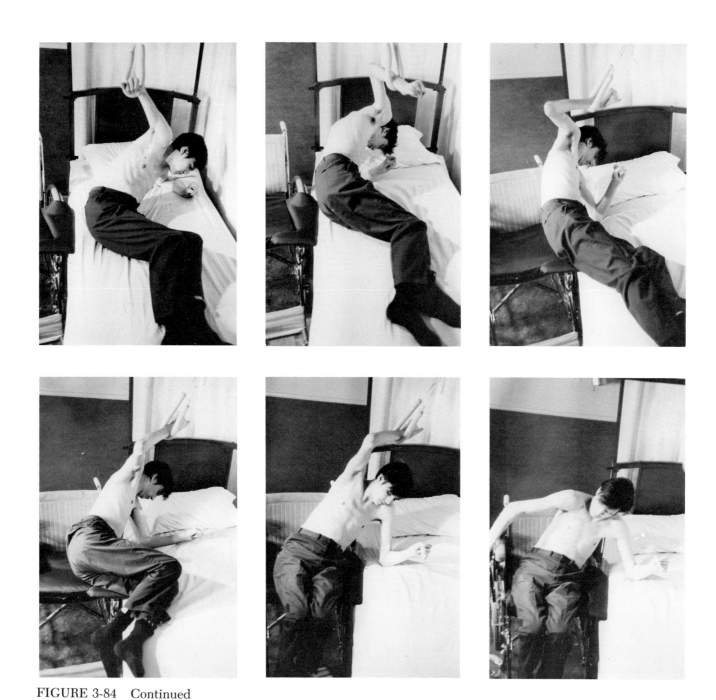

FIGURE 3-84   Continued

Method 5.   The patient who uses a front approach to transfer onto the bed will reverse the method to transfer back (Fig. 3-85). He positions himself so that he faces away from the chair. He allows his trunk to flex forward and reaches behind to hook his extended wrists over the edge of the mattress. Using his elbow flexors, he pulls his buttocks back onto the seat of the chair. He now releases the locks on the chair and wheels back far enough to swing the footrests back and lower his feet. The patient who uses this method of exit, but another method of entry, must learn to reposition his chair while on the bed.

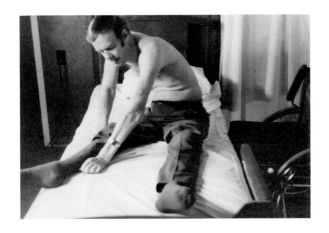 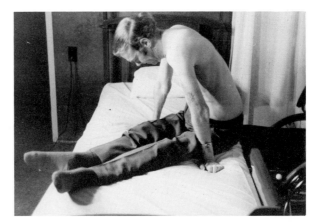

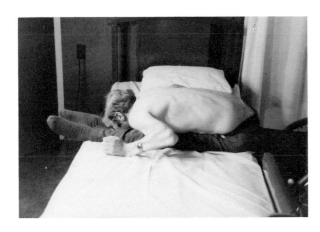 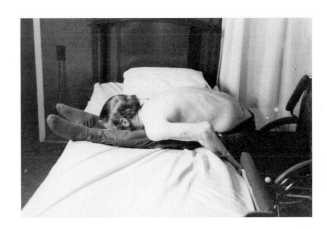

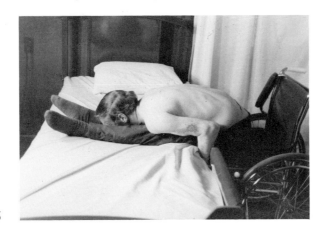 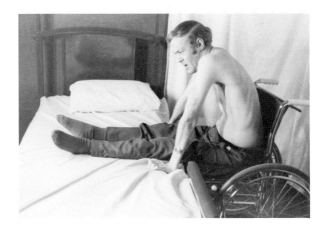

FIGURE 3-85

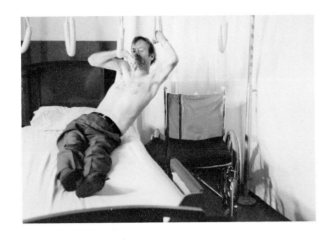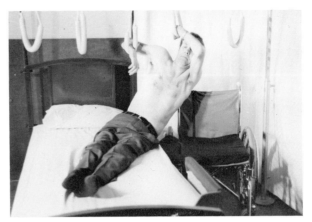

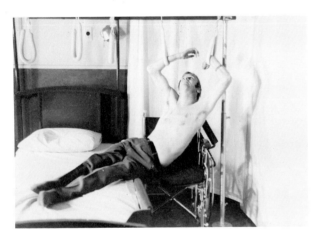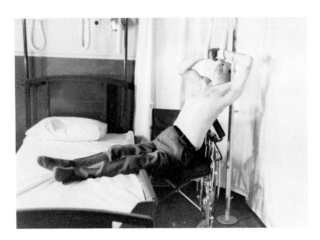

FIGURE 3-86

Method 6.   In this method, the patient uses an outrigger (described in "Bed and Equipment") and a padded nylon covered bridgeboard (Fig. 3-86). He sits up with both wrists in floating overhead straps and moves them towards the chair as far as possible. As he pulls bilaterally, his buttocks are raised and slide over towards the chair seat. This maneuver can be repeated until the patient is seated in the chair. The transfer method may be useful for those with elbow contractures or lack of hip flexion, but is not a first choice for mechanical advantages.

Bedmaking to Permit Handling of the Covers

When the patient is adept at transferring herself into bed, it is time for her to put her skill into practical use. This is accomplished when she can complete the task of going to bed by pulling up the bed covers.

The bed must be made so that it permits easy entry. It should be made in the normal way, except that covers are tucked in on one side only. The top corner is rolled diagonally across the bed from the untucked side. This will leave the bed unobstructed from the top corner of the footboard to the top of the tucked in side of the bed. After she has transferred to the bed, the patient can very easily use her wrist to unroll the bed clothes and cover herself (Fig. 3-87).

Continental quilts or duvets are easy to manage, and are warm. Electric blankets may also be useful, as they are light.

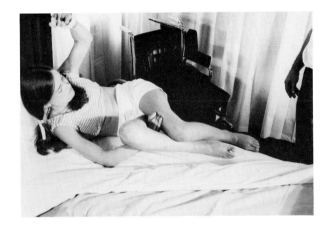
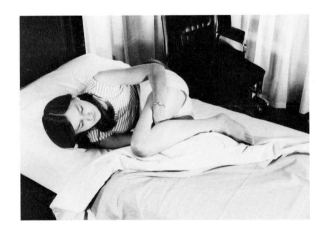
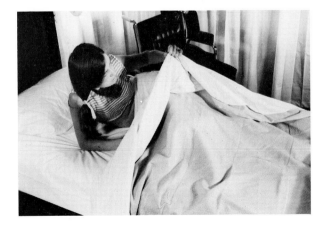
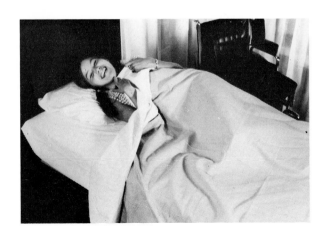

FIGURE 3-87

4

Toilet Transfers

A raised toilet seat is far more practical than a raised toilet bowl in the patient's home or residence. It is also more practical in an institution where people with differing disabilities reside. The open area beneath the seat permits access for cleaning and, when necessary, bowel stimulation or menstrual management. In addition, the raised toilet seat may be detached for use when traveling.

A permanently raised fixture can be most inconvenient for commode wheelchair users, since the commode seat may not fit over the raised toilet bowl (see Fig. 4-31).

VARIETIES OF RAISED TOILET SEATS

RAISED TOILET SEAT

A raised toilet seat (Fig. 4-1) should be the height of the compressed wheelchair cushion.

Toilet seats can be constructed with a small hole so that the patient does not sink down too far. The small hole also prevents spreading of the buttocks, thus helping to prevent natal cleft tears. The patient who slides one way easily, but has difficulty sliding in the other direction, may have slight modifications in toilet seat tilt or height.

A FLAT SEAT

A flat seat (Fig. 4-2) facilitates sliding.

PADDED TOILET SEAT

A padded toilet seat (Fig. 4-3) protects the skin, and is recommended for all quadriplegic people, particularly if the patient is very thin or is prone to decubitus ulcers. This seat is covered (both top and edges) with 1-inch (2.54 cm) foam and is upholstered with naugahyde.

TOILET SEAT WITH PROJECTION

A projection, incorporated with the seat, acts as a sliding board and leaves room for hand positioning (Fig. 4-4).

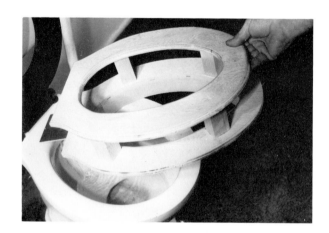

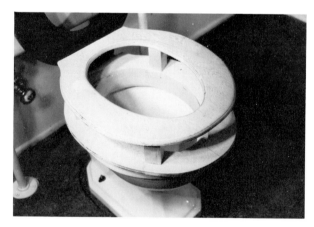

FIGURE 4-1

FIGURE 4-2

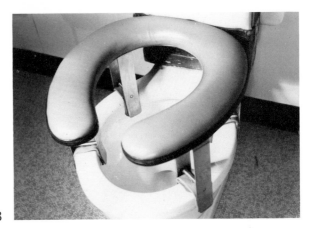

FIGURE 4-3

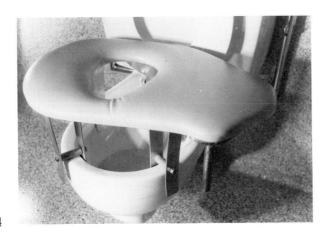

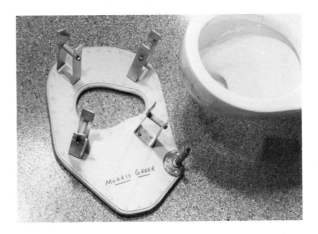

FIGURE 4-4

"Delta Wing" Toilet Seat

A delta wing toilet seat (see Appendix) provides the maximum in stability and in surface area for convenient placement of hands (Fig. 4-5). For these reasons the seat is extremely useful in early training. The seat has a minimum-size keyhole opening. Because the patient does not sink down into this hole he does not have to lift to slide off the seat. If the patient's knees should abduct they will be retained by the shape of the seat front. The rubber-tipped post is placed into the wheelchair arm socket. The wheelchair is then turned towards the toilet so that the post catches behind a lip on the under edge of the lifted wing, locking the wheelchair to the toilet seat when the seat is lowered. The leg is screwed into a floor flange on the underside of the toilet seat on the side away from the wheelchair. This is reversible so that transfers may be practiced from either side, or, if it is used permanently, it may be used in different situations.

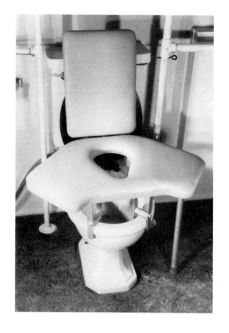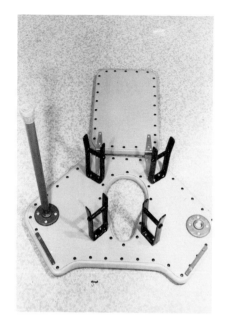

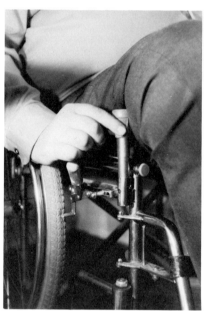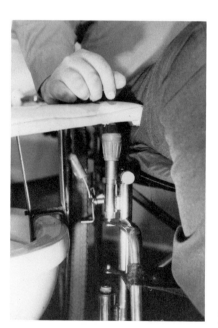

FIGURE 4-5

160

ANGLED TOILET SEAT

A raised toilet seat may be placed at an angle on the toilet bowl to accommodate a wide angle approach (Fig. 4-6).

ADDITIONAL EQUIPMENT

FOOTSTOOL

A footstool will compensate for the added height of the raised toilet seat. The footstool should have nonskid material underneath to stabilize it. A reversible footstool (Fig. 4-7) is useful for patients with different height requirements.

PADDED BACKREST

A padded backrest (Fig. 4-8) assists in posturing the patient and adds to his security and comfort, a prerequisite in bowel training.

GRAB BAR

A grab bar alongside the toilet at approximately 33 inches (83 cm) from the floor is often necessary for stability during transfer and bowel training. A table can be substituted for a grab bar for some patients, providing room for equipment. The grab bar may be attached to the wall (Fig. 4-9A), or may be a swing-away or swing-up bar with the height adjustable, as shown in Figure 4-9B.

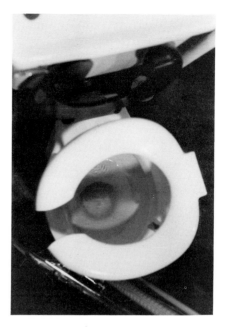

FIGURE 4-6

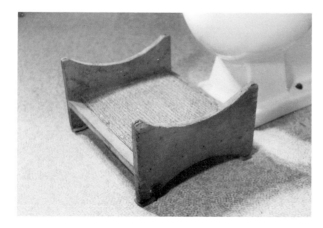

FIGURE 4-7

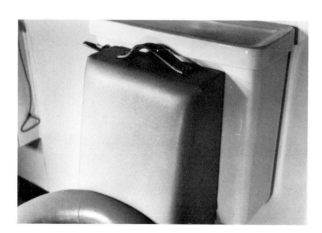

FIGURE 4-8

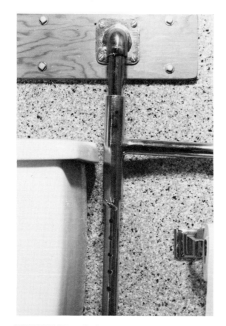

FIGURE 4-9 A

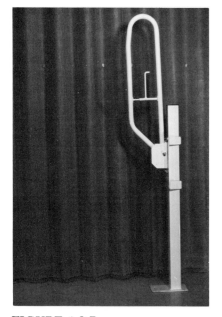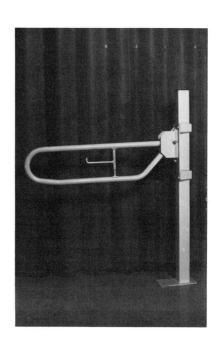

FIGURE 4-9 B

OVERHEAD STRAPS

Fixed or floating straps on an overhead bar frequently are necessary. These straps may be useful for transfers and also for mobility and stability during bowel care. The bar may be fixed or adjustable (Fig. 4-10).

162

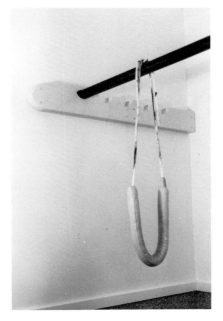

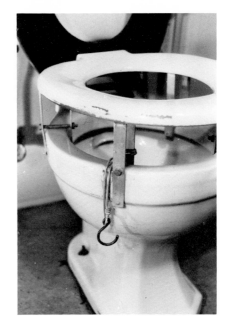

FIGURE 4-10   FIGURE 4-11

WHEELCHAIR HOOK

A rope or strap with a hook may be attached to the toilet if a castor lock is not enough to stabilize the wheelchair (Fig. 4-11).

PADDED TRANSFER BOARD

A padded sliding board with a post and flange may be made, so that it can be used for transfer to either side (Fig. 4-12) (see Appendix).

FIGURE 4-12
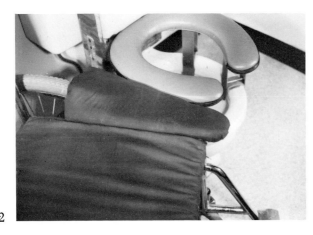

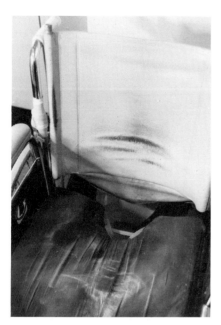

FIGURE 4-13

CUSHION CUT-OUT

The cutaway cushion and wheelchair seat may be used with either a swing-away back, or a back with a zipper on either side, opening halfway up the back from the bottom. This is for use with a semi-transfer through the wheelchair back. The cutout seat will not always be necessary. The U-shaped cutaway in the wheelchair seat must be closed at the top of the "U" with a strong washable (plastic covered) reinforcement strip to prevent the back of the wheelchair seat from sagging. (Fig. 4-13)

TRANSFERRING

WHEELCHAIR TO TOILET

During early transfer training, pants should be worn by the patient until he becomes proficient at transferring onto the toilet. A bowel regimen should be established before the patient starts learning toilet transfers, so that he uses the toilet before dressing in the morning or after undressing at night. This eliminates extra transfers onto the bed for taking off and putting on pants and underwear.

During early training it is important that the raised toilet seat should be level with the compressed wheelchair cushion; later the patient will be more able to tolerate small discrepancies.

A footstool will generally be needed to compensate for the extra height of the toilet seat, but the tall patient may not require one. Placing of the feet depends upon the balance, degree of spasticity, flaccidity, and build of the patient. Experimentation may be required to arrive at the optimum position for each individual. The feet may be moved at any stage of a transfer. The foot positions may be one of the following: both feet on the footrests, both feet on the footrest near the toilet, one foot on a footrest and one on the footstool, or both feet on the footstool.

To get into position for any of the side transfers the patient places the footstool in position and then backs his wheelchair alongside the toilet. He swings the front of the wheelchair in against the toilet bowl, angling the wheelchair at about 35 degrees. He locks the brakes and the castor locks, leaving the castors forward for stability. After sliding his buttocks forward in the wheelchair clear of the front of the wheel, he removes the chair arm.

Method 1. (Fig. 4-14) The patient places one hand on the grab bar or a table on the far side of the toilet and the other hand on the cushion close to his buttock. He leans forward, so placing his center of gravity more over his knees. He internally rotates the arm on the bar, enabling him to use the strong elbow and shoulder flexors to lift him and help the other arm to rotate him onto the toilet, while bending his head and upper trunk down and away from the direction of travel. He now positions his legs for maximum comfort and stability.

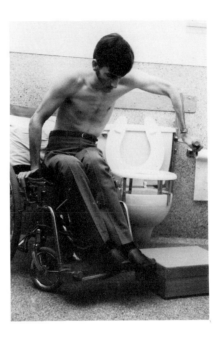 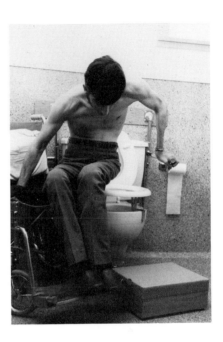

FIGURE 4-14

Method 2. (Fig. 4-15)   The patient places one hand close to his buttock and the other hand on the toilet seat. He locks his elbows and leans forward until he reaches a point of balance. A pushup with both arms together with a sharp head and shoulder movement down and away from the direction of travel should cause his buttocks to swing towards the toilet.

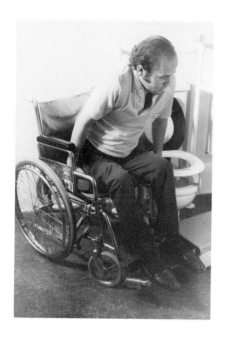 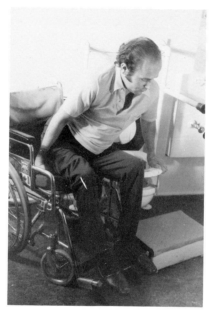 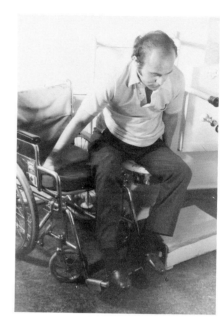

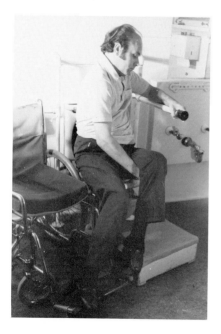 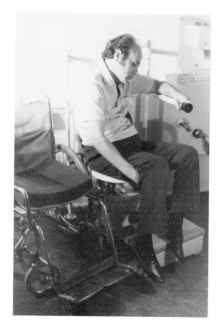

FIGURE 4-15

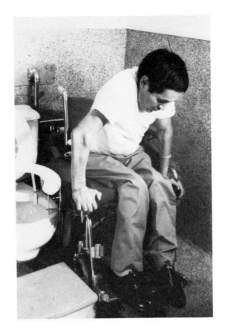
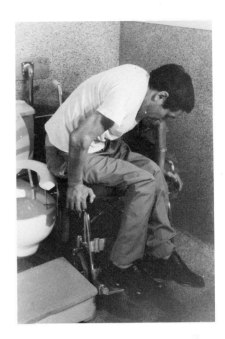

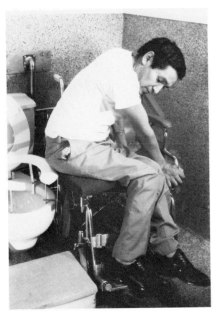
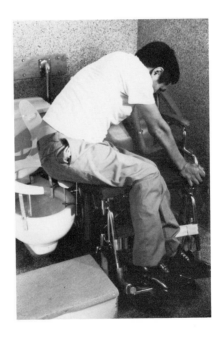
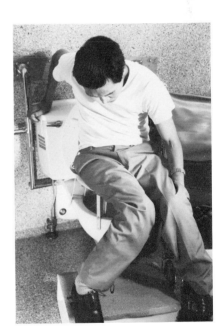

FIGURE 4-16

At first the patient may move for only a short distance, but as balance and strength improve, the transfer will be accomplished in only one or two moves.

Method 3. (Fig. 4-16)   In this technique the patient moves forward in the wheelchair and turns away from the toilet. He places one hand against the front of the wheelchair arm and the other on the cushion against the back of the wheel-

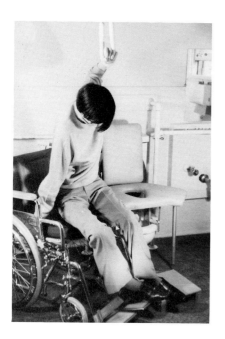

chair arm. He locks both arms and leans forward, pushing himself backwards onto the toilet seat. Note that as he moves back he looks to make sure that he is correctly positioned. Once he is on the toilet he picks up the leg nearest to it and lifts his foot onto the footstool; this leaves the other hand at the back of the wheelchair, a position that helps him twist to face forward. This action is completed when the other leg is lifted over onto the footrest. Either arm may be used to lift the second leg over, but a greater degree of twist is developed if the arm near the wheelchair is used.

Method 4. (Fig. 4-17)   The patient moves forward in the chair and places the wrist nearest the toilet in a floating overhead strap. He may now lift one or both feet across onto the footstool. He locks the other arm with the hand close to his buttock and leans over it away from the toilet. By pulling with the arm in the strap and pushing with the locked arm, he moves part of the way onto the toilet. He shifts the floating strap away from him as far as possible and repeats the action until he is on the toilet. He now positions his feet.

Method 5. (Fig. 4-18)   The patient moves forward in the chair and places his feet on the footstool. He puts his wrist in an overhead strap fixed in position halfway between the toilet and the chair. (If necessary, two straps may be used in this

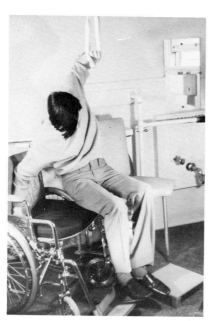
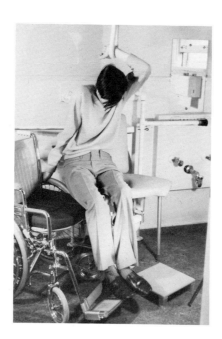
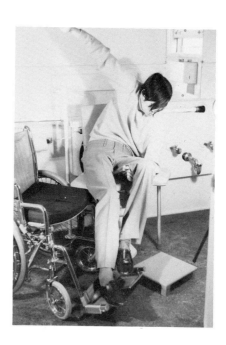

FIGURE 4-17

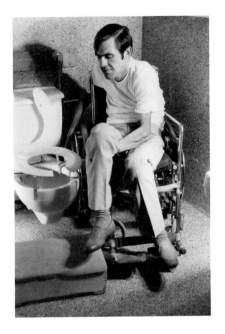
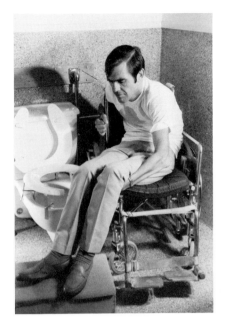

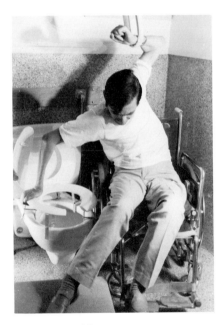
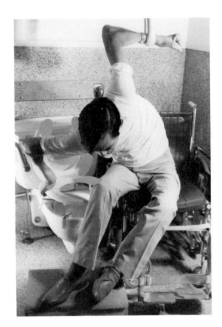
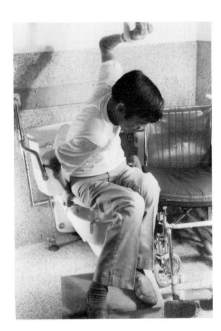

FIGURE 4-18

transfer: one directly over the toilet to assist in getting onto the toilet and one over the chair to assist in getting onto the chair.) The other hand is placed on the far side of the toilet seat with the shoulder internally rotated. Leaning well forward to place some of his weight over his feet, he adducts his shoulders and flexes his elbows strongly to lift and swing onto the toilet.

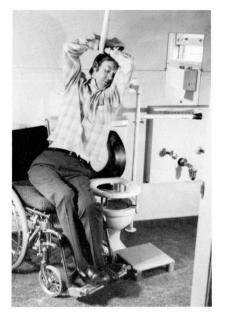
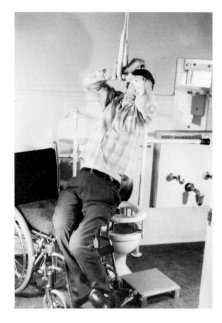
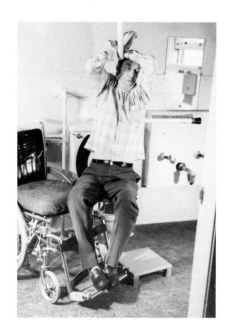

FIGURE 4-19

Method 6. (Fig. 4-19)   The patient positions his feet and places both forearms in an overhead fixed strap positioned directly over the toilet seat. By pulling strongly with both arms he lifts himself and swings onto the toilet seat. Care must be taken to ensure that the wheel does not graze the buttocks while the patient is learning this transfer.

Method 7.   The forward approach is a practical transfer method for a patient who is sufficiently flaccid to allow the knees to abduct without pressure and may be used permanently, or occasionally where space is restricted (Fig. 4-20). Sometimes it is advisable to cut off part of each side of the toilet seat and pad the seat; this eliminates the need for extreme abduction. In this technique the patient

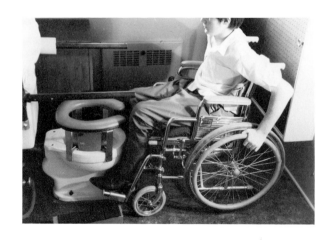
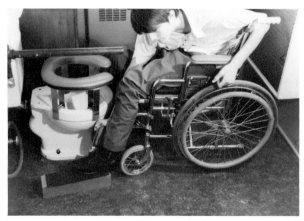

FIGURE 4-20

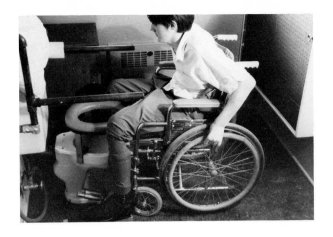
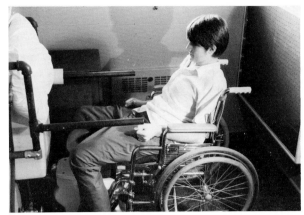
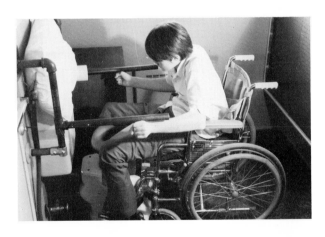
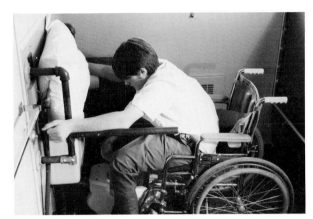
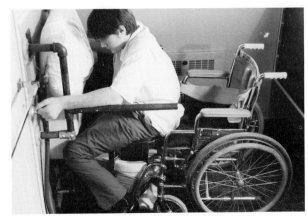
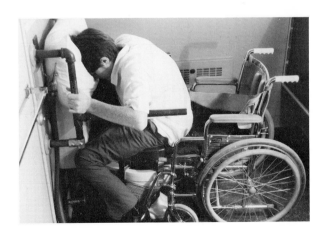

FIGURE 4-20   Continued

171

approaches the toilet from the front and lifts his feet to the outside of the footrests enabling him to wheel up to the toilet so that his cushion is butted to the toilet seat.

He applies his brakes and slides forward in his chair. He now reaches forward to hook his wrists around the grab bars to pull himself onto the toilet. The grab bars may be provided with knobs to prevent slipping. He may reposition his feet and rest his head on a pillow which has been placed on the water tank. This provides comfort and balance and leaves one or both hands free.

Method 8. A swivel-back chair may be used in a rear approach to the toilet (Fig. 4-21). The patient backs the chair over the toilet and places her feet on the midcalf straps. Leaning forward she pushes with the thumb web against the front upright of the chair arm. The patient's buttocks will slide out of the back of the chair, the swivel back allowing her room as it tips forward. Obesity, tight hamstrings, and spasticity preclude the use of this method. A cutout in cushion and seat may be necessary for the patient who is unable to slide far enough out of the chair (Fig. 4-13). Women who are bladder trained and who urinate frequently may use this method of transfer because of facility and the short time required. These women may find it more convenient to wear a skirt but no panties. In this case the swivel back must have an extension flap at the base.

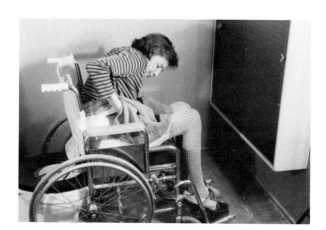
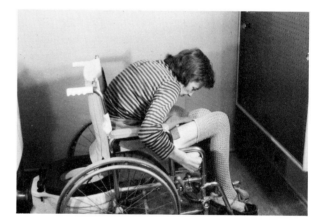
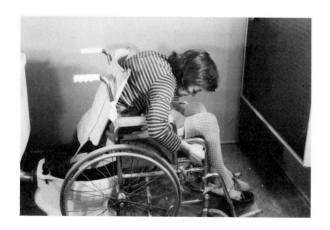
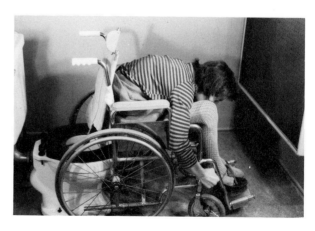

FIGURE 4-21

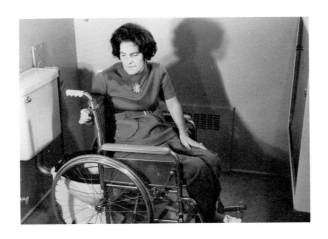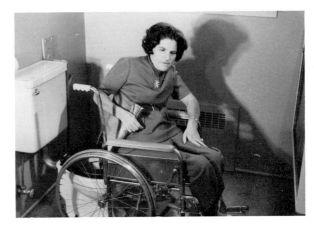

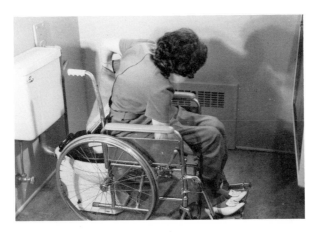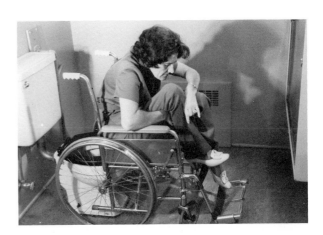

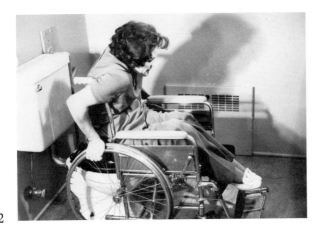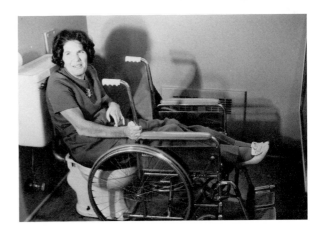

FIGURE 4-22

Method 9.   A rear approach transfer may be a practical transfer and of particular use in a restricted area (Fig. 4-22). Any tightness in the hamstrings will preclude the use of this method. The patient backs over the toilet until the crossbar of the wheelchair touches and then she locks the brakes. She opens the detachable back and flips it out of the way. She lifts her feet onto a strap half way up the leg rest and leans forward to push herself onto the toilet seat, using the wheel or the front upright of the wheelchair arms. Most patients will require a raised toilet seat and a backrest, but the raised toilet seat will be lower than usual, since the back of the wheelchair seat is lower than the front.

TOILET TO WHEELCHAIR

Method 1. (Fig. 4-23)   The patient places one hand on the wheelchair cushion on the far side and one hand on the grab bar or table beside him. He leans forward and pushes up to lift and swivel over onto the wheelchair seat. As he lifts, he ducks his head and shoulders, and turns them away from the direction of travel.

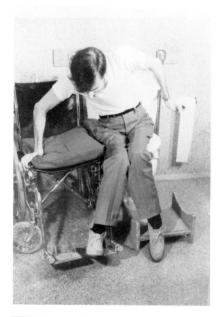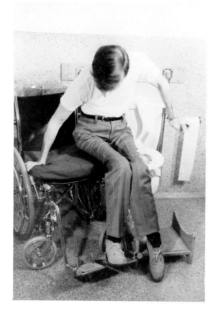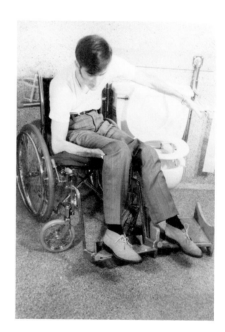

FIGURE 4-23

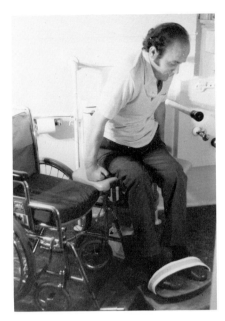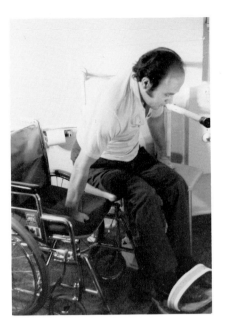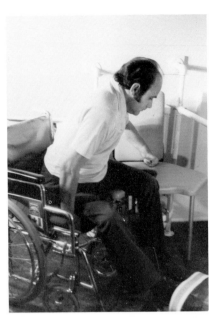

FIGURE 4-24

Method 2. (Fig. 4-24)   The patient places one hand on the toilet seat by his buttock and the other on the wheelchair cushion. He locks his elbows and leans forward until he reaches his point of balance. If he now does a pushup, his buttocks will swing towards the wheelchair seat. This pendulum action will be increased if he ducks his head and shoulders away from the wheelchair. At first the patient may move only a short distance, and must then repeat the maneuver several times to reach the wheelchair. This method is more successful with a patient who is of stocky build, rather than one with a "concertina" spine.

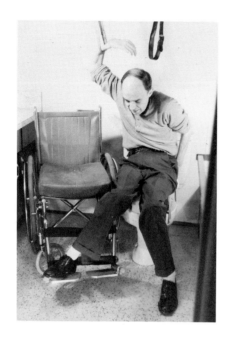 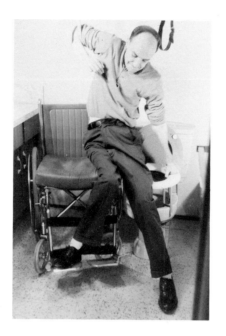

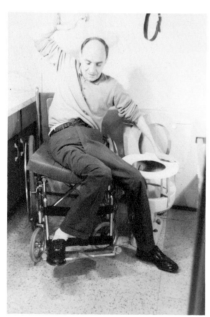 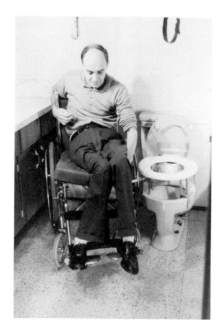

FIGURE 4-25

Method 3. (Fig. 4-25)   The patient puts the wrist nearest the wheelchair into a floating overhead strap, or a fixed strap over the wheelchair, and repositions his feet. He places the other hand on the toilet seat close to his buttock and locks the arm. Leaning forward and over the locked arm, he lifts with the arm in the overhead strap and pushes with the arm on the toilet seat. This shifts him toward the chair or onto it. It may be necessary to flick a floating strap closer to the wheelchair and repeat the maneuver.

Method 4. (Fig. 4-26)   The patient places his feet in position and then inserts both arms into the strap, which is in a fixed position over the wheelchair seat. He lifts with both arms and swings into the chair. This transfer requires careful placement of the feet to prevent the patient being shifted too far forward; precise timing in lowering to sitting is necessary to prevent a return pendulum action.

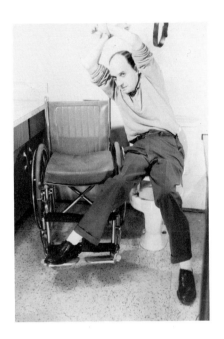
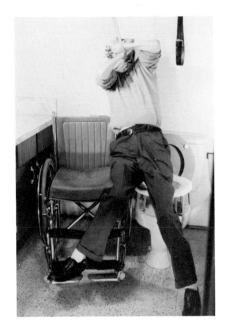
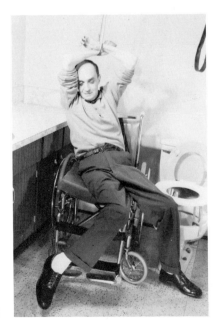
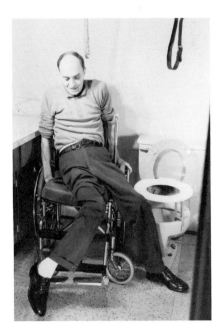

FIGURE 4-26

Method 5. (Fig. 4-27)   To move from the toilet to the wheelchair from a forward position, the patient remains in his forward position and pushes together or alternately with his hands against the wall, water tank, or grab bars. To develop this push he must internally rotate his shoulders, raising his elbows. Since his

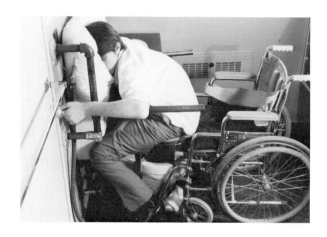
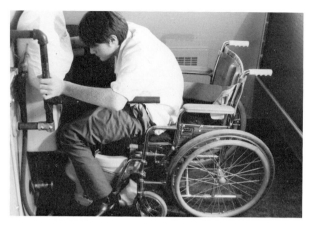

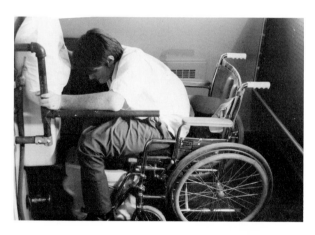
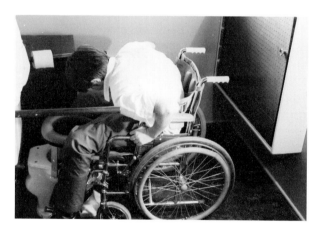

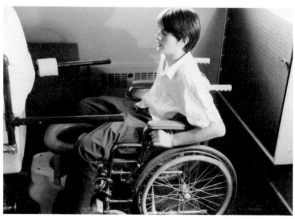

FIGURE 4-27

trunk is flexed he can use a hugging action which pushes his buttocks onto the chair.

Method 6. (Fig. 4-28)   The patient lowers her feet from the heel strap to the

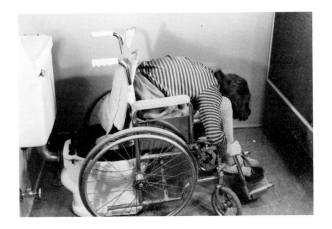 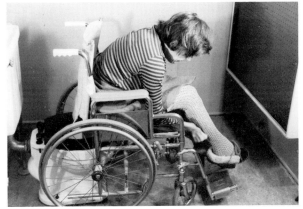

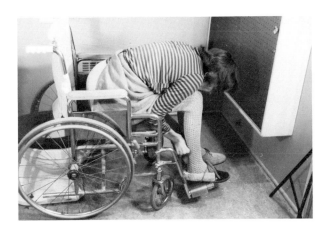 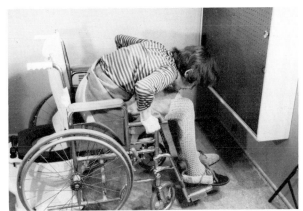

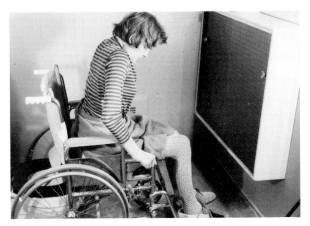

FIGURE 4-28

footrests. Leaning well forward, she places her elbows against the chair cushion and uses shoulder extension to pull herself forward in the chair before sitting up.

Method 7. (Fig. 4-29)   The patient reaches forward to hook her arms around

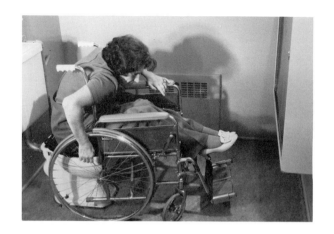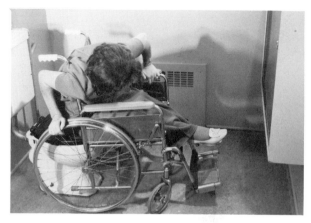

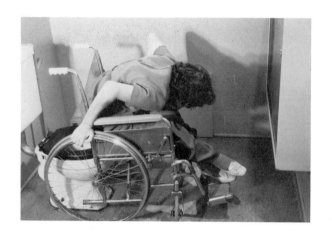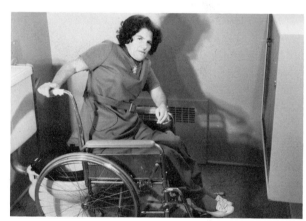

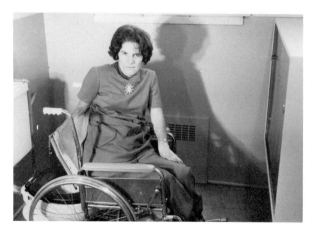

FIGURE 4-29

the chair back uprights. She initiates forward sliding by pulling with her arms and throwing her head forward sharply. The forward movement is assisted by the progressive weight of the lower legs as the feet near the footrests. Additional forward movement may be gained by pushing on the wheels or against the cushion or armrests while the trunk stays well flexed forward. An alternate or simultaneous arm movement may be used to push the patient well forward since adequate room must be left to fasten the chair back.

The gutter on the side of the wheelchair back should be positioned against the back upright at the bottom and pushed into place. The safety pin is pushed through the hole far enough to allow the locking dog to drop into the locked position. For convenience, the safety pin is fastened to the wheelchair (Fig. 4-30).

WHEELCHAIR COMMODE

A commode may be used when the bathroom is too small to place a wheelchair alongside the toilet in a conventional transferring position, when the patient is unable to transfer conveniently to the toilet, or when skin problems make fewer transfers desirable.

A commode with drive wheels at the rear and removable arms, brakes, and footrests is the choice for a patient who is able to transfer from bed to wheelchair. This may also serve as a shower wheelchair, which may be used directly after the toilet to save transfers and energy, and to prevent skin problems.

Many patients will need to have their commode, bed, and wheelchair the same height. The choice of wheelchair may therefore be limited by the height of commercially available commodes, or the expense of adapting a commode to the required height.

FIGURE 4-30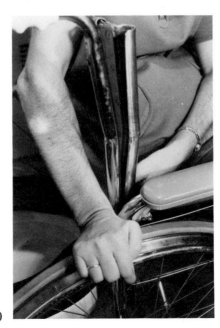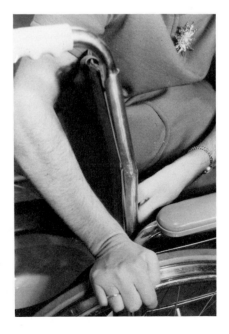

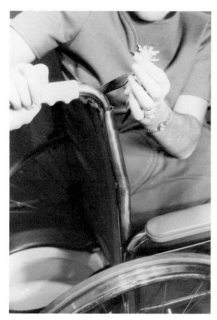 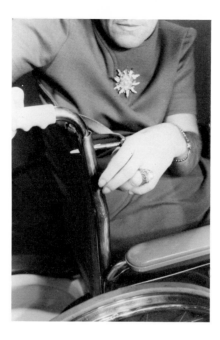 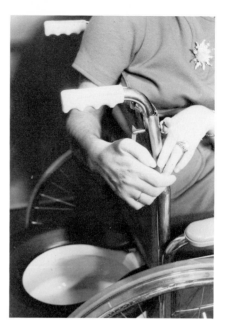

FIGURE 4-30 Continued

A commercially available commode wheelchair which is collapsible does not provide a side or front opening seat for bowel care. A side opening on a commode would not be as convenient for bowel stimulation by the patient as a raised toilet seat because of the obstruction caused by the wheel and the frame. If the front

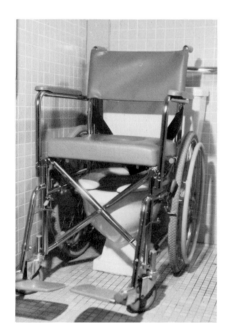 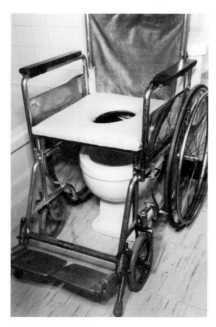

FIGURE 4-31   FIGURE 4-32

182

opening is required, a commode wheelchair is comparable to the front opening toilet seat, but the seat would have to be custom made (Fig. 4-31).

The collapsible feature of the commercial commode wheelchair makes it transportable; however, a raised toilet seat requires less baggage space.

If a commercially available commode is not obtainable a custom commode may be made by converting an old wheelchair (Fig. 4-32).

The center crossbars are removed and a length of tubing is welded across the front of the wheelchair at the junction of the front upright and the bottom bar. Additional stability is gained from the wooden padded seat, which attaches to the original seat rails. Because the crossbars are removed, the commode can be backed directly over the toilet.

The level of the commode seat should be raised to the height of the wheelchair seat, plus the height of the compressed cushion. For some patients, it is advisable to make a seat with a hole of smaller circumference and an open front to facilitate digital stimulation (See Chapter 7). Anti-tipping legs may be installed at the front of the commode.

BED TO COMMODE TRANSFERS

This transfer is made from bed to commode, not from wheelchair to commode, and is made in the same manner as a bed to wheelchair transfer.

Method 1. The transfer may be made to the opposite side of the bed from the usual wheelchair transfer. The brakes must be applied and the castors turned forwards and locked.

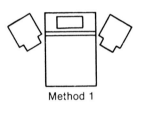

Method 1

Method 2. The wheelchair may be pushed out of the way and the commode put in its place. This requires good reaching ability, or a long stick with a shepherds crook to retrieve the needed chair and apply the brakes.

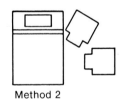

Method 2

Method 3. The commode may be placed further down on the same side of the bed as the wheelchair facing the bed. In this case the patient must be able to swivel and back out of the bed.

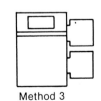

Method 3

183

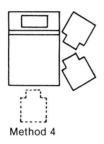

Method 4

Method 4.   The commode may be placed on the same side of the bed as the wheelchair or at the foot of the bed, but facing in the opposite direction to the wheelchair. The patient must be able to completely reverse positions in bed before transferring.

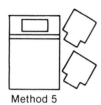

Method 5

Method 5.   Only a very small patient will be able to position the commode chair further down the bed, but facing in the same direction as the wheelchair.

5

Bathing

EQUIPMENT	DAILY SKIN CHECK
Shower Hose	BATHTUB TRANSFER
Taps	THE WHEEL-IN SHOWER
Bath Mitts, Brush, Soap	THE BATHSEAT SHOWER
Container Adaptations	TRANSFERRING TO BATHSEAT
Mirrors	TRANSFERRING FROM
Brush Adaptations	BATHSEAT TO CHAIR
DAILY WASH	CABINET SHOWER

Cleanliness is particularly important for the quadriplegic patient, to prevent skin problems and unpleasant odors. Despite the efficiency of the patient, occasional drops of urine may escape during changing or emptying urine collecting apparatus or during self-catheters. The patient may become accustomed to this smell and, therefore, be oblivious to its effect on others.

EQUIPMENT

SHOWER HOSE

A shower hose permits thorough washing and rinsing. The water must be turned on and tested before being directed at any anesthetic part of the patient's body. Particular care must be taken if there is no mixing or safety valve, and the water must be allowed to run for an adequate length of time to ensure a steady temperature. Ideally, the water temperature should be checked at the tap before directing the water through the shower head.

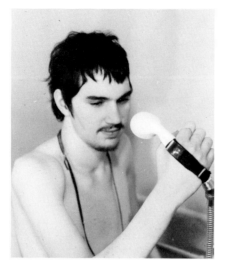

FIGURE 5-1

The telephone type handle of a flexible metal shower hose (Fig. 5-1) may be adapted if necessary by building up the handle, by attaching a velcro D-ring strap, or by attaching a hook handle.

TAPS

Taps may be adapted if necessary by rivetting, brazing, or gluing a lever arm to them (Fig. 5-2A). A long lever tap may be purchased to replace an unsuitable tap (Fig. 5-2B).

A tap which regulates heat and flow using a single lever is ideal for many patients (Fig. 5-2C).

BATH MITTS, BRUSH, SOAP

Bath mitts may be made of towelling or a lighter material sewn around three sides, and the cuff may be loose or closed with velcro. The soap may be slipped into the mitt for washing and removed for rinsing, or it may be drilled to take a

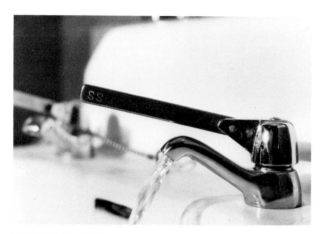

FIGURE 5-2 A

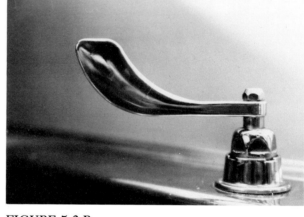

FIGURE 5-2 B

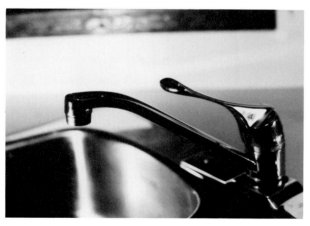

FIGURE 5-2 C

186

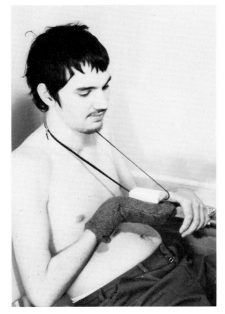

FIGURE 5-3

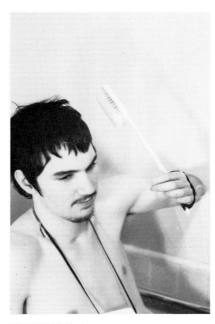

FIGURE 5-4

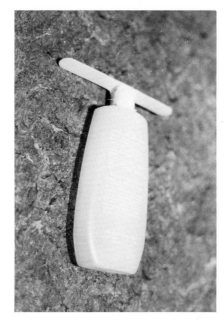

FIGURE 5-5

length of cord so that it can be hung around the neck, remaining within reach (Fig. 5-3). A bath brush may be adapted so that it can be firmly held to enable the patient to reach the back and legs (Fig. 5-4).

CONTAINER ADAPTATIONS

Shampoo should be placed in an easy-to-reach position. The dispenser may be adapted if necessary, or a small amount placed in a tin lid or equivalent. Screw-top bottles (preferably plastic bottles) may be loosely fastened and, if necessary, a lever such as a tongue depressor taped to the cap (Fig. 5-5).

A spray bottle may be placed in a box made to fit with a lid hinged to the top so that it acts as a lever to depress the valve (Fig. 5-6). A two-inch (5 cm) diameter hole may be made on the hinged side so that the spray can be directed through it.

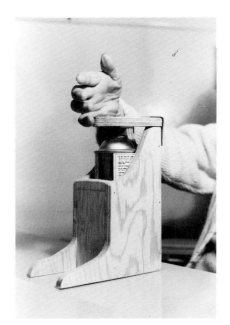

FIGURE 5-6

187

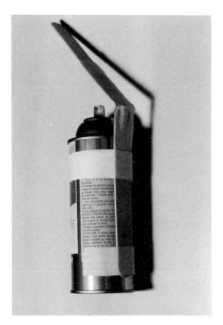

FIGURE 5-7

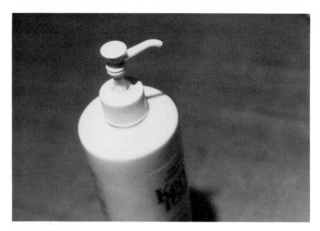

FIGURE 5-8

An adaptation may be made quickly by taping two tongue depressors together end to end. One is then taped to the spray can with the tape "hinge" level with the valve (Fig. 5-7). The free end of the tongue depressor acts as a lever to depress the valve with little effort required.

Press down caps are very convenient for many people (Fig. 5-8).

Commercially available handles can be attached to any spray can and often are easy for a quadriplegic patient to handle (Fig. 5-9).

MIRRORS

The mirror for daily skin inspection may require an adapted handle (Fig. 5-10).

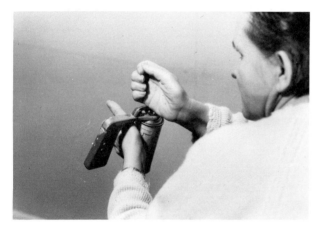

FIGURE 5-9

188

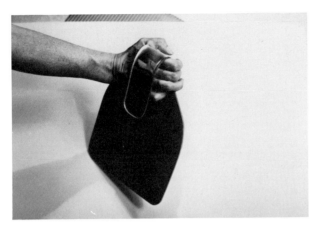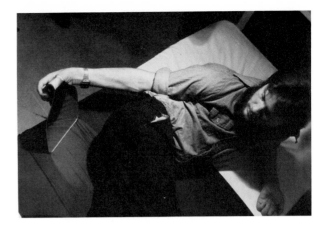

FIGURE 5-10

BRUSH ADAPTATIONS

Frequently shampoo brushes are manufactured with a loop handle, making them ideal as hair brushes or shampoo brushes for many patients.

DAILY WASH

If the patient can approach the wash basin so that his knees are underneath, the bottom of the basin and the drain pipe must be insulated. A side approach may be necessary for some patients because of bathroom design. In both cases the patient must be able to reach the taps, which should be lever type, or adapted to the patient's needs. It is safer to fill the basin with water and check the temperature, rather than letting the tap run. All equipment, including the soap and wash cloth, must be organized so that it is within reach. The wash cloth or bath mitt may be wrung out by squeezing it between the heels of the hands, by pressing it against the wash basin, or by pressing it into a small bowl with drainage holes. All areas can be washed while seated, except the buttock area. Feet may be washed with the leg resting on the opposite knee, with the feet on the footrest, or with the feet on a footstool of convenient height. The patient dries himself as thoroughly as possible using a towel, a dry bath mitt, or a towel with pockets sewn into the ends. He then transfers onto a flannelette sheet on the bed. This will absorb any additional moisture. His buttocks and perineum are easier to wash on the bed. The daily skin check must not be overlooked on completion of this routine.

DAILY SKIN CHECK

A convenient time for the daily skin inspection is after bathing and before dressing. A mirror may be adapted so that it can be firmly held. The areas that must be inspected are the skin over the spinous processes of the back, the hips, the crest of the pelvis, the sacrum, and the ischial tuberosities. Special care must be taken to check the natal cleft. The knees, the ankles, heels, soles, and toes must also be checked. Toenails should be trimmed regularly and checked to see that

189

they do not become ingrown. Elbows must also be checked for abrasions, particularly if elbows are used during transfers or shifts. Early detection of skin problems often can save weeks of treatment—weeks which would have caused time loss at work and would have interfered with social activities.

BATHTUB TRANSFER

Method 1.   A quadriplegic who can get from the floor to his chair will probably be able to get into the tub and out. A grab bar may be required, firmly fastened to the far wall of the bathtub, far enough from the wall to permit a hand to grip it. The height must be worked out for each individual; it is usually 6 inches (15.24 cm) above the tub rim.

In the technique for getting into the tub (Fig. 5-11) the patient may approach the bathtub with his chair at a 30° angle to the tub, or more commonly he may use a front approach with both footrests swung away. He slides forward in the chair, lifts both feet into the tub, and slides to the edge of the bathtub before reaching for the grab bar. He places both feet on the bottom of the tub to take part

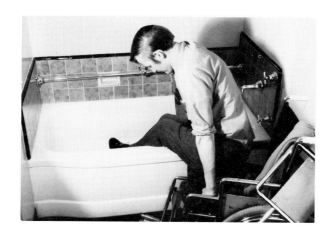
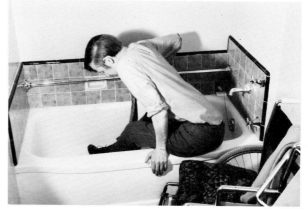
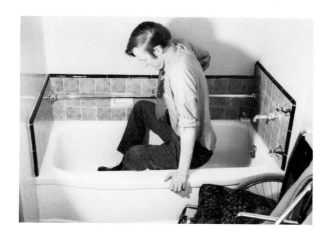
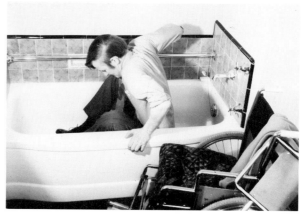

FIGURE 5-11

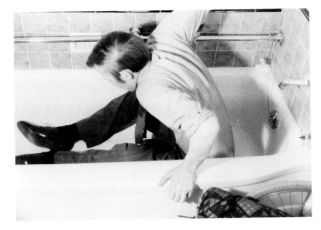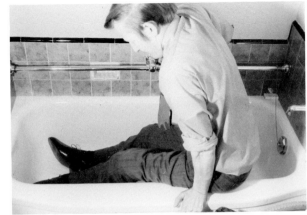

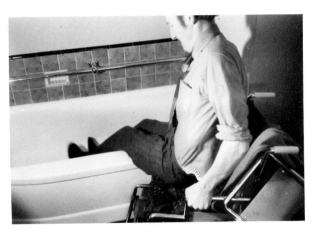

FIGURE 5-12

of his weight, but makes sure that his feet point towards the foot of the tub so that his legs will not buckle under him as he lowers himself.

To get out of the tub, the patient brings his knees up against his chest and leans forward, lifting himself up and then over to the bathtub edge (Fig. 5-12). This requires skill, balance, and a good deal of strength. When a patient is learning this skill, a helper can slip a towel around his waist or chest as a stand-in belt which can be controlled with one hand.

Method 2. The patient approaches the bathtub front on, and stops with the footrests a few inches away from the tub. He locks the wheelchair and lifts his feet onto the edge of the tub, before swinging the footrests away and wheeling the wheelchair closer. Stabilizing himself by placing his forearm in an overhead strap positioned so that it is centered over the outside edge of the tub, he places his feet so that they will slide towards the end of the tub. He lifts strongly with the arm in the overhead loop and pushes with the other hand on the wheelchair cushion to guide him out over the tub, before lowering himself into it (Fig. 5-13).

To get out of the tub, the patient reverses the procedure, using a very strong lift on the overhead strap and a push-up on the edge of the tub. The placement of the strap above the edge of the tub is important when getting out, because it helps to swing the buttocks toward the wheelchair. The patient places his hand so that he can pull himself toward the edge of the tub and rest his buttocks there momentarily while he replaces his hand on the wheelchair cushion. A further lift on the strap and pull on the wheelchair lifts him far enough onto the wheelchair seat so that he can let go of the overhead strap and lean back. He then pushes himself back into the wheelchair, using his hands on the wheels. The wheelchair is wheeled back to pull his feet up to the edge of the tub, before they are lowered to the footrests, which have been swung back into position (Fig. 5-14).

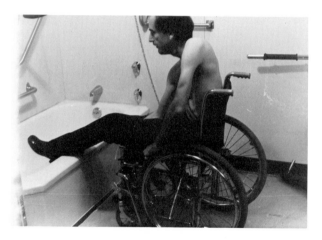
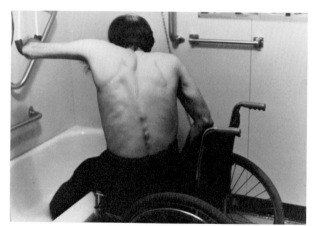
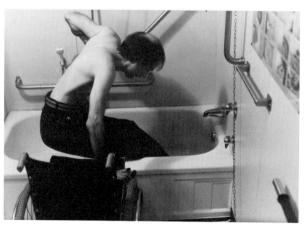
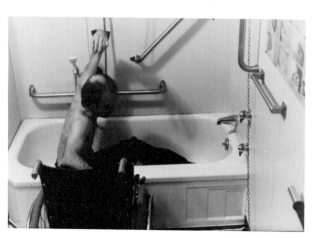

FIGURE 5-13

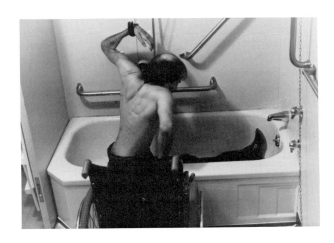
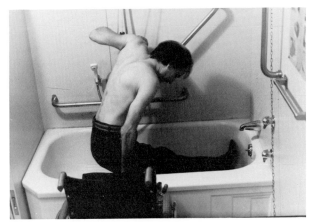

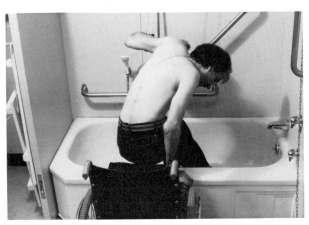
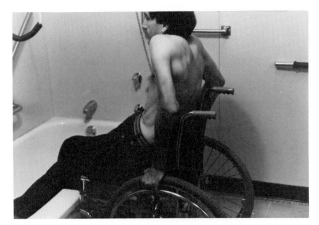

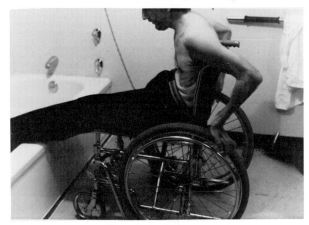

FIGURE 5-14

THE WHEEL-IN SHOWER (Fig. 5-15)

By far the most convenient situation is to have a shower area large enough to accommodate a commode wheelchair. The floor of the wheelchair shower should be recessed for drainage, and levelled to the regular floor by duckboards, close enough together so that the wheels will ride over them (Fig. 5-15C).

A tiled area sloped to the drain may be used if the bathroom is large. A small area will require too steep a slope, making it hard to wheel a wheelchair. The drain is best placed in a corner to reduce the degree of slope required (Fig. 5-15A&B) (See Appendix for bathroom plans).

The telephone shower, taps and washing aids must be within reach. A thermostat to cut the water off if it becomes too warm, or a safety mixing valve is required. Cut-off thermostats which can be inserted between the outlet and the hose are commercially available.

A folding commode chair is available which is versatile and transportable. An alternative is to use an older wheelchair, preferably of stainless steel. Any wheelchair used in a shower must have regular maintenance, particularly of the bearings, as the grease may be washed out. In an emergency, a plastic sheet may be used to protect a regular wheelchair. An air cushion may be used instead of a water absorbent cushion.

It is often convenient to shower immediately after toileting to ensure cleanliness and to save transfers. It is usual to transfer to the commode wheelchair from the bed, returning to the bed to dress after showering, if a morning routine is followed. Similarly, if an evening routine is preferred, a patient may first undress on the bed, and then transfer into the commode wheelchair.

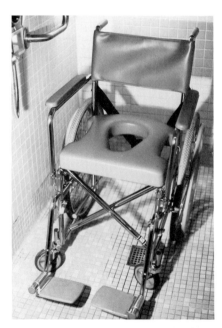

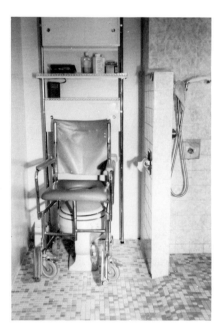

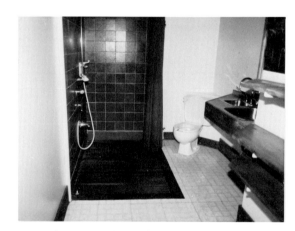

C.   Shower with duckboard flooring

FIGURE 5-15 A.   Large wheel-in shower with minimal slope to drain

B.   Adjoining toilet and shower in a bedroom

194

THE BATHSEAT SHOWER

Commercially made bathseats are available, which can often be used without modifications (Fig. 5-16). Some patients will require height adjustments for their model of wheelchair. Laterally or vertically extended backs may also be required if balance is poor. A footstool may be required in the bathtub to position the legs, or an extra bathboard may be placed near the foot of the tub so that a long sitting position with the legs up may be maintained. This enables a patient with poor balance to stabilize himself, or to wash his legs and feet more easily.

A custom-built bathseat, usually with a back, may be required (Fig. 5-17). Modifications such as cutouts for perineal washing, laterally extended backs for those with poor balance during transfers, or padded front ridges to prevent a person from sliding forward, may be useful. It is probable that the bathseat should be raised to the height of the wheelchair seat, or alternatively, the bathtub may be raised on a pedestal. All bathseats should be stable and they should be padded. They should preferably also be collapsible for easy transport, and adjustable to fit different bathtubs.

If necessary the seat may have a padded cutout on a hinged section to fit over the wheel of a commode or a wheelchair for use as a transfer board (Fig. 5-18).

An overhead strap may be used not only for transfer, but also so that the patient can lean and maneuver to wash underneath himself on the bathseat. A grab bar may also be required. This must be far enough from the wall to allow a hand to be inserted and should be at elbow height when the patient is sitting on the seat. The taps should be lever type for easy turning and must be within reach. As the bath seat may be moved forward or back this is easy to ensure. The taps may be behind the seat or in front, depending upon the balance and reach of the patient and the layout of the bathroom.

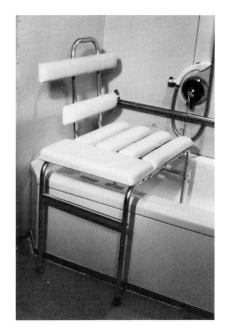

FIGURE 5-16

TRANSFERRING TO BATHSEAT

Frequently the patient will use the same methods and overhead equipment in this transfer as in his bed transfer. The main difference between a bed transfer and

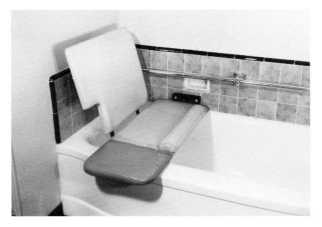

FIGURE 5-17

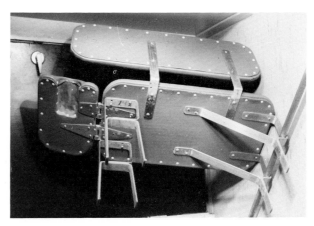

FIGURE 5-18

195

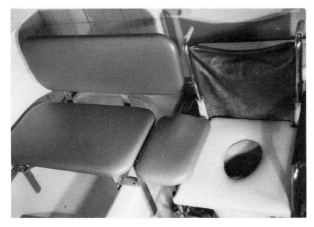
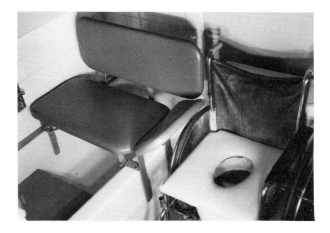

FIGURE 5-18   Continued

a bathseat transfer is in the positioning of the legs and the use of the side of the bathtub to assist in the transfer. It is advisable for the patient to learn the method of transfer wearing his slacks to provide skin protection and ease of sliding. When the patient has progressed to a wet run, talcum powder or silicone spray may be used to make the dry seat slippery. He may place a damp facecloth for any nonslip hand positions.

Method 1. (Fig. 5-19)   The patient lifts one leg into the bathtub and leaves the other on the footrest near the bathtub. This wide base gives him stability. The leg inside the bathtub will tend to pull his buttocks towards the bathtub until his

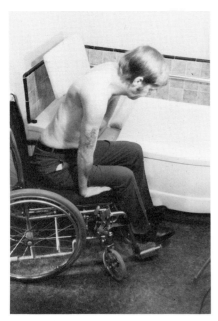
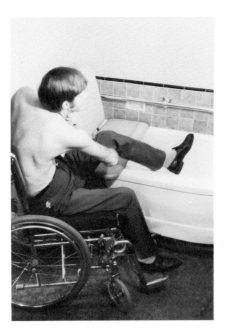
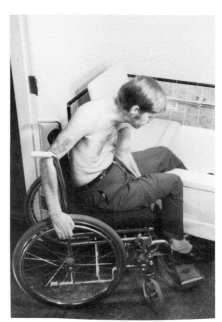

FIGURE 5-19

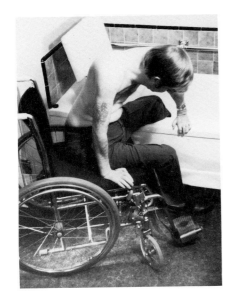 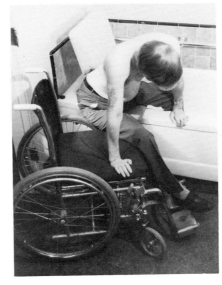 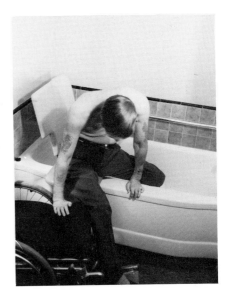

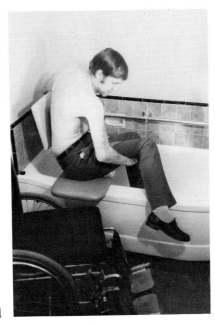 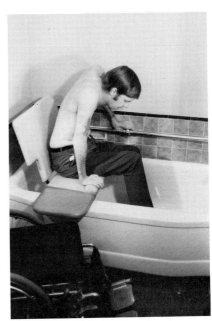

FIGURE 5-19   Continued

foot makes contact with the bottom. He must now pivot his shoulders towards the chair until the knee is stopped against the side of the tub. Further effort to pivot will lever him onto the bath seat with minimum effort because the knee creates a fulcrum against the bathtub side. As soon as the leg on the outside of the tub prevents further progress, it is lifted in.

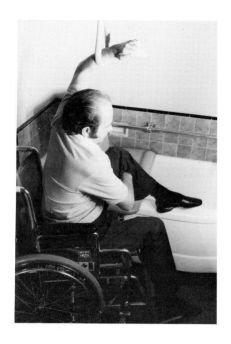
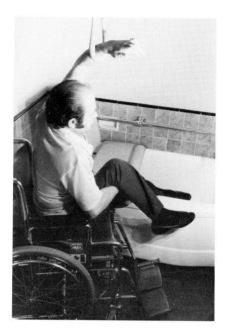

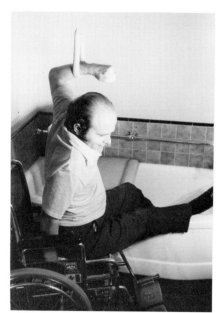
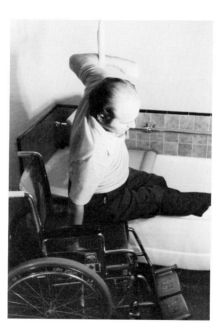
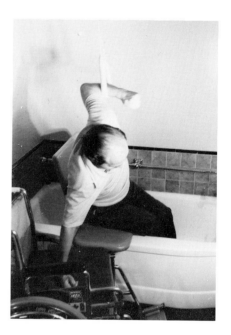

FIGURE 5-20

Method 2. (Fig. 5-20)   Both legs may be lifted into the bathtub first to provide additional help, because the extra weight of the legs will pull the patient onto the bathseat more easily, although he sacrifices some stability. As in the first method, the knees become a fulcrum against the side of the tub after the feet have reached the bottom of the bathtub. The shorter patient may require a footstool inside the bathtub to prevent the weight of his legs pulling him forward off the bathseat and to provide a secure sitting position. It is not recommended that the patient leave both legs on the footrests of the wheelchair while moving onto the bathseat, because he loses stability and leverage and could push the chair away unless it is locked to the bathseat.

Method 3. (Fig. 5-21)   The patient turns her wheelchair at a right angle to the bathtub in line with the bathseat. She locks her chair about a foot from the bathseat, leaving her room to lift her legs and place them on the seat. She swings the footrests away to allow her to wheel forward and bring her cushion into contact with the lip of the bathseat. She shifts forward until her feet nearly touch the far wall. She then lowers her legs and moves further onto the seat. Although the patient gains little leverage from the side of the bathtub, this method provides great security and stability, particularly for the patient with flaccid lower extremities.

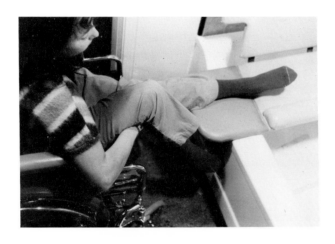
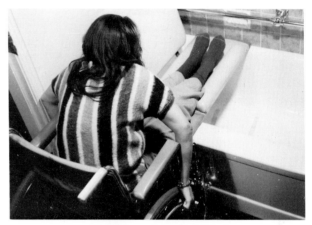
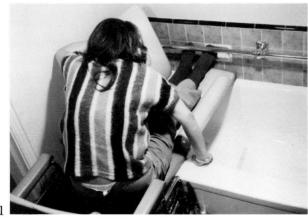
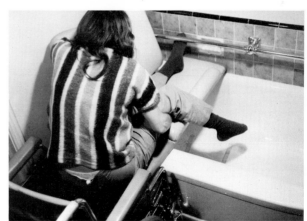

FIGURE 5-21

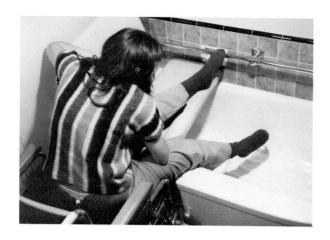
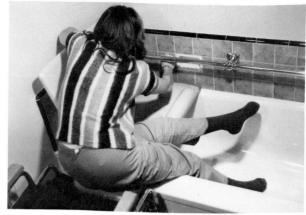
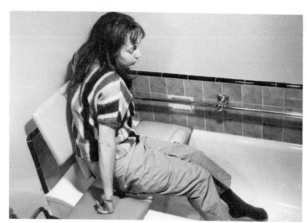
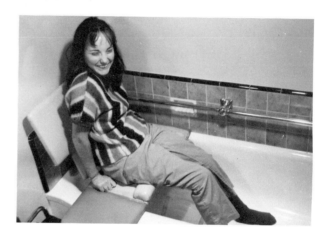

FIGURE 5-21   Continued

TRANSFERRING FROM BATHSEAT TO CHAIR

When the patient is ready to transfer from the bathseat to chair he spreads a flannelette sheet over his chair to absorb all moisture, particularly from the perineal area which would be difficult to dry otherwise.

Method 1. (Fig. 5-22)   The patient who must lean forward in order to move back will leave both legs in the bathtub for stability. Since a good deal of his weight is taken through his legs when he leans forward, the effort used to move back is lessened. He moves back until his legs meet the side of the bathtub; at this point he may lift one leg out and move back further before lifting the second leg out, or he may lift both legs out. If the patient lifts both legs out, his buttocks will twist towards the chair. If he then turns his trunk towards the bathtub, his knees will act as a fulcrum against the side of the bathtub and help to pivot him into the chair.

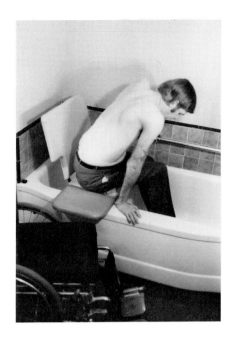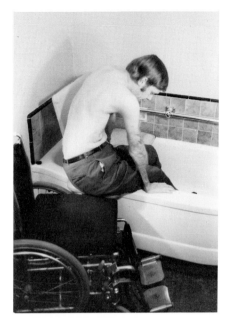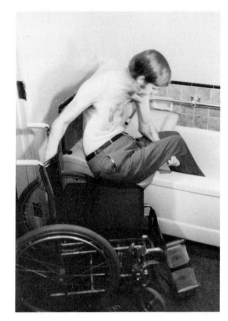
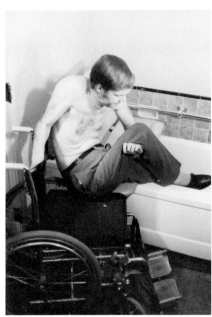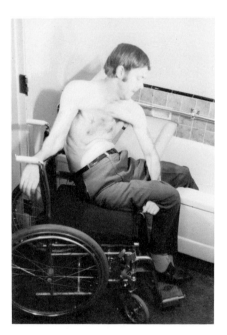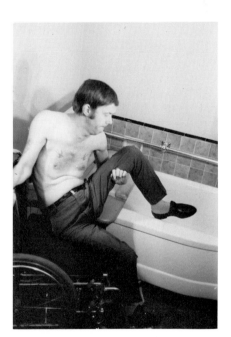

FIGURE 5-22

201

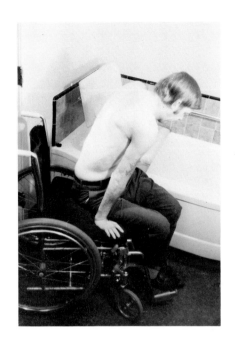
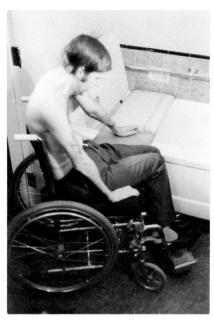

FIGURE 5-22 Continued

Method 2. (Fig. 5-23) An alternative method is to leave both legs in the bathtub and, by continuing to move back, the legs straighten and slide onto the bathtub rim. They are lowered when the patient is back in his chair. This method is suitable for the patient with flaccid legs, who is able to maintain stability while he leans forward, but is unable to lift the legs in this position.

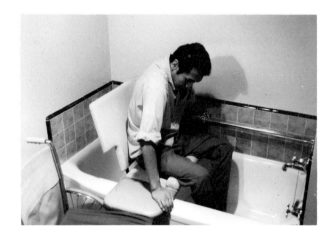
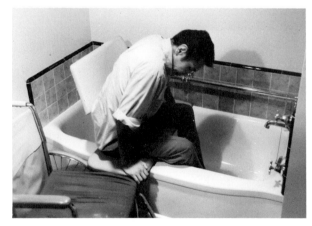

FIGURE 5-23

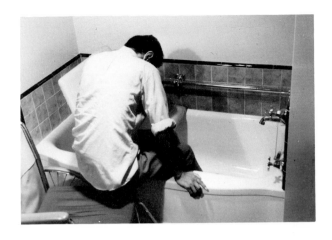 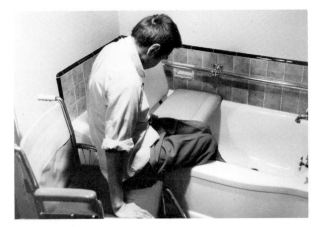

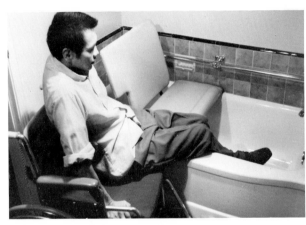 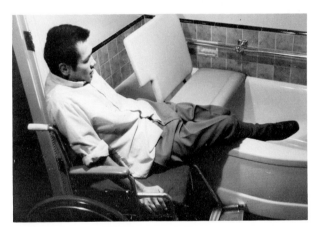

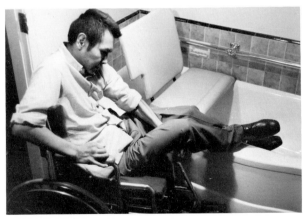 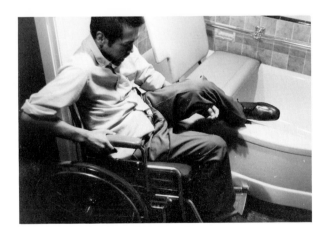

FIGURE 5-23   Continued

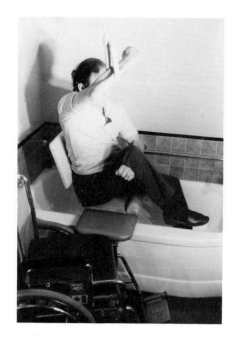
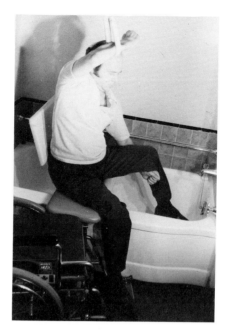
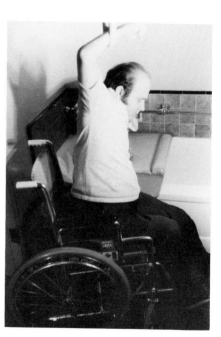

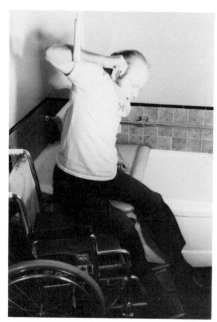
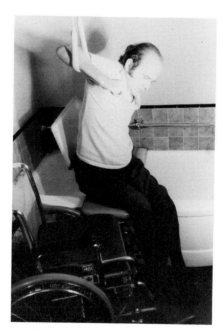

FIGURE 5-24

Method 3. (Fig. 5-24)   Lifting both feet out of the bathtub first provides a pulling action, which helps to move the patient towards the chair. As he turns away from the chair, the knees become a fulcrum against the bathtub so that further movement will pivot him into the chair.

Method 4. (Fig. 5-25)   The patient shifts along the bathseat and turns her back towards the chair. She lifts her legs onto the seat and moves further back towards the chair. When lifting her legs she may place her feet against the wall with her knees flexed. This will assist her to move back. When she is seated in the chair she unlocks the brakes, wheels back far enough to swing the footrests into position, and lowers her legs.

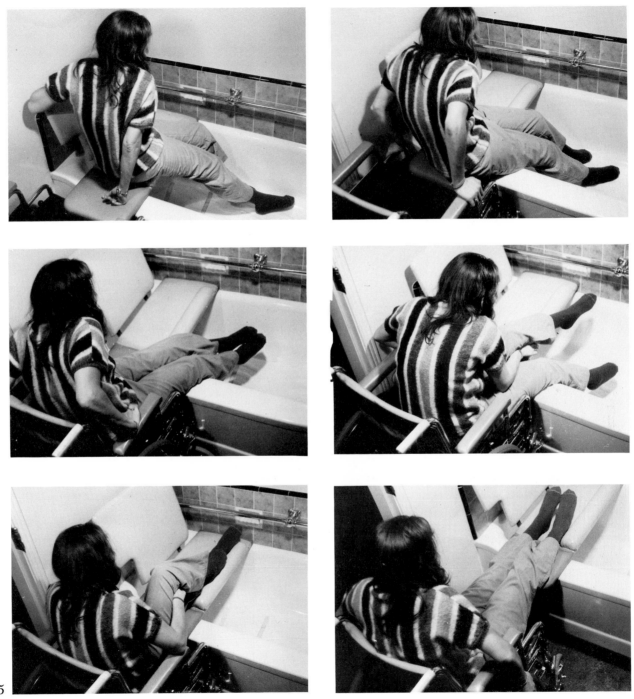

FIGURE 5-25

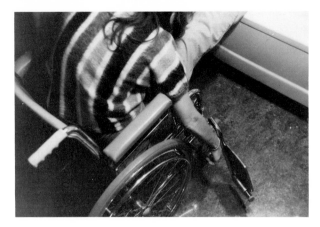 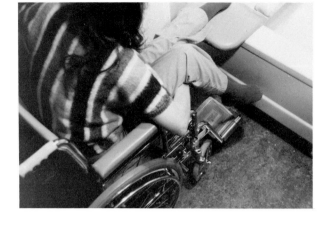

FIGURE 5-25   Continued

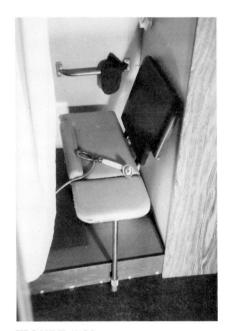

FIGURE 5-26

CABINET SHOWER

A bathseat, as previously described, adapted for use in a commercially available cabinet shower, must protrude through the doorway of the shower providing a bridge board from the wheelchair into the shower (Fig. 5-26). The shower seat must be provided with legs to bring it to the correct height.

6

Dressing and Undressing

The quadriplegic patient should clothe his upper half while sitting in the wheelchair because this position provides better balance than does long sitting on the bed. Feet can remain on the bed or on the footrests of the wheelchair, depending on the ability of the patient to stabilize himself. The order of dressing must be worked out in order to eliminate unnecessary maneuvering. For instance, if the patient goes to the toilet in the morning, he should dress his upper body in the chair, go to the bathroom, and then dress his lower body back on the bed. If he has his legs in position to put his pants over his feet but uses another position to pull them over his buttocks, he should put both underpants and pants on over his feet before changing the position.

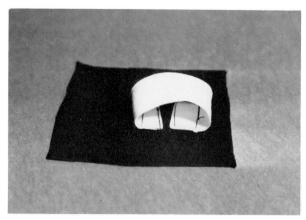

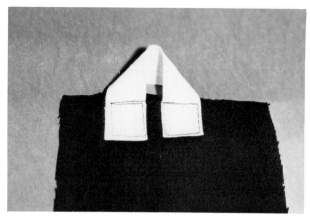

FIGURE 6-1 A. Center loop   B. Edge loop

EQUIPMENT

A loop may be sewn onto a garment to enable the patient to pull by hooking a thumb or finger into it. The loop should be sewn so that it remains open (Fig. 6-1). Loops should match the material as closely as possible for cosmesis.

A dressing stick may be useful for the patient who lacks range, strength, or balance to reach extremities (Fig. 6-2). The length must be adjusted to the individual, but be as short as possible. The handle may have to be adapted so that it can be firmly held. Sticks for pulling require a hook; sticks for pushing require a V cut

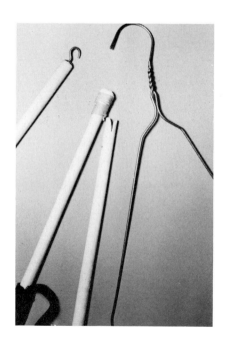

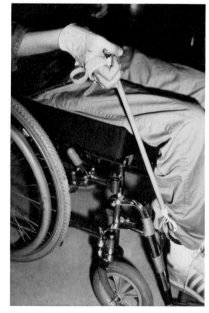

FIGURE 6-2

or a padded nonslip end such as a rubber thimble. A wire coat hanger, pulled so that it is elongated, may often suffice as a temporary but effective pulling stick. Usually dressing sticks are used only in the early stages of training.

SHIRTS AND BLOUSES

Putting On

Shirts should have large armholes and loose cuffs. Women will be unable to manage blouses with back openings. Strong material is necessary, particularly while the patient is learning to dress. Sport shirts worn outside the pants are easiest to put on for general wear, as they eliminate tucking in.

The method chosen depends upon the patient's ability to balance and the time spent on fastening the shirt. The reach-around-the-back method will be used by the patient with excellent balance and good shoulder musculature. Methods employing a throwing action require fair balance and practice. Although a buttoned or T-shirt must be larger and can be harder to put on and take off, this may be compensated for by the time saved in fastening and unfastening.

Method 1. The very low-lesion patient may be able to put a shirt on in a normal fashion, slipping one arm into a sleeve and reaching behind his back with the other arm to the second sleeve.

Method 2. (Fig. 6-3) The patient pushes the sleeve of the shirt completely into position on the arm and shoulder, using tenodesis or a thumb of the other hand hooked into the material. She leans forward to allow the shirt to fall behind the shoulder, working it as far round her back as possible. She reaches behind her neck and hooks thumb or fingers into the collar to pull the shirt further round the back. Leaning forward and balancing with an elbow on the knee or a hand against the front arm upright of the wheelchair, she reaches down behind her back to put the hand into the other armhole and straightens her arm, shaking the sleeve on. She now sits up to arrange the collar and front of the shirt.

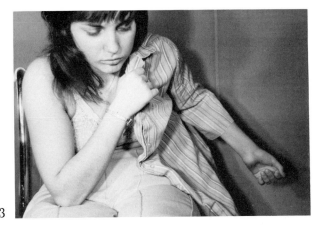 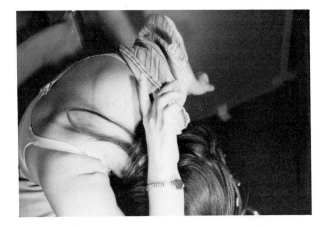

FIGURE 6-3

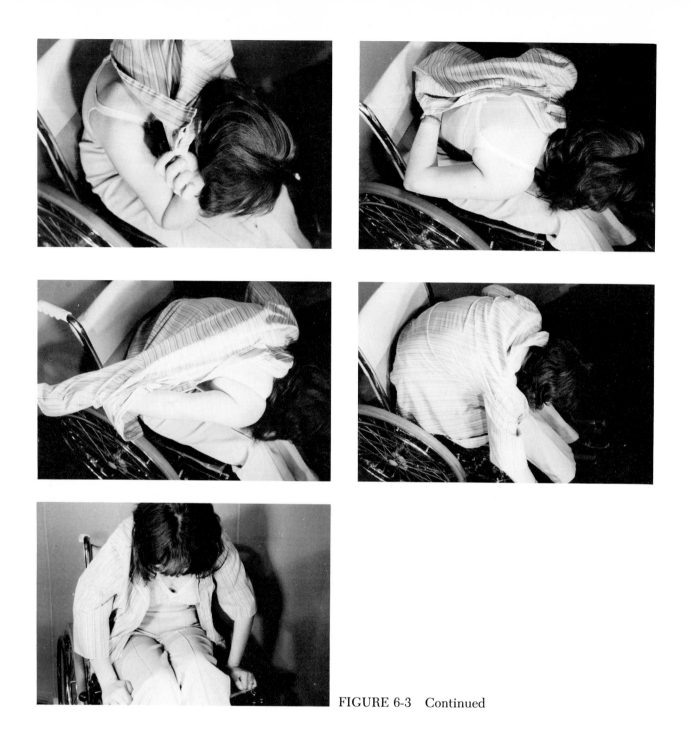

FIGURE 6-3   Continued

Method 3. (Fig. 6-4)   The patient places the back of the shirt on his knees with collar towards him and the front of the shirt opened out. He inserts his arms into the sleeves until the armholes are above the elbows and his hands are free. Placing his hands under the bulk of the shirt across his chest, he pushes the shirt away from his chest and flings it up and over his ducked head. At the moment that the shirt reaches the back of the neck, the arms straighten, allowing the shirt to drop into position on the shoulders. He leans forward to allow the back of the shirt to slip down between his trunk and the chair back.

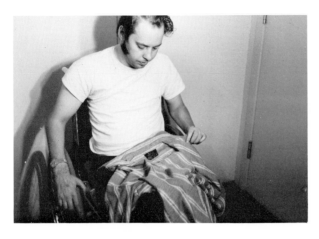

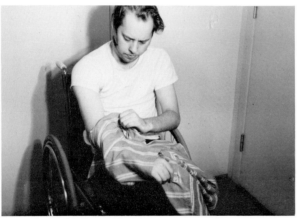

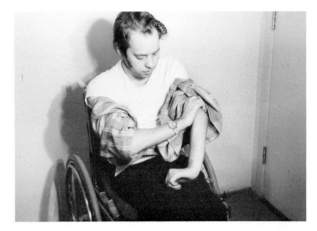

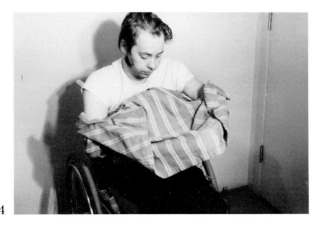

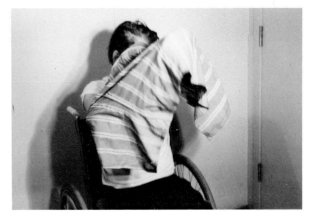

FIGURE 6-4

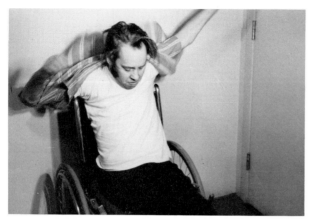

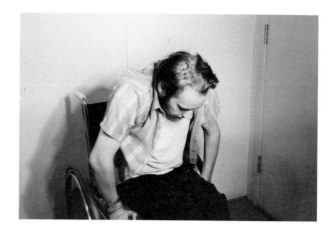

FIGURE 6-4 Continued

Method 4. (Fig. 6-5) In this method the patient places the shirt on his knees with the front down and the collar facing him. He crosses his arms to insert his hands into the armholes. He throws his arms up to flip the shirt over his head, uncrossing his arms as he does so. Uncrossing his arms adds momentum and flares the shirt out in a smooth flow to drop in place over the back as he straightens his arms. He leans forward and wiggles his trunk to let the shirt drop down his back.

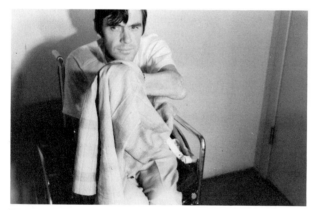

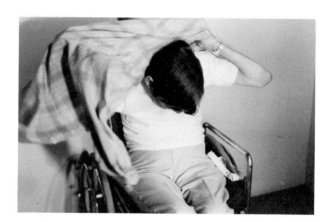

FIGURE 6-5

212

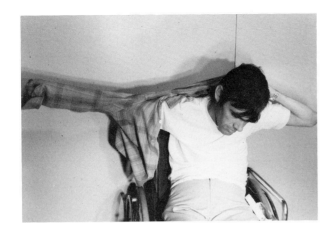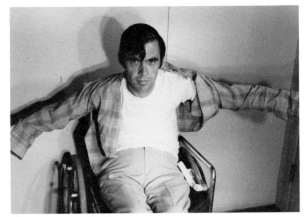

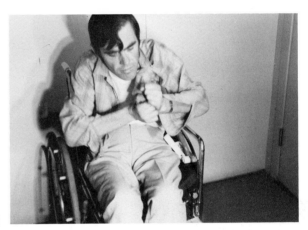

FIGURE 6-5   Continued

Method 5. (Fig. 6-6)   The patient places the buttoned shirt or T-shirt on his knees inside out and front down, with the collar facing him. He inserts his arms until the armholes are above his elbows. He bunches the back of the shirt on his hand and thumb web. He throws his arms up and back so that the collar slips over his head. As he drops his arms down again, the collar is pulled down over his head and he slips his hand inside to pull the shirt into position.

This method may also be used when the shirt is right side out. In this case the shirt is placed front down and with the collar away from the patient. If the shirt has long sleeves this is the easier method.

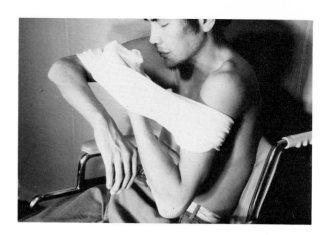
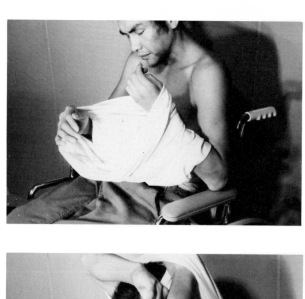
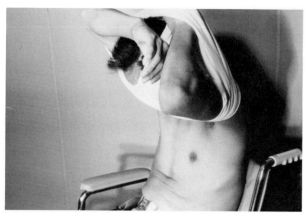
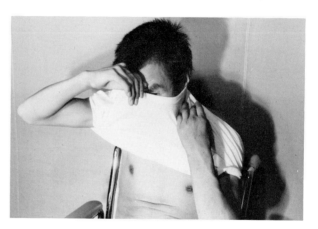
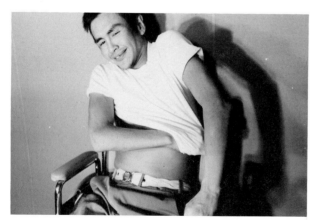

FIGURE 6-6

Method 6. (Fig. 6-7)   The patient places the buttoned shirt or T-shirt front down on his knees with the collar facing away from him. He puts his arms into the sleeves, and abducting and externally rotating his straight arms, he pushes his

214

hands through the cuffs. He then puts one or both thumbs into the collar opening and bunches the back of the shirt onto his thumb web. He can push the shirt onto the crown of his head by pushing up and ducking his head. He forces the shirt to

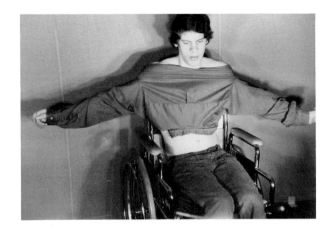 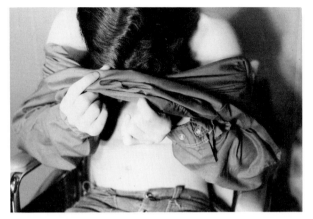

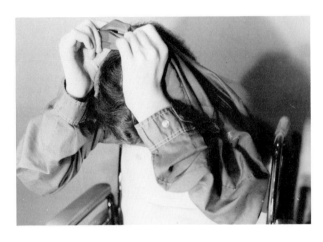 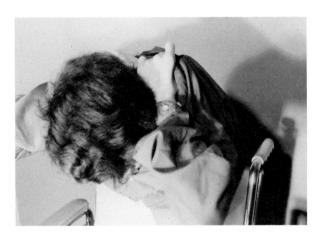

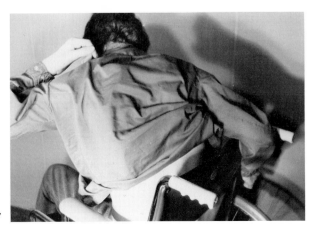 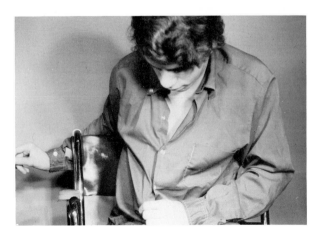

FIGURE 6-7

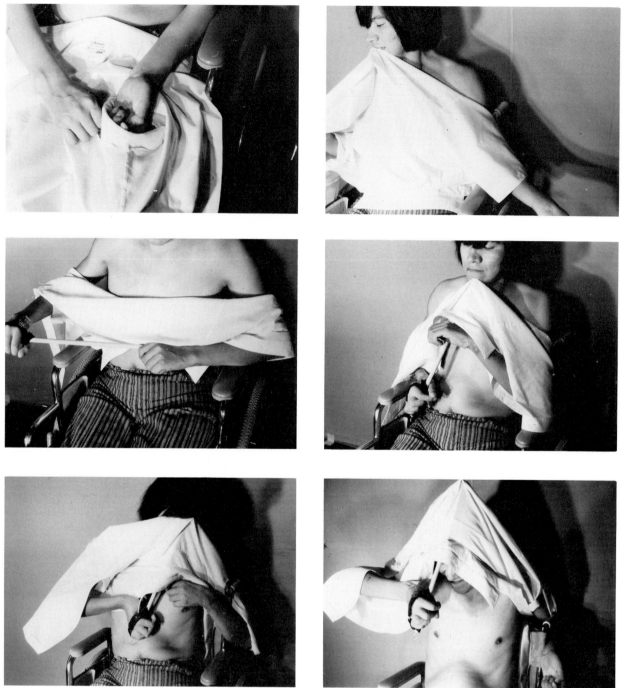

FIGURE 6-8

216

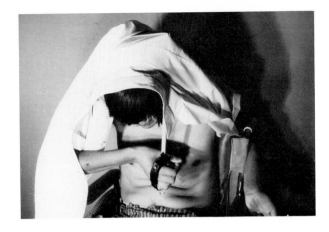
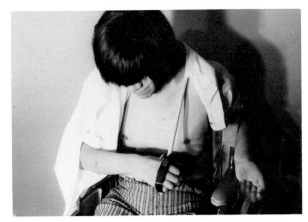
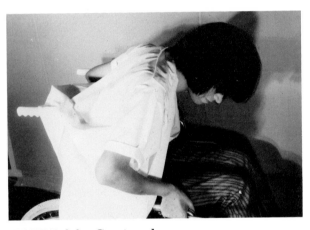
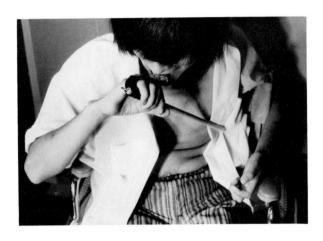

FIGURE 6-8   Continued

the back of his neck by alternately flexing and extending his neck and then moving his arms down and back. He now leans forward to let the shirt drop down his back.

Method 7. (Fig. 6-8)   The dressing stick may be used if the patient lacks range or strength to push the shirt over his head with his hands. In this case he places the shirt on his knees with the collar towards him. He inserts his arms using hands or teeth to pull until the armholes are above his elbows. He now straps the dressing stick to his hand, using a velcro D-ring or loop, and puts the end under the bulk of the shirt. He works the shirt over his head, flexing and extending his neck while maintaining the pushing action with the dressing stick until the shirt reaches the back of his neck. If necessary, balance may be maintained by hooking an arm around the back of the chair. The shirt will drop down the back when the patient leans forward. He can then hook a thumb into the facing to arrange the front of the shirt.

217

Method 1. (Fig. 6-9) The shirt must be unbuttoned and opened out. The thumb on the dominant side is inserted under the shirt near the opposite shoulder and pushes the material off the shoulder and down the arm past the elbow. The shoulder is shrugged to assist in this maneuver. When the elbow is flexed and the shoulder is extended, the sleeve will slide down the arm until it can be shaken off the hand. The bulk of the shirt is thrown behind the chair, and the sleeve is pushed off the other arm in a similar manner.

Method 2. (Fig. 6-10) This method may be used with shirts with roomy armholes, T-shirts, or sweaters. The patient puts his hand inside the shirt and pulls the armhole down to slip it over the flexed elbow and pulls his arm out of the sleeve. He takes the other sleeve off in a similar manner. He pulls the shirt from his head by bunching the front of the shirt round his hands and pulling up and forwards.

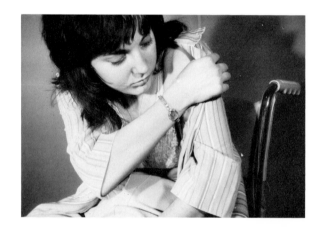
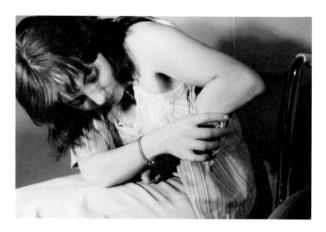
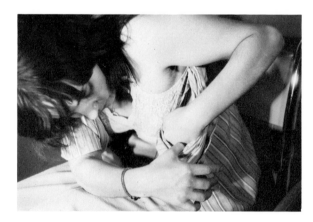
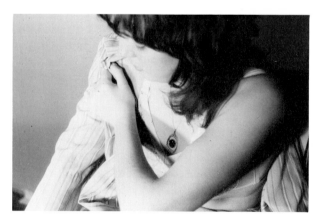

FIGURE 6-9

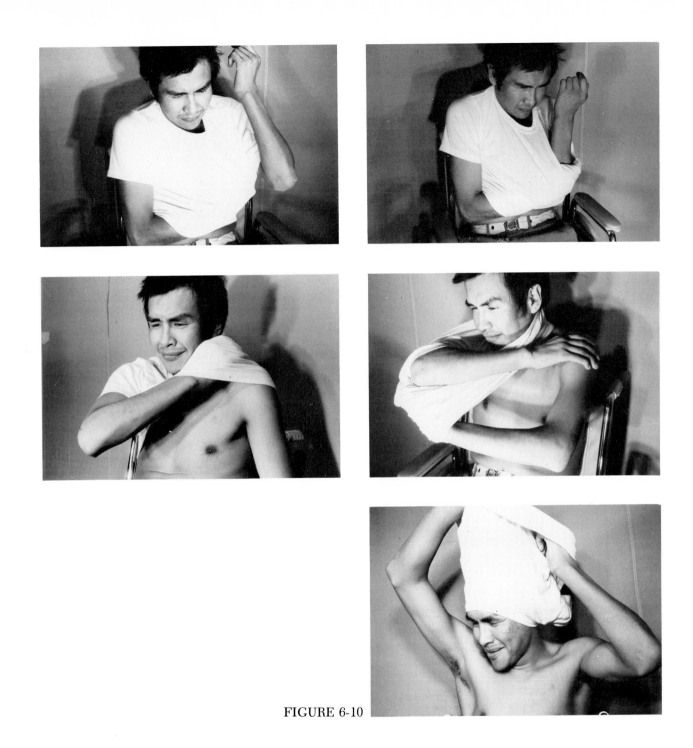

FIGURE 6-10

Method 3. (Fig. 6-11)   The shirt is unbuttoned, and the thumb is hooked into the facing on the lower part of the shirt front. He flings this arm over the back of the chair and catches the armhole of the shirt on the pushing handle of the

219

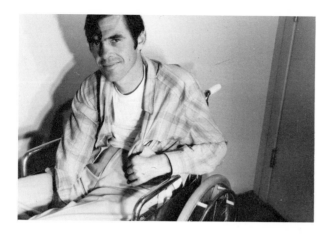
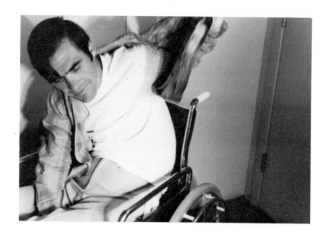

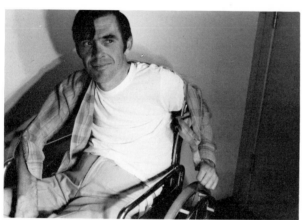
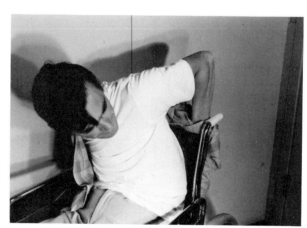

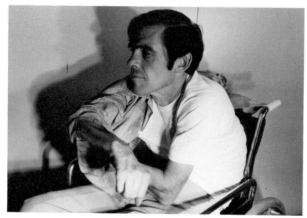

FIGURE 6-11

wheelchair. By leaning forward and lifting the elbow, he removes his arm from the sleeve. As he pushes the remaining sleeve off, a forward bouncing action of the trunk may be necessary to release the shirt back from between his trunk and the wheelchair.

Method 4. (Fig. 6-12)   The patient pushes the front of the buttoned shirt or T-shirt up until it is bunched across his chest at armpit level. He inserts his thumb or thumbs under the material so that the front of the shirt rests on his thumb web. He then pushes it over his head, flexing and extending his neck to work the mate-

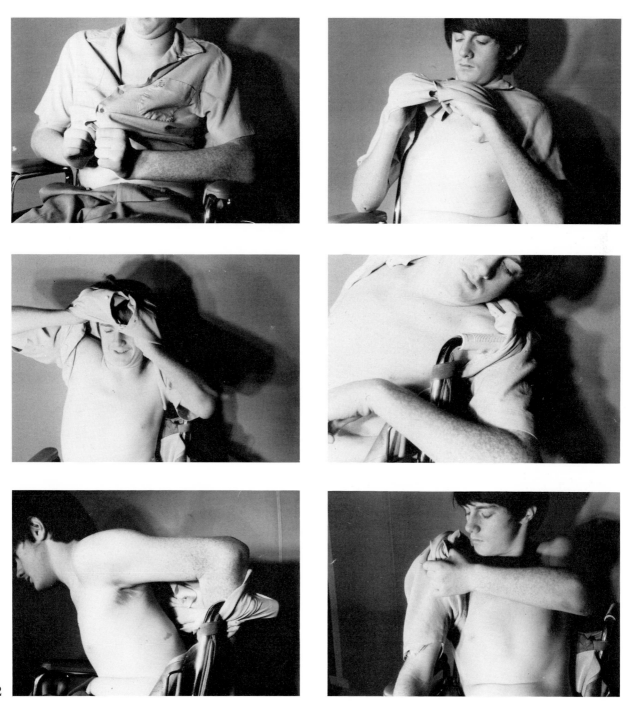

FIGURE 6-12

221

rial to the back of his neck. He places one arm over the back of the chair and hooks the armhole of the shirt onto the pushing handle of the wheelchair. By leaning forward, he pulls the sleeve down the arm until it is below the elbow. The sleeve can then be shaken off this arm. The other sleeve is easily removed by hooking the free hand into the armhole and pulling it downward.

Method 5. (Fig. 6-13)   This method may be used with a buttoned shirt or with a pullover. The patient hooks one arm behind the pushing handle of the wheelchair for stability. He reaches behind his neck with the other hand, and hooks under the collar with his thumb. A loop across the inside collar back, sewn so that it remains open, may be required during the learning process. The patient ducks his head and pulls forward while allowing his trunk to swing slightly forward to release the back of the shirt. He maintains his pull on the collar while alternately flexing and extending his neck. He continues this until the shirt is pulled over his head. It is now simple to pull the sleeves off by using his hands or teeth.

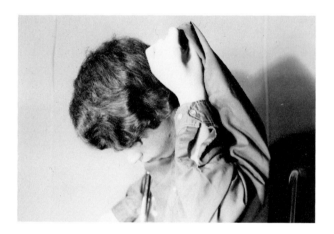
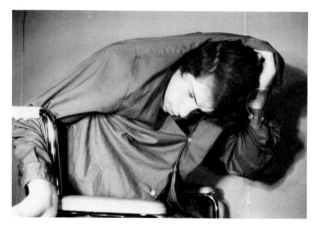
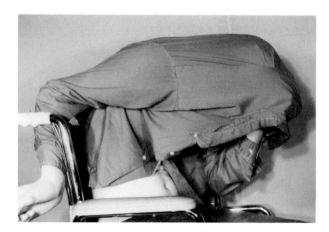
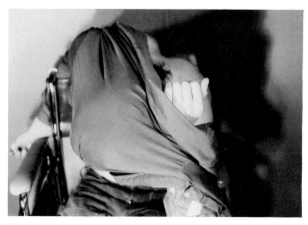

FIGURE 6-13

222

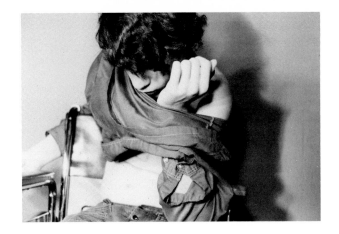
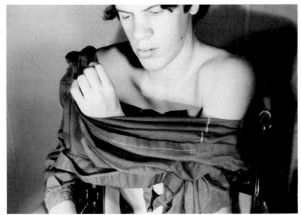

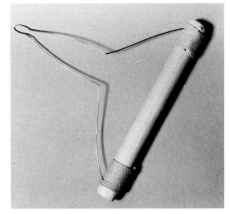

FIGURE 6-13   Continued

Buttonholes should be vertical and large enough to permit easy insertion of the button. A flat button is easiest to manage, particularly if it has a sewn shank.

Equipment

Very simple aids to dressing may be easily made. Several types of buttonhooks are described here.

A 4¹/₂-inch (11.43 cm) length of a ¹/₂-inch (1.27 cm) hardwood dowel and about 11 inches (28 cm) of 12 gauge piano wire are used in this hook. The wire should be bent to shape and the ends inserted through holes drilled near the end of the dowel and bent back (Fig. 6-14). Whipping of the bent ends serves two purposes: covering the sharp ends and preventing them from moving. The design permits the throat of the buttonhook to accommodate any size buttonhole without strain. The handle may require adaptation for a firm hold.

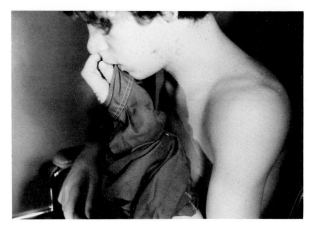

FIGURE 6-14

223

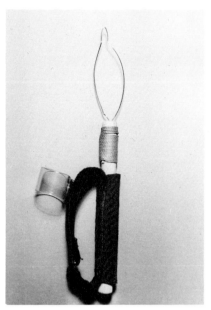

FIGURE 6-15 A

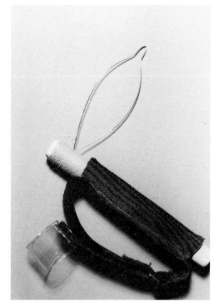

B

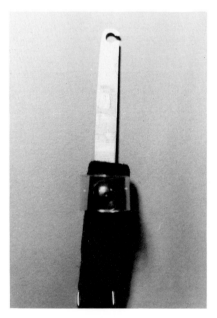

FIGURE 6-16

A length of ¹/₄-inch (0.64 cm) hardwood dowel and about 7 inches (18 cm) of 12-gauge piano wire are required for a second type of hook. Two holes are drilled down at opposite obtuse angles from the center of the dowel, so that the drill breaks through the sides about ³/₄-inch (2 cm) down. The wire is bent to shape and the ends inserted into the holes. After bending the ends upward, the wire and dowel may be covered with whipping. The handle may require adaptation (Fig. 6-15A). The angle may be varied if required (Fig. 6-15B). Commercially available buttonhooks may be used. These are generally more rigid, fitting fewer sizes of buttonhole, but they do not twist out of shape easily.

A 5-inch (12.70 cm) length of ¹/₂-inch (1.27 cm) 14 gauge stainless steel or tempered aluminum is cut. Ten inches (25.40 cm) will be required if it is to be bent into a loop handle. The tip is ground to half the gauge, and a ¹/₄-inch (.64 cm) hole is drilled in the center, leaving ¹/₈-inch (.32 cm) of material at the end. A cut ¹/₈-inch (.32 cm) wide is made from the edge to the hole, and all edges are smoothed. The handle may be bent into a loop to fit the hand, or otherwise adapted for a firm hold (Fig. 6-16). This buttonhook is most useful for unbuttoning.

One-inch (2.54 cm) velcro squares may be substituted for buttons (Fig. 6-17). The top velcro is invisibly sewn and the button is resewn in the buttonhole so that the shirt appears to be buttoned.

Open-ended zippers, such as those on jackets, are very hard to start and may require velcro strips as a substitute.

Methods for Fastening

Method 1—Without Equipment. The shirt button may be held, using tenodesis or remaining finger function, and worked through a buttonhole held in the same manner (Fig. 6-18A).

Teeth may be used to hold the facing taut while buttoning (Fig. 6-18B).

Many Western style shirts have press studs instead of buttons. These may be easier for some patients to manage. The heel of the hand may be pressed against a rigid thumb, chest wall, or the heel of the other hand (Fig. 6-18C).

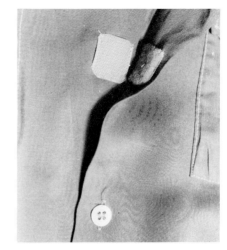

FIGURE 6-17

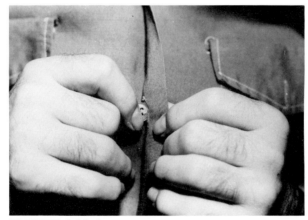

FIGURE 6-18 A

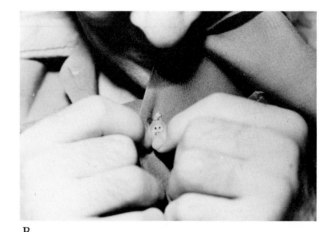

B

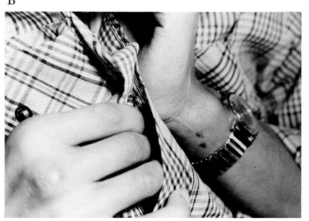

C

Method 2—With a Flexible Hook.   The patient who can control his arm best when it is by his side, making it possible for him to pull in a horizontal plane, will use the hook shown in Fig. 6-19A. The handle may require adaptation for a firm hold.

The patient who can abduct his arms to reach the higher buttons may prefer the buttonhook shown in Fig. 6-19B.

Method 3—With a Rigid Hook.   The stainless steel or aluminum buttonhook is not as easy to use as the wire buttonhook for buttoning but is easier to use for unbuttoning (Fig. 6-20).

Method 4—Adaptation.   Velcro squares may be pressed together by using tenodesis, the heels of the hands, or a rigid finger (Fig. 6-21).

Cuff Buttons

Cuff buttons are more difficult to manage than shirt front buttons because only one hand and the teeth are available for fastening and unfastening. The simplest method is having a cuff loose enough to permit the hand to pass through

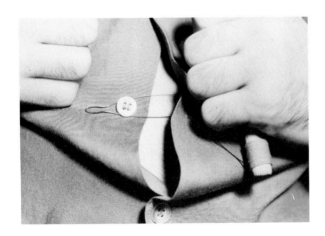
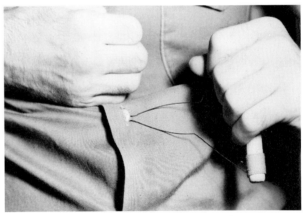

FIGURE 6-19 A

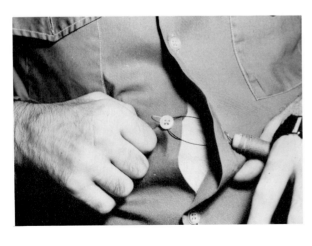
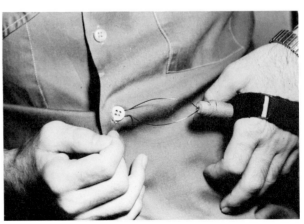

B

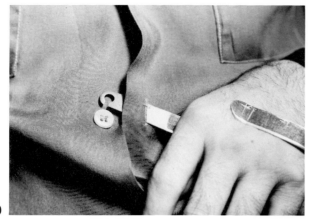
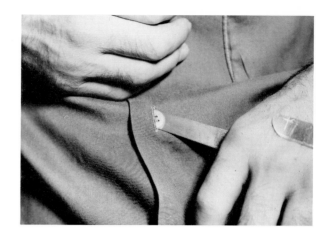

FIGURE 6-20

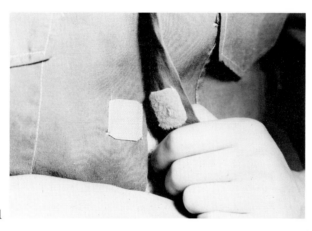
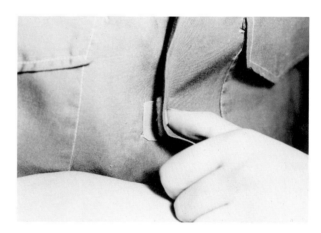

FIGURE 6-21

without fastening. If it is not loose enough, the button may be moved closer to the edge, or may be sewn with an elastic shank to permit the cuff to expand. If cuff links are used, they may be replaced with a cuff link made of two buttons sewn with an elastic shank between them.

The cuff may be fastened by using a buttonhook in one hand while the teeth are used to pull the buttonhole over the button. A velcro fastening may also be used on the cuff.

UNFASTENING

Method 1—Using No Equipment. In one technique, a thumb or finger is inserted into the shirt front opening under the button and holds the button in position, while the other hand pulls the buttonhole down over it (Fig. 6-22A). Another means is to insert a thumb or finger into the shirt front opening and hold the buttonhole firm while the button is pushed out with a finger or fingernail of the other hand (Fig. 6-22B).

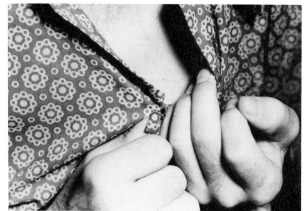

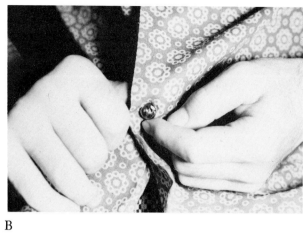

FIGURE 6-22 A   B

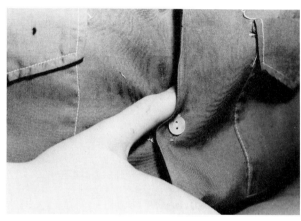

FIGURE 6-23 A

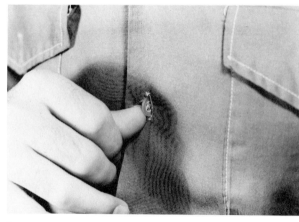

B

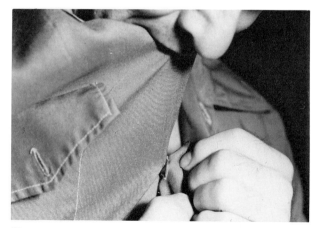

C

228

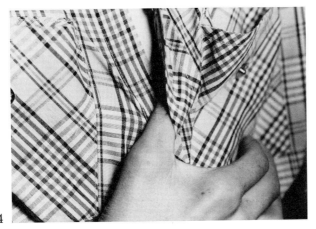 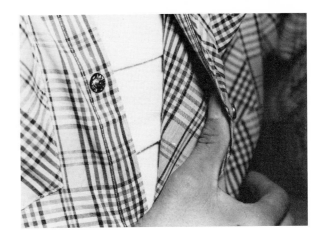

FIGURE 6-24

If the buttonhole is quite loose, it may be worked over the button with one thumb behind the facing (Fig. 6-23A). Additionally, a thumbnail may be used to lift one side of the button, forcing the other side down through the buttonhole (Fig. 6-23B). The teeth may be used to hold the facing taut while the button is undone (Fig. 6-23C).

Press studs are very simple to pull apart with the thumb or a finger (Fig. 6-24).

Method 2—Using a Flexible Hook. If a buttonhook is used, it is pushed into the buttonhole and then turned so that it lies half over the button. This lifts the buttonhole on one side and permits the button to slide out (Fig. 6-25).

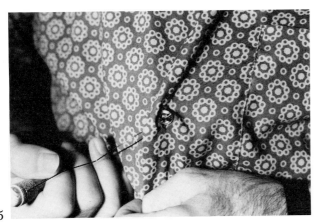 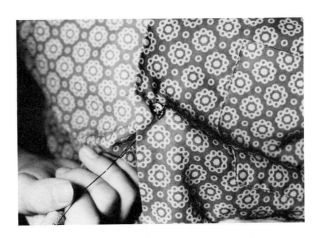

FIGURE 6-25

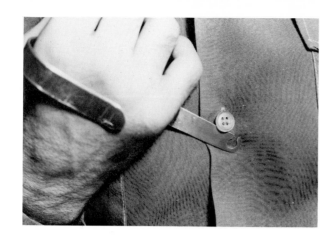

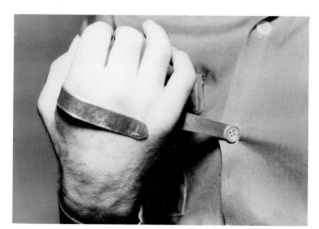

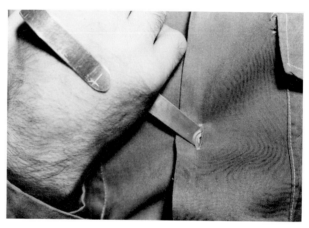

FIGURE 6-26

Method 3—Using a Rigid Hook. If a patient has more difficulty unbuttoning than buttoning, the stainless steel or aluminum hook should be used (Fig. 6-26).

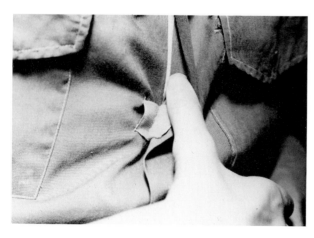

FIGURE 6-27

Method 4—Adaptation. Velcro squares may be pulled apart easily with thumb or fingers (Fig. 6-27). The velcro should be closed before laundering or lint will accumulate preventing closure.

BRASSIERES

Brassieres should have a narrow band and should be a fairly loose fit for easier fastening. Back-hooked brassieres will always be fastened in front and then turned to the back. An advantage of this brassiere is the small number of hooks necessary for a good fit. Front-hooked brassieres may be used by preference, or because the patient is unable to turn a conventional brassiere fastening to the back. Difficulty in turning the brassiere may be aggravated by the excessive perspiration that sometimes occurs in quadriplegics, especially in the early stages of rehabilitation. A brassiere that hooks in the front is usually fastened around the waist before positioning the straps, because the waist is usually the smallest section of the torso in circumference and vision is less obscured. Stretch brassieres are difficult for many patients to manage because, if the brassieres are not fairly tight, small women find they slide up during activity. Larger women may have trouble positioning this type of brassiere.

ADAPTATIONS

A large hook such as a pants hook may be substituted for normal hooks (Fig. 6-28A). This hook must be used only in a front-hooking brassiere because it will create a pressure area on the back when the patient leans against the chair. Loops may be sewn to the brassiere under the hooks and eyes so that the thumbs can be inserted (Fig. 6-28B). The hooks may need to be opened a little. A loop may be sewn or temporarily tied to one of the loops, long enough so that it may be hooked over the chair arm. Thumb pockets may be sewn so that the fastening can be seen easily, as it protrudes beyond the thumb tips. The thumbs are held in a fairly rigid position by the small pockets, which act rather like splints (Fig. 6-28C).

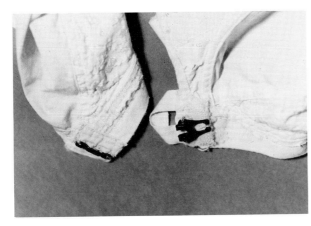
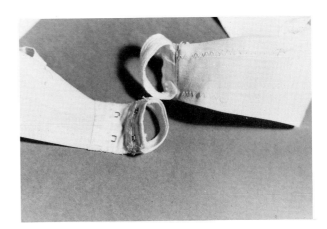

FIGURE 6-28 A　　　　　　　　　　　　　　B

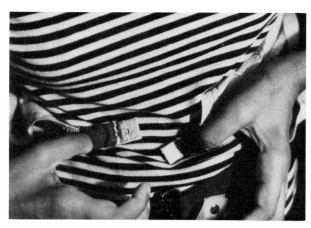

FIGURE 6-28 C

A front-hooked brassiere may be adapted, or a brassiere with a hooked back may be converted to a front-hooked brassiere, by cutting and binding the seam between the cups. The band is fastened with a velcro D-ring, the hook velcro facing out, and a thumb loop is attached near the free end (Fig. 6-29A). The upper part may be fastened with large or small hooks with thumb loops under the hooks and under the eyes (Fig. 6-29B). A velcro D-ring fastening is easy to align, and is a firm fastening. It should not be used at the back because of the probability of creating a pressure area. A velcro closure with no D-ring is not a reliable fastening for a brassiere. A length of elastic may be inserted into the brassiere shoulder straps to enable the patient to push them onto her shoulders and to assist in keeping them in place.

PUTTING ON BRASSIERES

Method 1. (Fig. 6-30) The patient places the brassiere on her knee with the top towards her and the outside up. She hooks thumb or fingers of one hand into

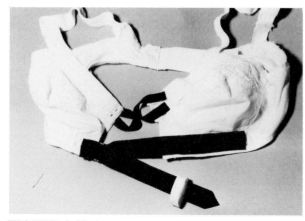

FIGURE 6-29 A

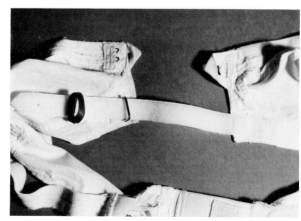

B

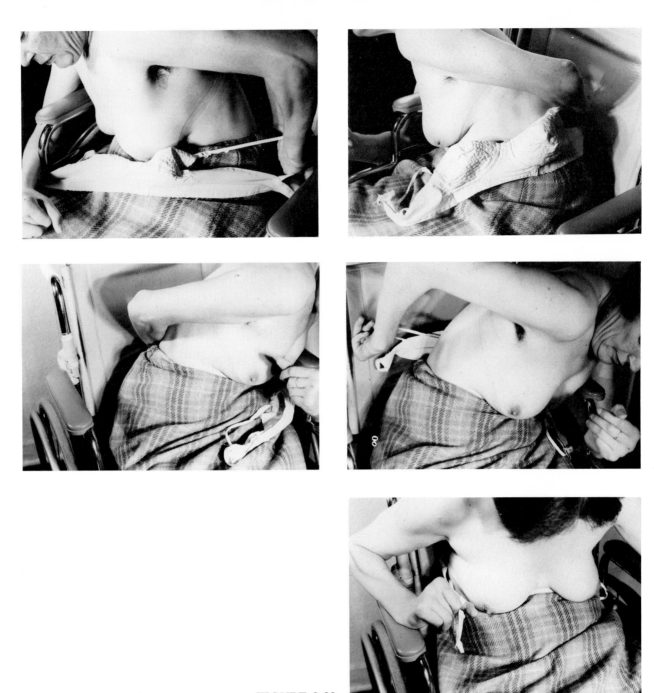

FIGURE 6-30

the strap on that side and leans forward, maintaining balance with the other arm.
She now pushes the brassiere around her back as far as possible. She changes arms
and, leaning forward again, she reaches behind her back for the released strap.

When there is lack of sensation or position sense in the hand, this may take practice, and she may have to observe movement in the part of the brassiere which remains at the front, indicating that she has caught the loose end. Care must be taken not to pull the strap too far around.

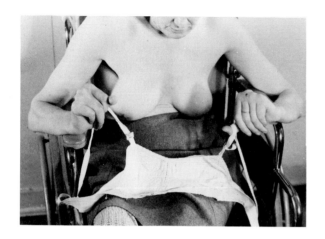
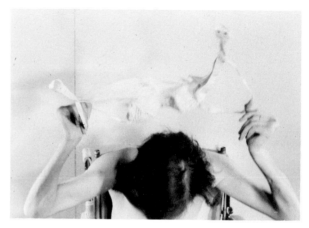
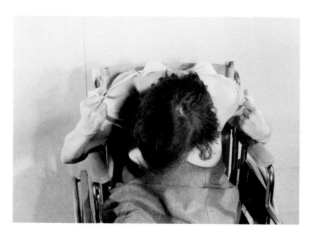
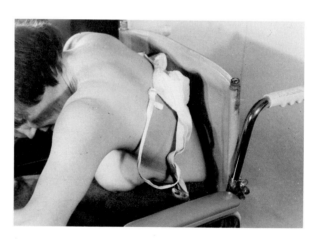
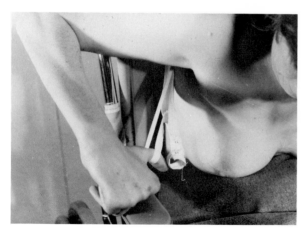
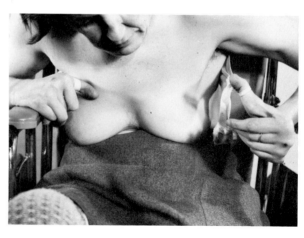

FIGURE 6-31

234

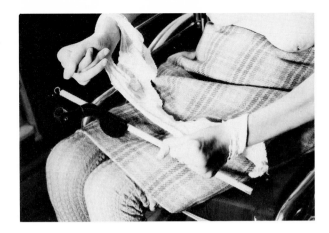

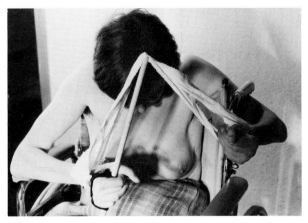

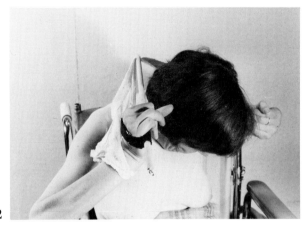

FIGURE 6-32

Method 2. (Fig. 6-31)   The brassiere is placed on the lap with the inside facing upward and the shoulder straps toward the patient. The patient hooks the straps into thumbs or fingers and flings the brassiere over her head, releasing one strap only when the brassiere is down her back and level with the wheelchair pushing handles. She reaches under her shoulder to retrieve the straps and pulls the brassiere down her back by bouncing her trunk forward in the chair and using a sawing motion with her hands. Some patients are unable to bounce forward while their hands are in use. These patients must let go of the straps and pull themselves forward. The brassiere, if well placed, then slides down the back.

Method 3. (Fig. 6-32)   The patient places the brassiere on her lap with the top towards her and the inside up, and slides her wrists down through the straps. She now hooks her thumbs under the brassiere and pushes it over her head. If she lacks range or power she may require a dressing stick to accomplish this. Without releasing the straps she works the brassiere down her back.

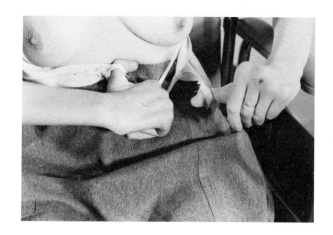 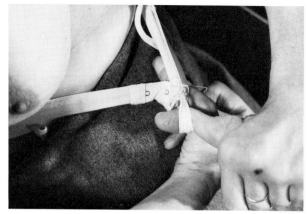

FIGURE 6-33

FASTENING BRASSIERES

Method 1. (Fig. 6-33)   The thumbs are inserted into the thumb loops and the ends are brought together for fastening. If the thumbs are rigid, the hooks and eyes can be placed on the base of the backs of the thumbs so they can be easily opposed.

Method 2. (Fig. 6-34)   If only one hand can be effectively used, the thumb may be hooked into one thumb loop, while the other longer loop is hooked over the armrest. The free hand is placed under the fastening to bring it forward into position for fastening.

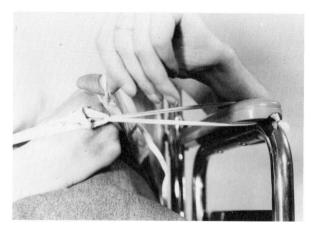

FIGURE 6-34

Method 3. (Fig. 6-35)   The end of the velcro strap is threaded through the D-ring using the heels of both hands or a thumb hooked through a loop placed an inch or so back from the tip of the strap. The tip is then pulled using the heels of the hands until the loop is through the D-ring. The lower band of the brassiere is placed in position with the other thumb and the strap is pulled by the loop until the opening is closed, before allowing the velcro strap to touch the opposing hook velcro. Once the bottom band is secure, the top hook is easy to fasten, since there is no strain on it. This may be accomplished using thumb loops under hooks and eyes, or a short velcro D-ring fastening.

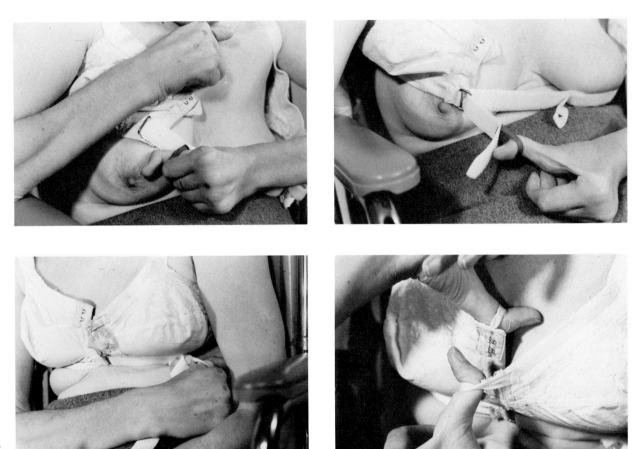

FIGURE 6-35

237

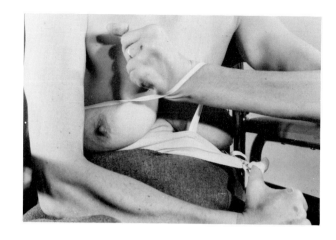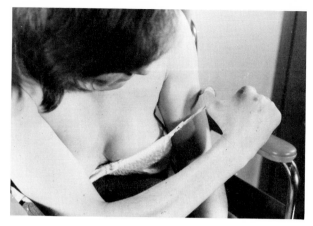
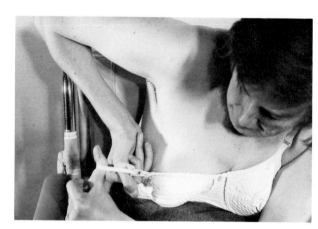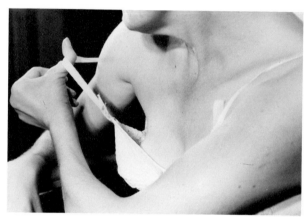

FIGURE 6-36

TURNING A BACK-HOOKED BRASSIERE AND PLACING STRAPS

After the hooks are fastened, the brassiere is turned around into position by pulling and pushing on the shoulder straps (Fig. 6-36). If possible, it should be turned so that the hooks pull into the eyes, i.e., to the left. When the brassiere is straight, one strap is hooked onto the opposite thumb web, and either the elbow or the hand inserted through the strap. The other arm is inserted also, and both straps are pushed up onto the shoulders. A dressing stick is occasionally required to enable a woman who does not have sufficient strength, who has restricted movement, or who is obese, to push the straps onto the shoulder.

REMOVING BRASSIERES

The brassiere strap is removed from the shoulder by hooking a thumb or pushing stick into it, and pushing out and down (Fig. 6-37). The shoulder is extended when the strap reaches the elbow to slip the forearm and hand out of the strap. When the strap is nearly at the elbow, some patients flex the elbow and remove the hand from the strap. The strap slides off the arm when the arm is straightened. Then the other strap is removed. A brassiere with back hooks is turned by the straps so that the opening is at the front, ready to be unfastened.

UNDERPANTS AND PANTS

Jockey shorts may be used by male patients, because they do not wrinkle or bunch in the crotch as boxer shorts do. They provide good support, which assists in keeping the urine collection apparatus in position. Obese patients may be able to wear boxer shorts only. For ease in putting them on and taking them off, open loops may be sewn at the waistband, one on either side by the side seams. Sometimes an additional loop at the back will be necessary.

Some patients do not wear shorts because of the inconvenience of putting them on, though this is not recommended. If shorts are not worn, pants should be changed frequently. Patients who wear pants that are tight, or have raised seams, run a risk of pressure areas.

A loose-knit cotton type of pantie is recommended for women, to which loops

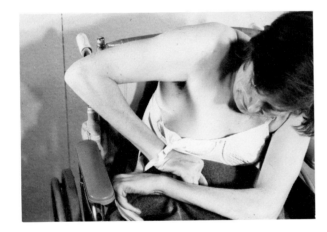
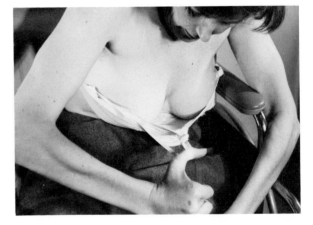
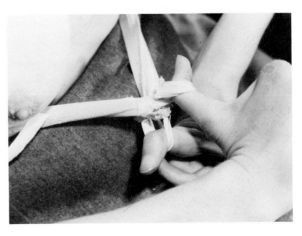

FIGURE 6-37

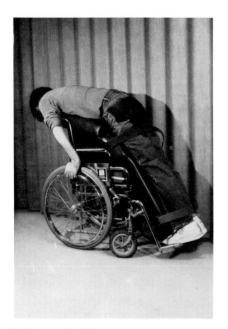

FIGURE 6-38

may be added if necessary. If there is difficulty in putting the cotton panties on, a slippery material may be used instead, although this will not absorb perspiration as well.

Outer pants should be on the large side, both for ease in putting on and for comfort when sitting. They should be made of a material that will enable the patient to slide easily, for instance, a cotton-terylene mix.

If slacks are made of a material such as denim or corduroy, which does not slide easily, a nylon patch, which does not normally show, can be sewn onto the seat of the slacks. Many patients will use these patches only while they are learning to transfer (Fig. 6-38).

Women will find a front-fastening zipper easier to manage than a side zipper. A back zipper is contraindicated because it will be most difficult to zip up and may cause a pressure area.

For comfort and cosmesis, dress pants may be tailored to fit a seated person.

PUTTING ON PANTS

Method 1. (Fig. 6-39)   The low-lesion patient may put his pants on while in the chair. To gain stability he may first slide forward in his chair. He begins by either crossing one leg over the other knee, or holding a leg up with his wrist to slide his foot into the pant leg and pull the waist over his knee. He puts his foot on the footrest and repeats the procedure with the other leg. He tucks his pants as far under his buttocks as possible, lifting his legs alternately to do so. He now holds his pants at the side, using tenodesis or an extended wrist inside and under the waist-band, and places his forearm on the armrest. As he does a quick pushup with the

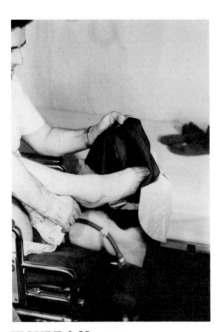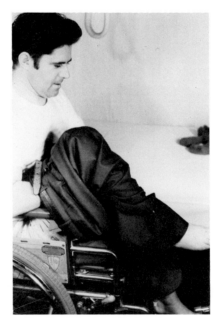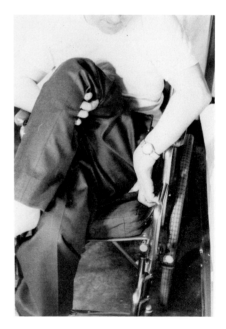

FIGURE 6-39

240

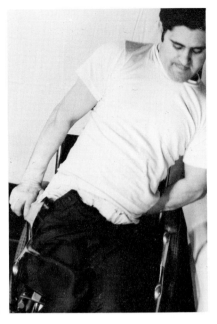
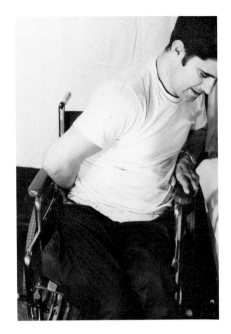

FIGURE 6-39   Continued

other arm, the armrest becomes a fulcrum, assisting his pull on the pants and also levering his buttocks up to enable the waistband to be pulled up.

Method 2. (Fig. 6-40)   In this method the patient sits in the chair with the chair in the transfer position by the bed. He places his pants on the bed with the waist open in position to receive a foot when he lifts it onto the bed. He now holds the pants so that they do not move while his foot slips into the pant leg. The foot may require more than the force of gravity to slide it into the pant leg; in this case leaning forward may cause the knee to straighten, or a push on the knee, internally or externally rotating the hip, will direct the foot down the correct pant leg. If necessary, the leg and pant leg may be lifted together, and then the pants held

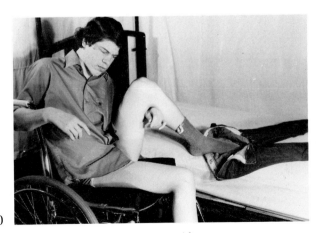
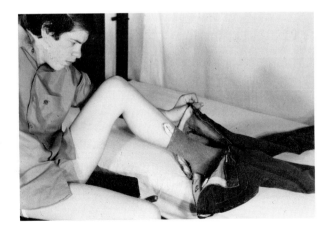

FIGURE 6-40

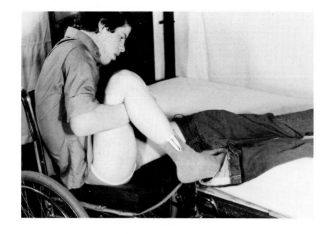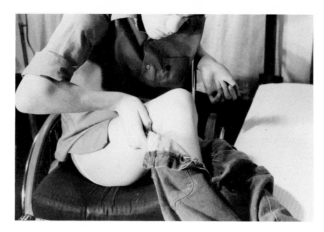

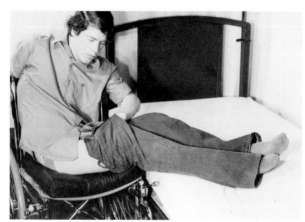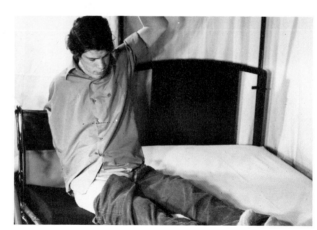

FIGURE 6-40   Continued

again while the leg slides further down the pant leg. The pant waist is pushed to below the knee so that the other leg can also be slipped into the pant leg. The pants are pulled up as far as possible before the patient transfers to the bed. He completes pulling his pants over his hips on the bed.

Method 3. (Fig. 6-41)   The patient sits on the bed and flicks his pants out so that they lie straight in front of him. He inserts a wrist under his calf from the inside, so that when he picks his leg up, it is externally rotated with the toe pointing toward the top of his pants. He works the pant leg opening over his foot with his free arm and then places his foot on the bed. While he holds the top of the pants, he allows the weight of the leg to force his foot down through the pant leg. The other leg is inserted in the same way. The pants are pulled up as far as possible by friction of the hands on the material and by a wrist pulling against the crotch. When the pants are pulled up to the buttocks, he leans back on alternate elbows to roll from side to side, using the free arm to pull the pants over the hips.

242

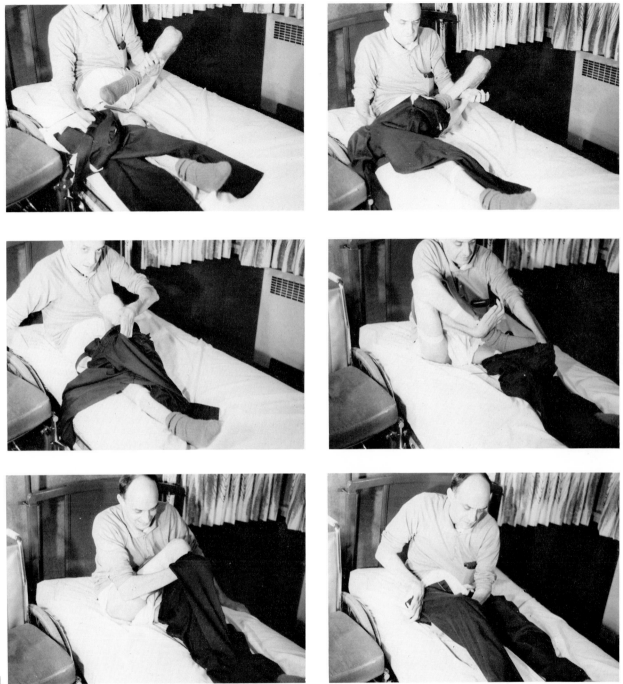

FIGURE 6-41

243

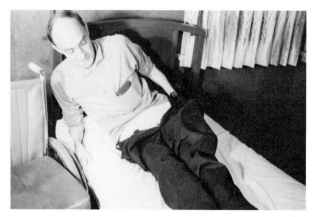 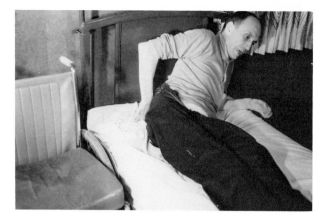

FIGURE 6-41   Continued

Method 4. (Fig. 6-42)   The patient lies on his side on the bed, leaning on an elbow. He reaches down with his free arm to pull his upper leg towards himself, and rests the knee on the extended wrist of the lower arm. The free arm is used to pull the pants over the foot and work the material up until the foot is free and the waistband is at the knee. Either the upper or the bottom leg may be inserted into the pants first. The top of the pants is opened so that the other leg can be directed towards the opening and the pants are pulled onto the leg. The pants are pulled up as far as possible by holding the material between the heels of the hands, or by using an extended wrist under the waistband and one at the crotch. Then the patient rolls from side to side to pull his pants up.

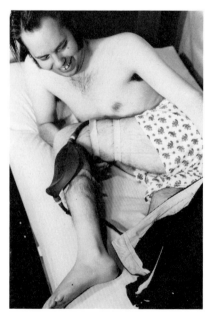 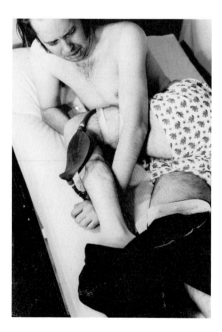 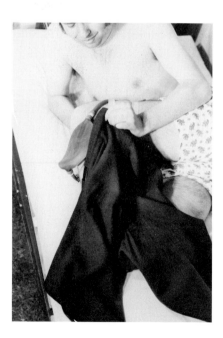

FIGURE 6-42

244

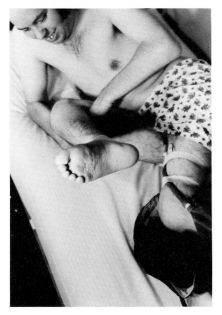
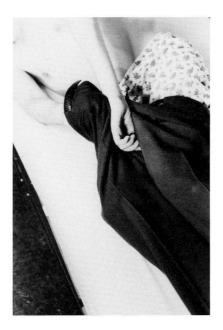
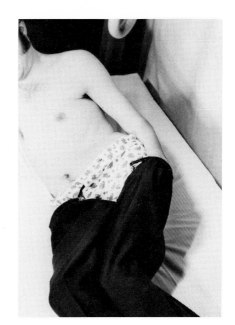

FIGURE 6-42   Continued

Method 5. (Fig. 6-43)   The patient leans forward with one elbow resting on the bed. He inserts a wrist under his calf and levers his foot off the bed. The other arm pulls the pants over the foot until the waistband is clear of the heel. Still resting on one elbow, he uses the friction of his two hands in opposition to pull the pant leg up and over his foot. He gathers his pant leg down around his knee to allow the waistband to be scooped around his other foot.

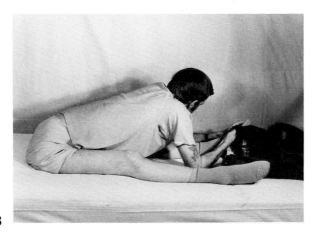
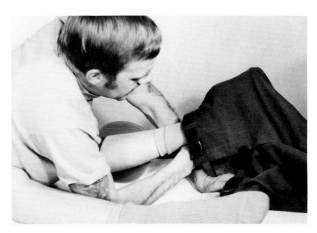

FIGURE 6-43

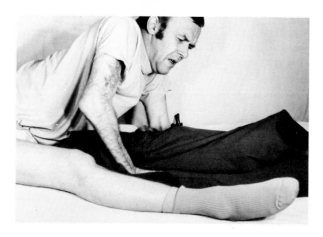

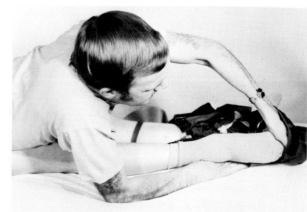

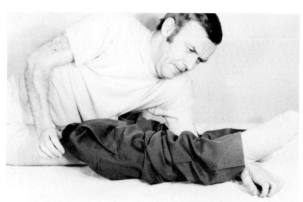

FIGURE 6-43   Continued

Method 6. (Fig. 6-44)   The patient sits up on the bed and hooks his knee with an extended wrist. When he drops back onto the bed his leg is raised towards his chest, enabling him to slip the pants over his foot with the free arm. He works the pants up the leg using hands and teeth. He sits up again and repeats the

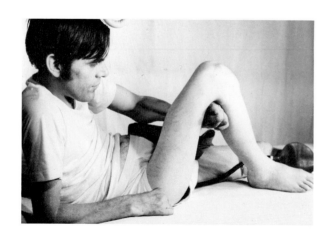

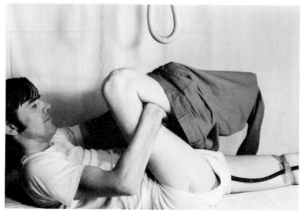

FIGURE 6-44

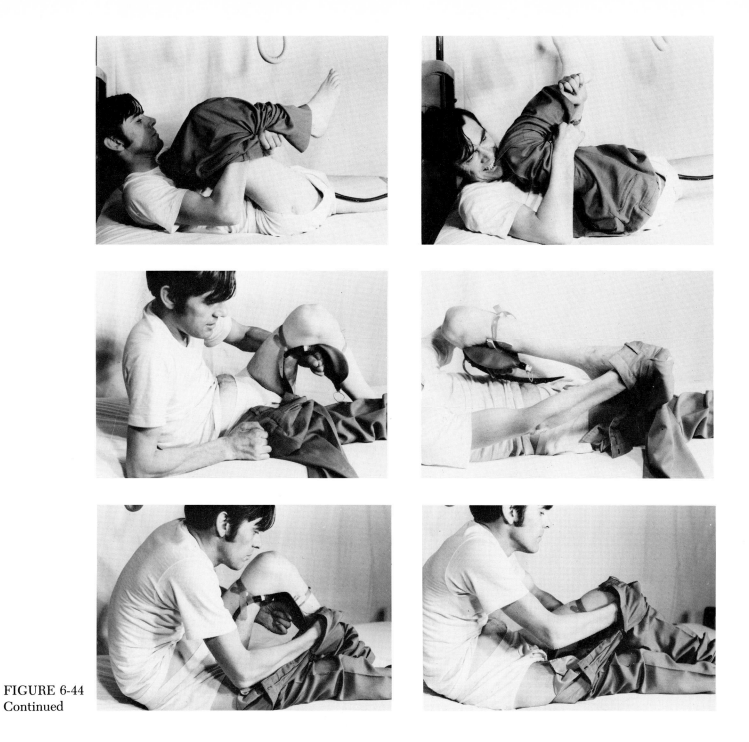

FIGURE 6-44
Continued

procedure with the other leg. The patient may put the pant leg on in the lying position, or he may sit up and allow the weight of the leg to help straighten itself and slide into the pant leg. He lies down to roll from side to side to work his pants over his hips.

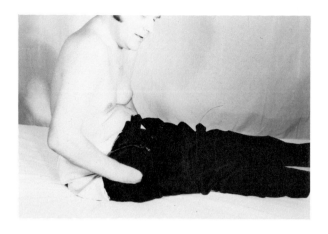
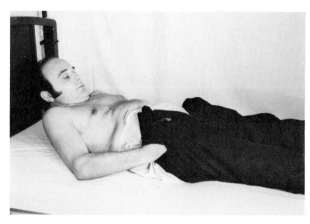
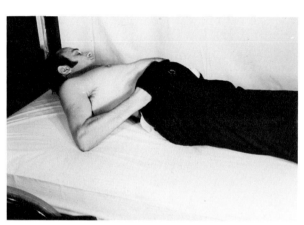
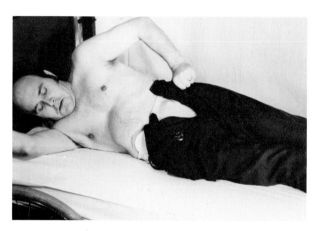

FIGURE 6-45

Method 7. (Fig. 6-45)   After the patient has his pants pulled over his legs, if he puts his hands in his pants pockets and drops back onto the elbows, this will pull the pants up so that when he rolls he can pull the pants clear of his hips easily. Reciprocal pulling with the hands in the pockets and the elbows on the bed after the pants are pulled up will align them for fastening.

Method 8. (Fig. 6-46)   The patient lies on his side and works his trunk into flexion. If he has flexor spasm, this position will encourage his legs to flex so that they are within easy reach. If he does not have flexor spasm, he must work his trunk into sufficient flexion so that he can place a wrist around the back of a leg to pull him into a jackknifed position. Using both hands, he threads his lower foot into the pant leg; then he straightens his leg by pushing on the knee or thigh, while keeping the waist of the pants in position with the other hand. The other knee is pulled up and the other pant leg is slipped on. The pants are worked up as far as possible before the patient rolls from side to side to pull them over his hips.

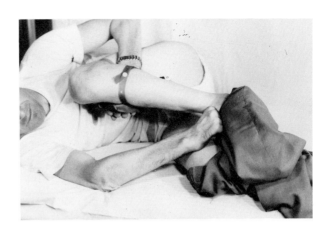

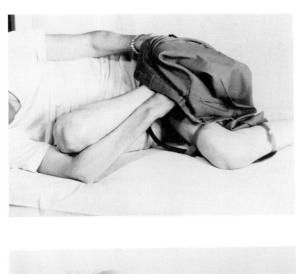

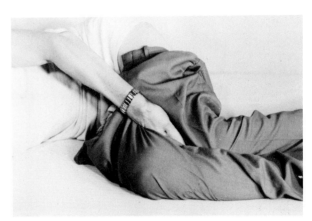

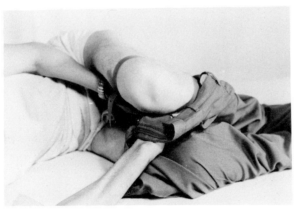

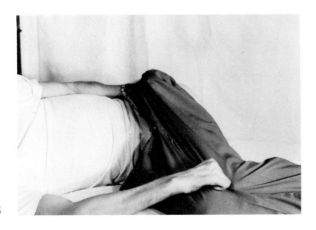

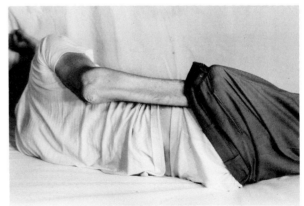

FIGURE 6-46

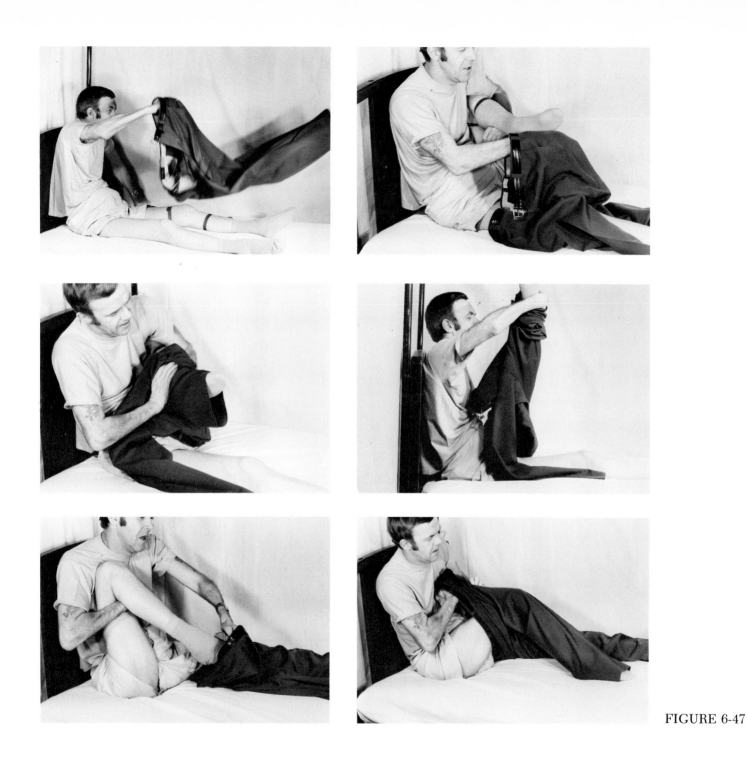

FIGURE 6-47

Method 9. (Fig. 6-47)   The patient sits against the head of the bed and flings his pants out so that they lie straight in front of him. He uses an extended wrist to pick up a knee and pulls it close to his chest so that the foot can be threaded easily into the pant leg. The pant leg is worked up using friction of the hands until the foot is free. If the patient is sufficiently flaccid, he can straighten his leg so that it is vertical, allowing the pants to fall into position. The other leg is now pulled up and inserted into the waistband. The pant leg may be pulled up the leg in the same manner as before, or the leg may be allowed to slip down into the pant leg by gravity while the pants are held in position at the waistband. The patient now moves down the bed so that he can roll from side to side to enable him to pull the pants over his hips.

Method 10. (Fig. 6-48)   A patient with extensor spasm may make use of this spasm by sitting against the head of the bed and holding his pants inside the waistband, or with his hands in his pockets. He pulls on the pants with extended wrists while initiating his extensor spasm. This will slide him down the bed and into his pants.

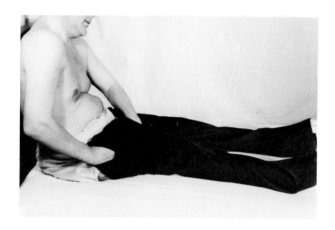
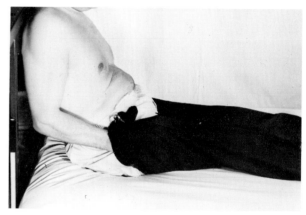
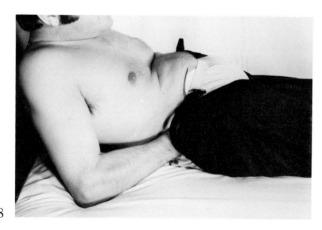
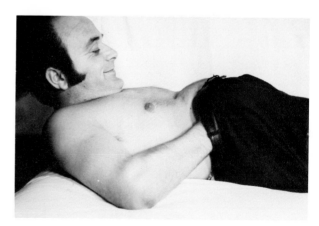

FIGURE 6-48

Method 11. A patient who must lean against the head of the bed, or the raised head gatch for balance, may be unable to pull his feet within reach, and therefore must use a dressing stick (Fig. 6-49). A patient with flexor or extensor type spasm, or a patient with tight hamstrings, may find that his heels dig into the mattress on any attempt to lean forward. This patient will need a dressing stick as a substitute for forward flexion. A dressing stick may be required in the early stages of training in any situation in which the patient cannot reach to slip his pants over his feet.

Method 12. A patient with excessive spasticity or tightness may require a bed with a gatch and a knee flexion component so that his heels do not dig into the mattress. The patient shown also requires loops from the foot of the bed to pull himself forward. While holding himself flexed forward, he uses a dressing stick to work his pants over his feet. Once the pants are high enough, he slips his wrist through the pants dressing loop, and holds himself forwards with this while he reaches for the pants loops on the other side. He works the pants well up over his knees and then lowers the gatch to complete pulling his pants up, by rocking from side to side (Fig. 6-50).

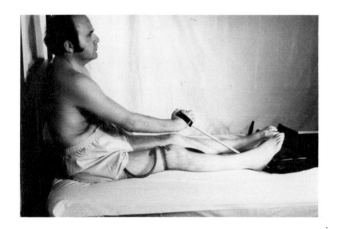
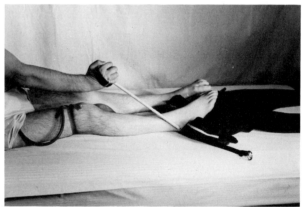
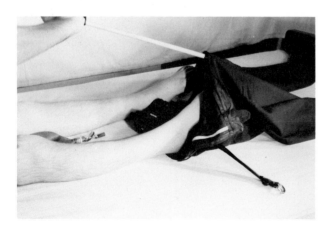
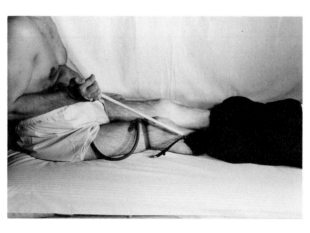

FIGURE 6-49

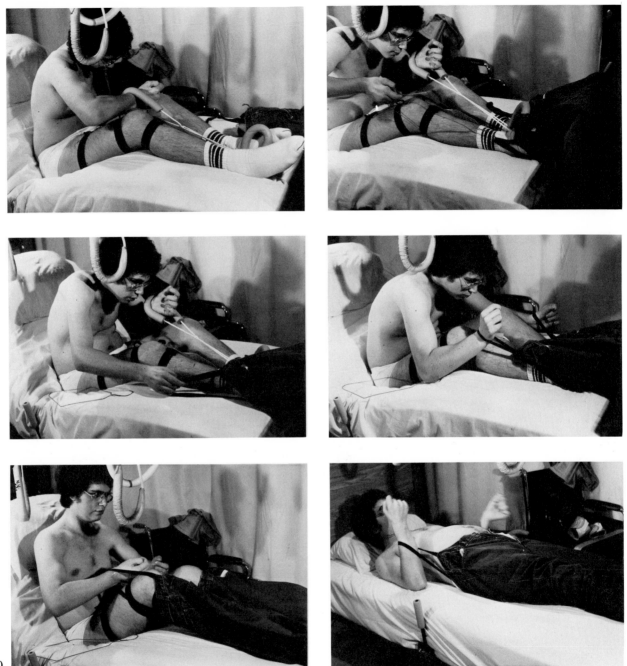

FIGURE 6-50

REMOVING PANTS

Method 1. (Fig. 6-51)   The patient sits in his chair and unfastens his pants. He places one hand inside his pants at the back and leans away from this side. While he leans over the arm of the chair, he synchronizes a pushup and a scoop of the hand under the freed buttock. He repeats this action on the other side. With practice the pants can be freed of the buttocks in two moves. The patient lifts one leg at a time to push the pant legs off.

Method 2. (Fig. 6-52)   The patient sits on the bed and unfastens his pants. He hooks his thumbs over the waistband of his pants, locks his elbows, and does a

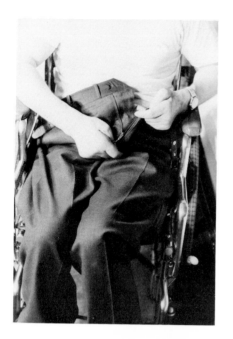

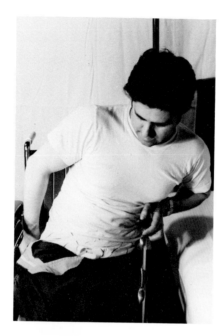

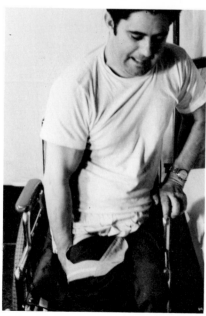

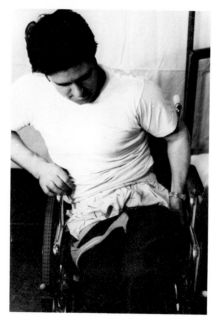

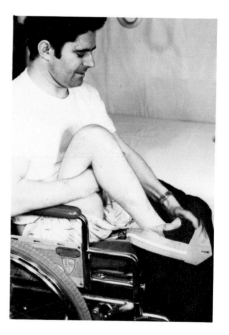

FIGURE 6-51

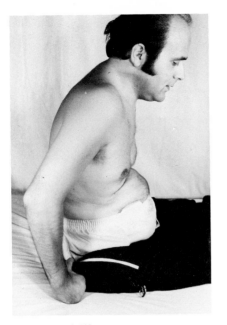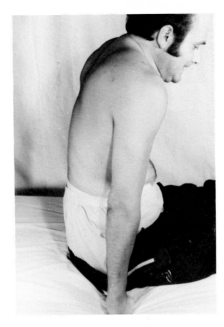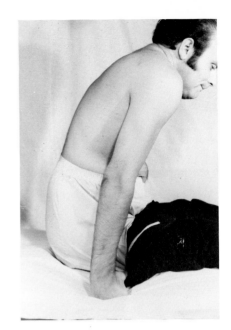

FIGURE 6-52

pushup. He flexes his trunk and head forward so that his buttocks move back and out of his pants.

 Method 3. (Fig. 6-53) The patient sits on the bed and hooks one arm into an overhead strap while the other hand catches the waistband at the back of the

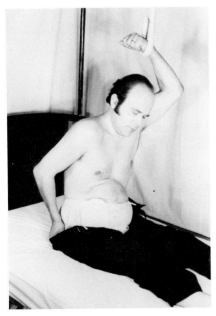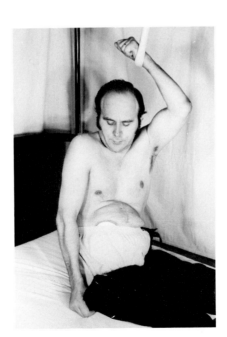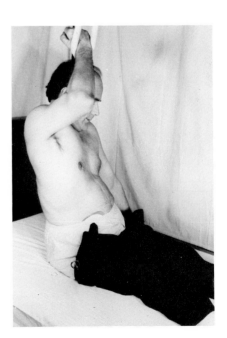

FIGURE 6-53

pants. He jerks up and pushes the pants under his buttock simultaneously. He switches arms to release the other side.

Method 4. (Fig. 6-54)   The patient sits on the bed and unfastens his pants.

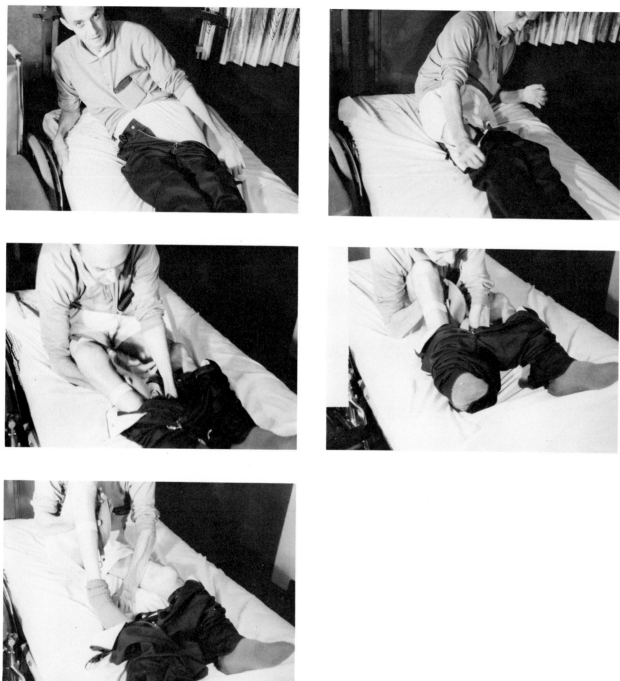

FIGURE 6-54

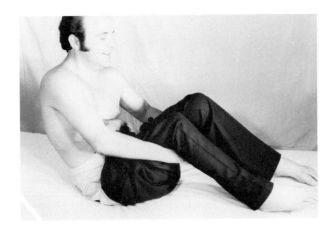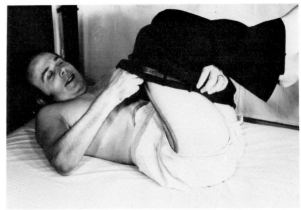

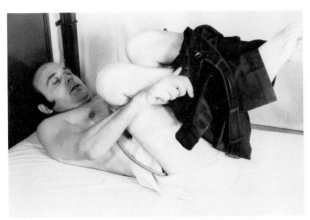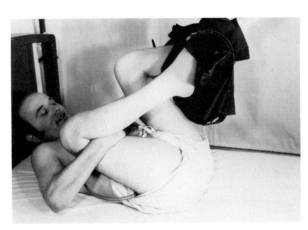

FIGURE 6-55

He leans back supported on one elbow while the other hand pushes the pants down over the freed buttock. He leans to alternate sides, repeating the process until the pants are below his hips. He sits up to push the pants below his knees. Holding the pants down with one hand, he pulls up a knee to lift a leg out of the pants. The process is repeated for the other side.

Method 5. (Fig. 6-55)   The patient hooks his wrists under his knees and pulls them up as he falls back onto the bed. He now hooks both knees with one arm while he pushes the pants down over his knees. He places a wrist under each knee and kicks them off by pulling alternately with his arms.

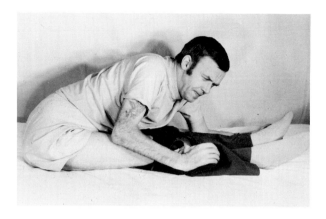

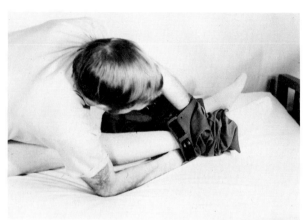
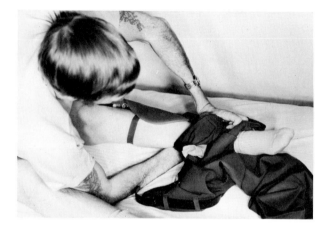

FIGURE 6-56

Method 6. (Fig. 6-56) The patient works his pants clear of his buttocks using one of the previous methods. He sits up and leans forward on one elbow and uses friction of both hands to work his pants down. He may lean on first one elbow and then on the other to push the pant legs down. When the pants are at his ankles, he inserts a wrist under the calf while still leaning on his elbow, and extends his wrist and flexes his elbow to lever his foot off the bed. The free arm pushes the pants away under the heel.

Method 7. (Fig. 6-57) The patient sits on the bed and leans back on alternate elbows to push the pants down past his hips. He remains in this position and hooks a wrist under a knee to pull it up. He pushes the pants down over his knee and then hooks a wrist under his bared knee. He pulls and slackens on the knee alternately to kick his leg partially out of the pants. He repeats the process with alternate legs until the pants are worked off.

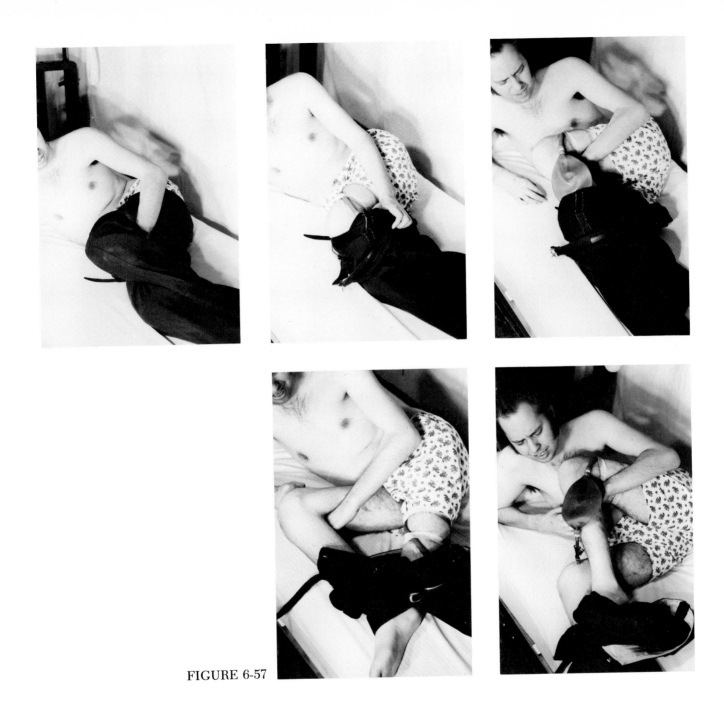

FIGURE 6-57

Method 8. (Fig. 6-58)　The patient lies on the bed and, rolling from side to side, pushes his pants down past his hips. He works his trunk into a flexed position so that he can hook a wrist behind his leg to pull it up to his chest. He uses one arm to maintain the position of the leg while the free arm pushes the pants down past his knee. He now hooks the bared knee with an extended wrist and pulls it up as far as possible so that he can push the pant leg off his foot with his free arm.

Method 9. (Fig. 6-59) The patient works his pants down over his hips using

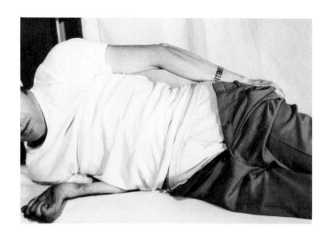
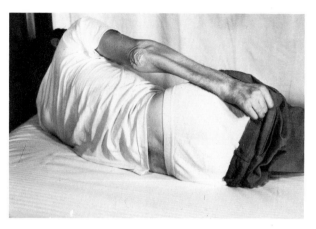
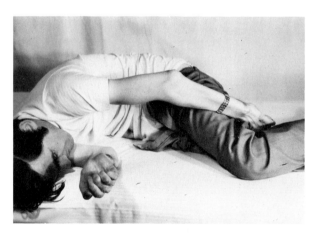
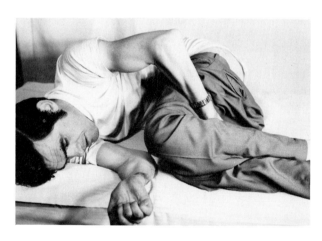
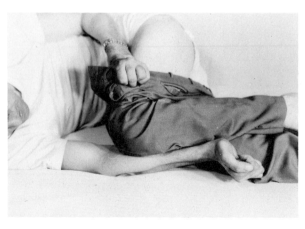
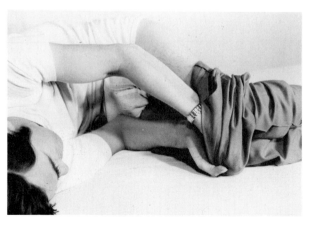

FIGURE 6-58

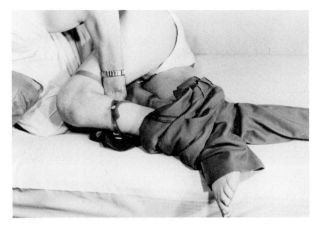
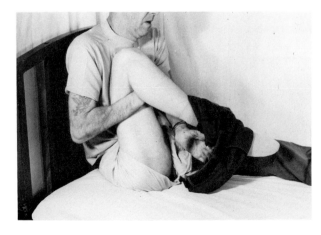

FIGURE 6-58
Continued

one of the previous methods and then sits close to the head of the bed and places his hand under a knee. He rocks back, picking up his knee, and leans against the head of the bed. This frees both hands so that one arm can hold the knee while the other works the pants off the leg.

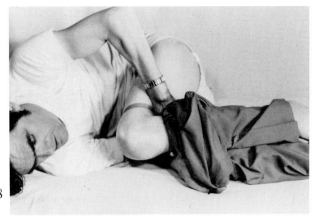
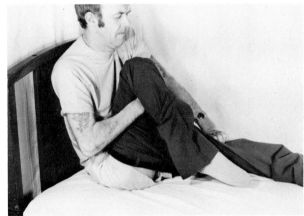
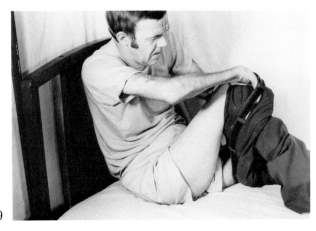
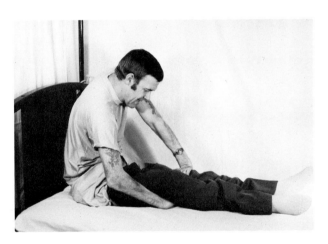

FIGURE 6-59

Method 10.   The patient lies on the bed to work his pants down over his hips using one of the previous methods. He now moves up to the head of the bed and leans against it so that both hands will be free (Fig. 6-60A). By moving up the bed he will drag the pants part way down his legs. If the patient is unable to lift his knee so that he can reach his feet, he will require a dressing stick to push his pants over his feet (Fig. 6-60B). Some patients may use this method reclining against a raised head gatch.

FASTENING PANTS

Waistband

An elastic waistband saves the necessity of fastening the pants, provided that it is not too difficult to pull the pants up. If elastic is not satisfactory, a hook fastening is easier to manage than either a press stud or a button.

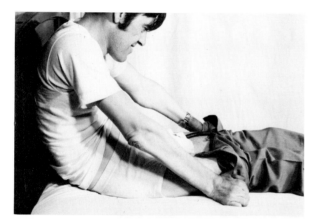

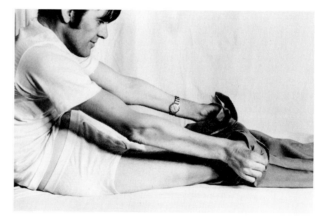

FIGURE 6-60 A

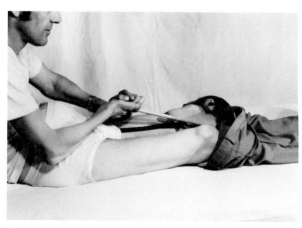

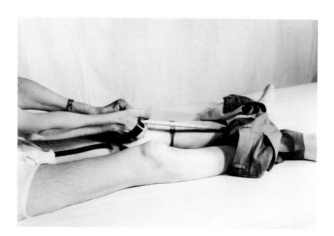

B

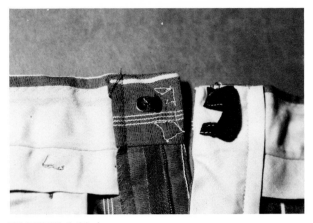
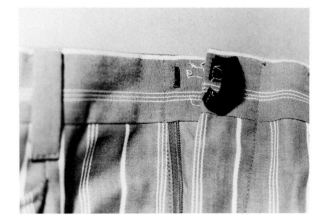

FIGURE 6-61 A   B

Adaptations

For ease in fastening, a loop just large enough to insert a thumb is sewn to the extreme edge of the hook side of the waistband (Fig. 6-61A). A similar loop is sewn to the inside of the waistband underneath the eye (Fig. 6-61B).

A D-ring may be sewn on the hook side of the waistband and 4 inches (10.16 cm) of hook velcro is sewn to the eye side on the waistband (Fig. 6-62A). Four inches (10.16 cm) of the opposing velcro is sewn to the hook velcro at the fly so that it will fasten when folded back. A thumb loop is sewn to the free end (Fig. 6-62B) or a thumb hole is cut near the tip. The velcro can be backed with leather to give the cosmetic effect of a belt when fastened.

Methods

A patient may hook the fastening of his pants by depressing the eye side into the abdomen with the heel of one hand. The other hand pushes the hook side over

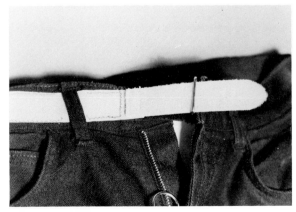
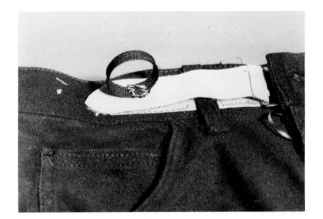

FIGURE 6-62

and down into position. The hand on the eye side is released to allow the abdomen to expand and snap the hook into the eye. A conventional hook-type fastener may be fastened using the belt loops of the pants. A thumb is inserted into the loops on either side of the fly and brought together until the hook is in position. If necessary, the hook may be spread for easier fastening. The leather-faced velcro is threaded through the D-ring and then pulled back, using the thumb loop. If this is difficult, a hook may be pushed through the D-ring to catch the loop and pull it through.

Zippers

Fly zippers may require a loop fastened to the tab. The loop must be large enough to accommodate a thumb. It can be made of shoelaces, split rings, key chain, leather thong—in fact, any material strong enough to withstand laundering and a strong pull, but at the same time able to meet cosmetic demands. A longer fly zipper may be sewn into the slacks to enable a patient to check his urine collecting apparatus, or to do self-catheters.

To pull up the zipper, one hand holds the material at the base of the zipper, while the thumb of the other hand, inserted in the loop, pulls the tab up. Usually the patient leans back if he is sitting in a wheelchair, thus eliminating the folds in the front of his pants and reducing his girth (Fig. 6-63).

Pant Leg Zippers. Pant leg zippers can be sewn to the inner seam of each pant leg unless there are adductor spasms or tightness; then they would be sewn into the outside seam to prevent possible pressure sores. The zippers are used for any of three reasons. First, they facilitate checking and emptying the urinal apparatus. In addition, they facilitate dressing. Also, it may be practical to use standing splints or braces to improve circulation and as a prophylactic for G.U. malfunction; if so, the zippers simplify applying and removing braces.

Zippers should reach to within 4 or 5 inches (10.16 cm or 12.70 cm) of the crotch. The zippers should be heavy duty and sewn so that they do not catch in the material. Dress pants should have a hidden zipper for cosmesis. The zippers must have a thumb loop of strong and unobtrusive material fastened to the tab. A small zipper opening in the pants will suffice if emptying the urinal bag is the only concern.

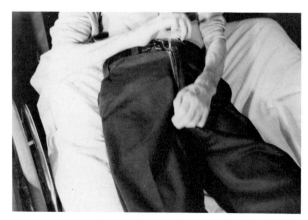

FIGURE 6-63

Managing the Zipper. The following method is for the patient who is able to flex forward at the hips so that his chest rests on his knees, and who then can return to the upright position. When leaning down, the patient places one thumb in the cuff of the pants by the zipper or, in lieu of a cuff, in an unobtrusive thumb loop. He places the other thumb or a finger in the zipper loop and pulls it up to the knee. In order to check the urinal apparatus, he will have to open the zipper completely. To do this, he sits upright and holds the material taut at the knee with the palm of one hand, while pulling the zipper up with the other hand. To close the zipper, the patient holds the material at the top of the zipper with one hand and pushes the zipper down past the knee. Holding on to the back of the wheelchair with one wrist, he leans forward and completes closing the zipper.

If the patient is unable to return to the sitting position after leaning forward, he may manage by raising his leg and placing his foot on a raised object, such as the leg strap on the wheelchair, the toilet bowl, or a footstool. This will place the zipper tab within reach.

If the patient must hold on to the back of the wheelchair with one wrist to maintain balance, the bottom of the pants must be held down in some manner. For instance, an elastic may be sewn under the instep, or an eye may be attached to the shoe and a corresponding hook on the pant cuff.

If the zipper is fixed at the pant cuff, a dressing stick may be hooked into the zipper tab loop to pull it up.

If zippers are not used, a looser pant leg may be pulled up by friction of the heels of the hands at either side of the knee. Pusher mitts may be useful for extra friction. A dressing stick may be used in combination with the friction of the hands.

SHOES, SOCKS, AND STOCKINGS

TYPES OF SHOES AND FASTENINGS

Shoes should fit well to prevent foot deformities. Inside seams should be smooth to avoid pressure areas.

FIGURE 6-64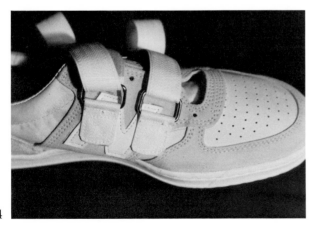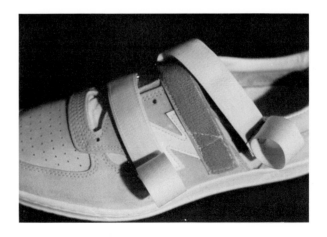

Slip-on shoes may require to be a larger fit for ease in putting on, but may be prone to slip off during transfers. If elastic laces are used to replace ordinary laces, the shoes become similar to a slip-on shoe.

Shoes may be adapted by adding a velcro D-ring with a finger loop, which is easily fastened, and provided the straps are long, the shoe can be opened wide. The straps should match the color and material of the shoe. Many types of shoes are commercially available which are normally fastened in this manner (Fig. 6-64).

Boots may be adapted with a second side opening zipper and with extra loops at the top of the back of the boot (Fig. 6-65). Because these boots open widely it is easy to slip the foot in, and the long back acts almost like a shoe horn. The heels of the boots may be ground down so they are smooth and rounded. This stops the heels from digging into the bed during transfers. It is very easy to fasten the zipper if a ring is placed in the zipper tab (Fig. 6-66).

An oxford-type shoe with a wide opening and front lacing may be suitable. The shoe should be large enough to permit the heel to be inserted without the use of a shoehorn, if possible. Cosmesis demands a work and a dress shoe, but women

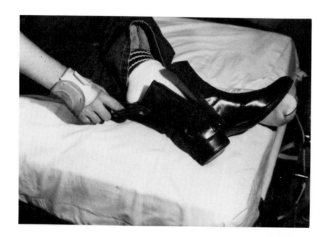
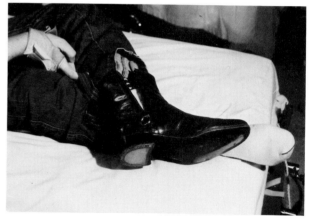
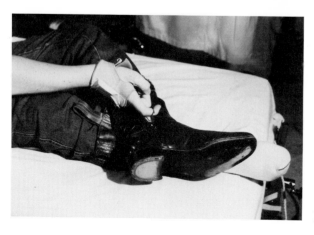

FIGURE 6-65

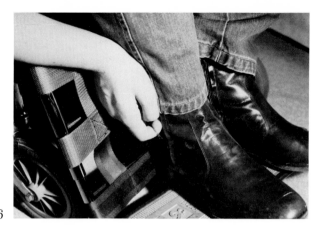

FIGURE 6-66

should avoid a high-heeled dress shoe because of the difficulty of positioning the feet on the footrests.

It is often necessary to stabilize the tongue of the shoe on one side. This can be done by making two holes in the tongue under the two top eyelets on one side of the shoe and threading the lace through them. A zipper is easily fastened, and may be sewn or laced into a shoe. A thumb loop should be fastened to the tab on the zipper.

A waist belt hook generally used on pants or skirts may be sewn to the side of the shoe, and an elastic lace inserted into the eyelets in place of the usual lacing (Fig. 6-67). A loop is formed at the top eyelet (see Appendix). The loop is released from the eyelet and drawn back to allow the shoe to open. The laces may be tightened more easily if a hook is used.

Some patients need a thumb loop at the back of the shoe to assist in donning the shoe (Fig. 6-68). This should be large enough for the thumb and of the same color leather as the shoe. It should be sewn neatly to the outside without bulky stitching on the inside.

A shoehorn may be required if the back of the shoe folds down when pushing the foot into the shoe. In this case it is usually too difficult to hold a shoehorn and

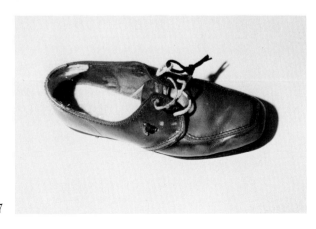

FIGURE 6-67

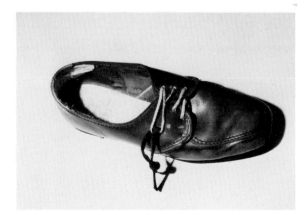

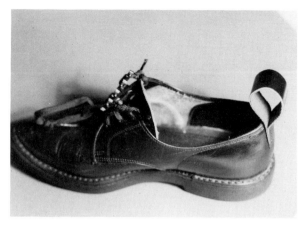

FIGURE 6-68

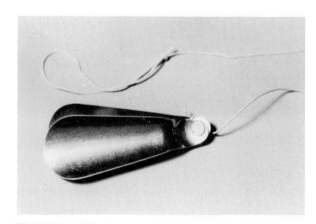

FIGURE 6-69 A

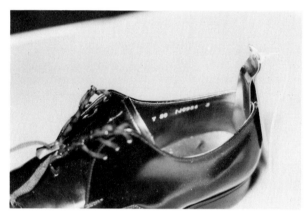

B

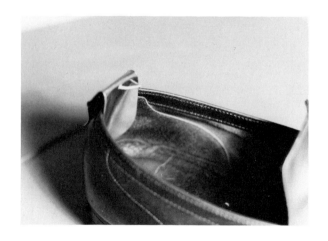

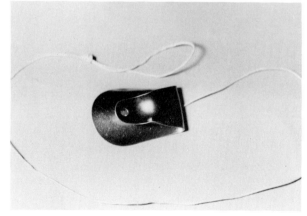

FIGURE 6-70

push the foot into the shoe at the same time. A homemade shoehorn may help. Two shoehorns may be placed one on the other and riveted together at the top with a washer between them to separate them (Fig. 6-69A). A length of cord may be fixed to the top so that the shoehorns may be easily pulled out after the shoe is on (Fig. 6-69B). A clip-on shoehorn can also be made by bending the top of a metal shoehorn back to clip over the back of the shoe (Fig. 6-70). A cord with a loop at the other end may be fixed at the bend for easy release. In either design of shoehorn, it is attached to the shoe before the shoe is positioned to receive the foot.

TYPES OF SOCKS AND ADAPTATIONS

Socks should be of a loose knit without tight tops. If there is elastic in the tops, some of it can be removed provided that the top elastic is left intact (otherwise the sock will unravel). Thumb loops may be required inside the top of the sock. Loops should be sewn so that they are open and protruding above the top of the sock; they should match the socks in color as closely as possible. A loop on either side of the sock is usually adequate.

Many types of stockings are manufactured with a semi-elastic top to hold them up, a factor which is very satisfactory provided the tops are not tight. Pantyhose will not be practical if a catheter is used, and they make it difficult to handle clothing during toiletting.

BASIC POSITIONS FOR PUTTING SHOES AND SOCKS ON

Various positions can be used by an individual patient; however, the aim is maximum stability so that, if possible, two hands are free to work and clear the heel from a surface. Socks are easiest to put on if two hands are used, but putting on shoes and taking off shoes and socks may often be accomplished with one hand only. Where possible, the position should enable counterpressure to be applied. The methods of handling socks and shoes are described following the description of positions. It is always necessary to work out the optimum position first, then the handling method.

Position 1. (Fig. 6-71)   A patient who has a good range of movement in the hip joint and good balance may slide forward in his chair for stability and then

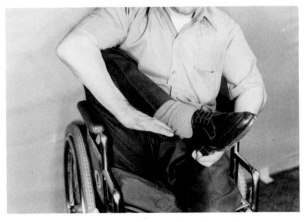

FIGURE 6-71

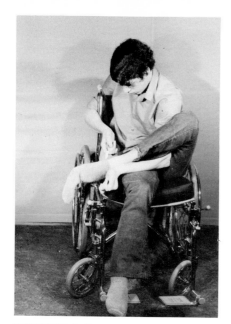

FIGURE 6-72

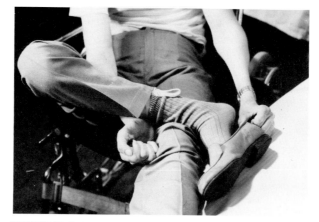

FIGURE 6-73

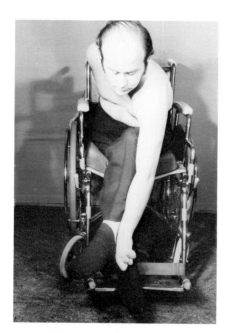

FIGURE 6-74

pick up his leg. He stabilizes it and applies counterpressure with one arm while working with the other.

Position 2. (Fig. 6-72)   If the patient sits in the chair with one ankle crossed over his knee he is in a very stable position which, in addition, secures the foot so that his two hands may be free to work. If the ankle is inclined to slip off the knee, an arm may be used to hold it, but the hand can still be left free to assist in dressing.

Position 3. (Fig. 6-73)   The patient sits in the chair in the transfer position and places one leg on the bed. He crosses the other leg over so that the foot is within reach. This position is extremely stable and will probably enable him to use both hands.

Position 4. (Fig. 6-74)   The patient sits in his chair with one knee crossed over the other. This position leaves the heel free and counterpressure applied by the other knee. Since the position usually leaves only one hand free, it is usually used for removing socks and shoes. Note that castors must be turned forwards for stability.

Position 5. (Fig. 6-75)   The patient sits in his chair with one arm hooked around the pushing handle for stability. He lifts his leg with the other arm hooked under his knee so that he can lower his foot into his shoe.

Position 6. (Fig. 6-76)   The patient, sitting in the chair, faces the bed about a foot away. He applies his brakes and lifts one leg to rest against the edge of the mattress. This position allows him to keep his leg flexed, freeing both hands while his foot remains within reach. If he wishes to apply pressure, any flexion of his arms will cause him to lean forward, pushing against his knee with his chest.

Position 7. (Fig. 6-77)   The patient sits on the bed with one calf crossed over the other leg. This raises the foot from the bed and leaves both hands free to work. Extra stability may be gained by leaning on one elbow.

270

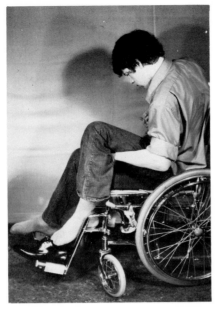

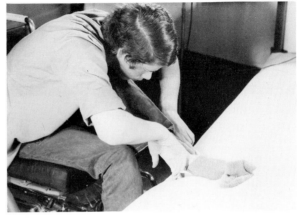

FIGURE 6-75

FIGURE 6-76

Position 8. (Fig. 6-78)   The patient sits on the bed with his elbow on the bed and lifts his heel, using wrist extensors and elbow flexors. This position leaves only one hand free. The leg cannot flex when pressure is applied to the sole of the foot because the chest and shoulder prevent it.

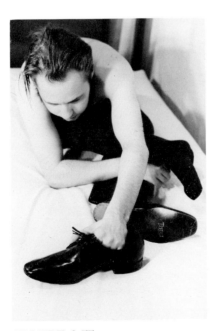

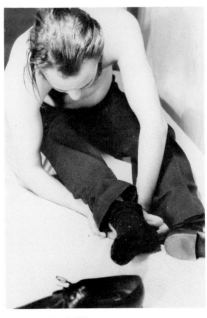

FIGURE 6-77

FIGURE 6-78

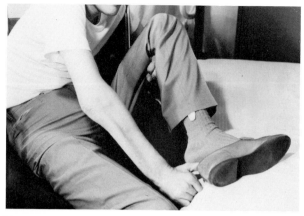

FIGURE 6-79

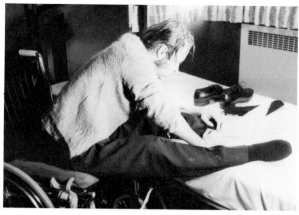

FIGURE 6-80

Position 9. (Fig. 6-79) The patient sits in the chair with the chair in transfer position and places one foot on the bed. He pulls the leg up and into outward rotation with a wrist under his knee. This position places the foot on its side, leaving the heel free. If necessary for extra stability, he may hook the arm near the bed around the chair back upright, pull the knee up with the other hand, and transfer the knee to the wrist of the arm holding on to the chair back.

Position 10. (Fig. 6-80) The patient sits in the chair in the transfer position with both legs on the bed. This position is very stable and permits the use of both hands.

Position 11. (Fig. 6-81) The patient lies on the bed with one knee pulled up to his chest. He holds it in external rotation with his arm inside the knee and over the lower leg. This position leaves both hands free and his heel within reach.

Position 12. (Fig. 6-82) The patient lies on the bed with his knees pulled up to his chest with his forearm, thus leaving one hand free to work.

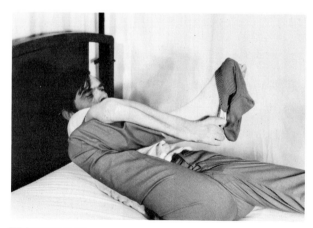

FIGURE 6-81

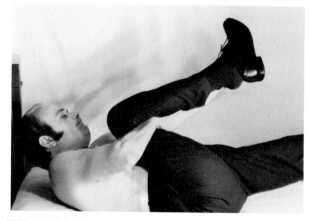

FIGURE 6-82

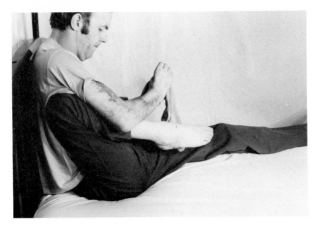

FIGURE 6-83

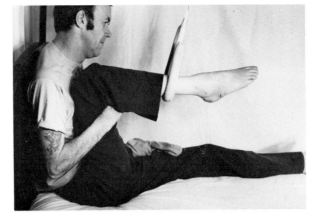

FIGURE 6-84

Position 13. (Fig. 6-83)   The patient sits against the head of the bed and pulls his knee up with his leg in external rotation. He holds it in position with an elbow in front of his knee, leaving two hands free to work.

Position 14. (Fig. 6-84)   The patient sits against the head of the bed and rests his foreleg in an appropriately placed sling. This position leaves both arms free to work.

Position 15. (Fig. 6-85)   The patient sits against the head of the bed and uses a dressing stick to reach his feet. This position is used if the heels dig into the bed on forward flexion of the trunk, or if the patient is unable to reach his feet.

Position 16. (Fig. 6-86)   The patient with excessive spasticity or tightness may require a gatch bed with a knee flexion component to prevent his heels from digging into the bed when he leans forward. He may also require a dressing stick.

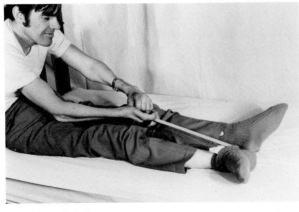

FIGURE 6-85

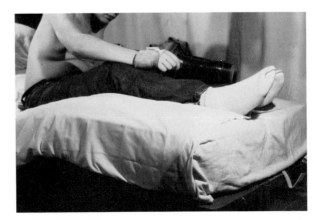

FIGURE 6-86

Putting Socks On

Method 1. (Fig. 6-87)   The top of the stock is stretched open using the thumbs and, if necessary, the teeth. The sock is slipped over the toes with a hand on each side of the foot so that the toes line up with the opening. As the sock is moved up the foot, the patient internally rotates his hands to maintain the thumb position as a hook in the sock, he slides his thumb to the back of the sock to clear the heel. Friction of the hands may be used to smooth the sock into position.

Method 2. (Fig. 6-88)   The fingers or thumbs are inserted into the sock loops and the socks are stretched out so that the opening lines up to accommodate the toes. The socks are pulled up and twisted so that the loop is pulled under the heel. If one hand must be used to maintain the position of the foot, or to lift the heel from a surface, the loops may be pulled alternately. The hands are turned so that the pull against the thumb occurs when the thumb is in extreme extension so that it will hold without any muscle action. (A pull on the back of the thumb will merely flex it and allow the loop to slip off, but a pull against the inside of the thumb will cause it to maintain its extended position). Talcum powder sprinkled inside the sock or on the foot will facilitate sliding the sock onto the foot.

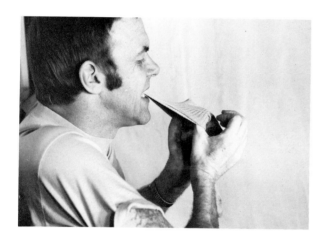

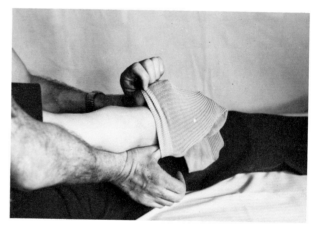

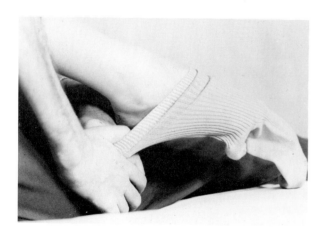

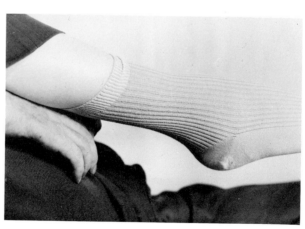

FIGURE 6-87

274

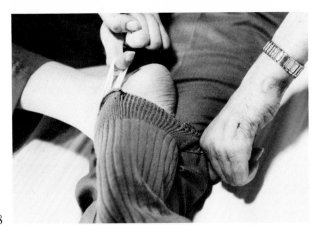
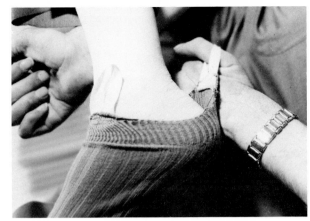

FIGURE 6-88

Method 3. (Fig. 6-89)   A dressing stick might be required to pull on the sock loops. This may be particularly useful if a patient's heels dig down into the mattress when he reaches for his feet. Since usually only one hand is free to use a

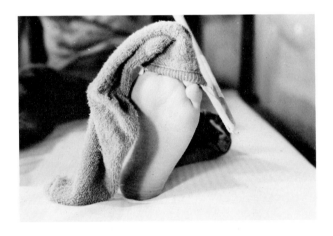
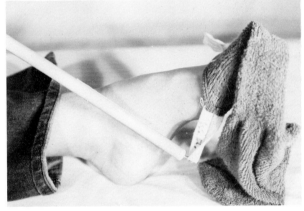

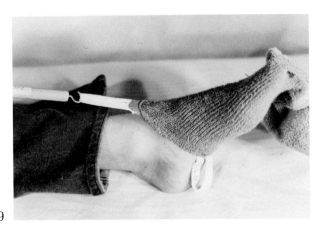
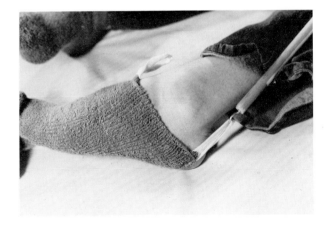

FIGURE 6-89

dressing stick, there is more difficulty starting the sock on the foot. The sock may be maneuvered onto the big toe, which will hold one side of the sock while the other side is stretched over the little toe.

Method 4. (Fig. 6-90)   A stocking gutter may be made of thin polypropylene or a similar material, and covered with slippery nylon taffeta. Loops will be required near the top back of the gutter. This gutter makes it easier to slip the socks

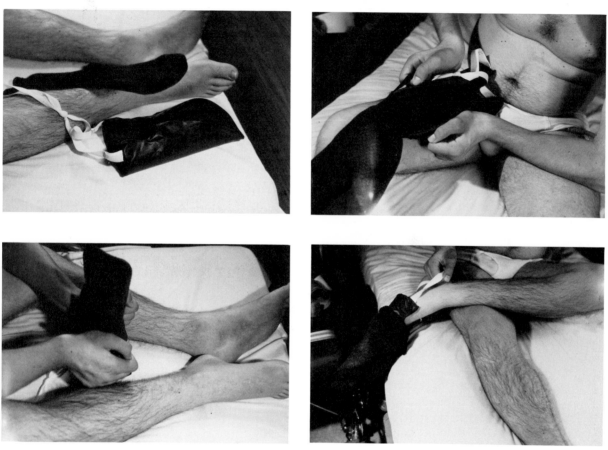

FIGURE 6-90

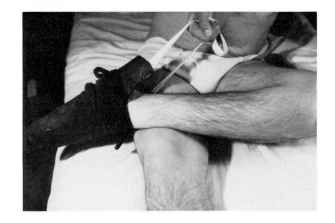 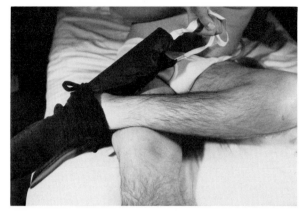

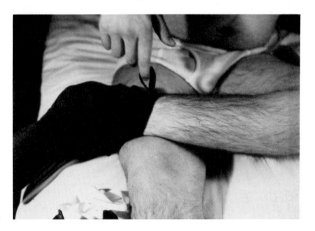

FIGURE 6-90   Continued

over the toes as far as the heel, after which it must be pulled out, and the socks pulled up using sock loops.

An advantage of this method is that the sock can be slipped onto the gutter as long as the patient is in a stable position and can use two hands; but only one hand is required to reach down to slip the opened sock over the toes.

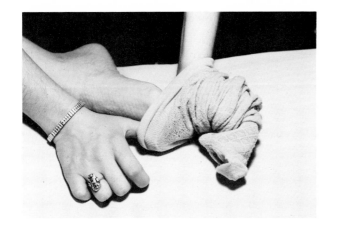
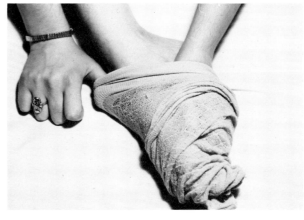

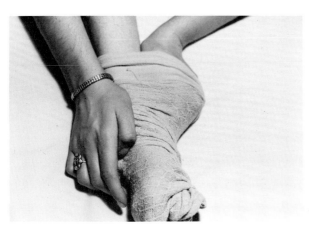
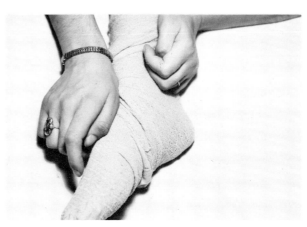

FIGURE 6-91

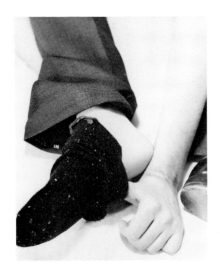

FIGURE 6-92

Putting Stockings On

The patient assumes her normal position for donning socks. She slips the stocking onto one hand and holds the other side, stretching it with her thumb (Fig. 6-91). She slides the stocking onto her foot, keeping her hand inside the stocking for as long as possible. She works the stocking up by alternately pulling on the top and stroking the stocking. Loops at the top of the stocking would probably cause it to ladder. Garters may be permanently attached to the tops at side or front with a pulling loop, but again will ladder all but the sturdiest hose. A stocking gutter, as shown in Method 4, may be useful, and does not harm the stocking. Pantyhose are hard to manage because of the need to slip them down for toiletting, and because of the difficulty in putting them on.

Removing Socks and Stockings

Socks are easy to push off, provided that the heel can be lifted slightly. The thumb or fingers form a natural hook when pushing under the sock top or in a

278

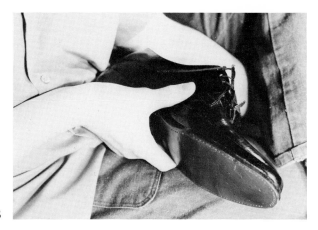
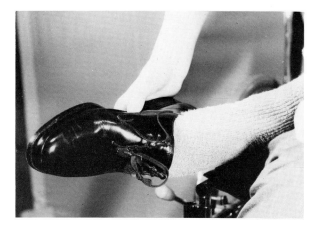

FIGURE 6-93

loop (Fig. 6-92). A dressing stick may be required if the heels dig down hard, or if the feet are not within reach. The dressing stick may be notched so that the base of the V catches the sock top (see Fig. 6-2).

Putting Shoes On

Method 1. (Fig. 6-93)   The patient uses tenodesis to pick up the shoe under the instep and pushes it onto his foot, using the side of his hand or thumb against the heel.

Method 2. (Fig. 6-94)   The patient picks up the shoe by placing a hand

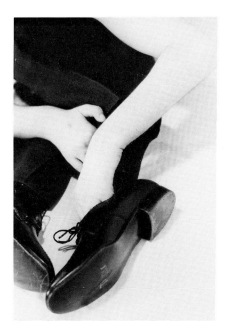
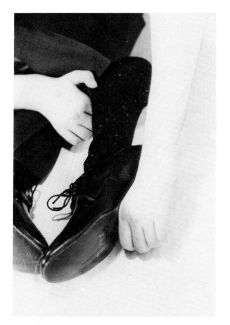
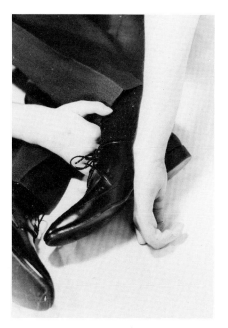

FIGURE 6-94

279

inside it and slips the shoe over his toes. He now catches the shoe under the instep against the heel. He pulls the shoe on by using the side of his hand. Counterpressure is applied by the other arm, against the knee or by the force of gravity.

Method 3. (Fig. 6-95) The patient sits in the wheelchair and, if necessary, stabilizes himself with one arm over the back of the chair. He moves his foot over, leaving room for the shoe to be placed on the footrest. He lifts his leg with a wrist

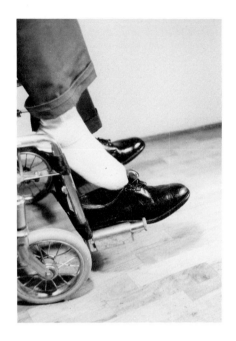
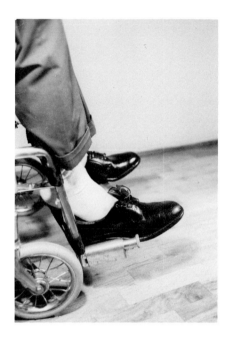
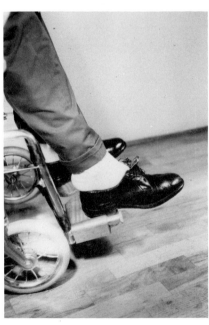
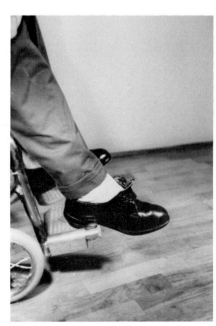

FIGURE 6-95

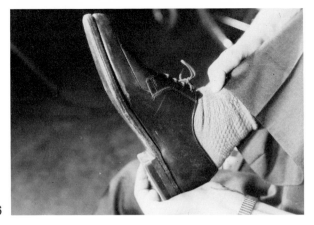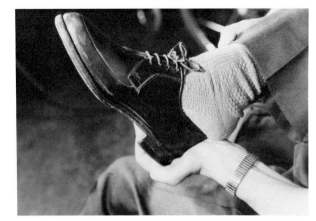

FIGURE 6-96

under the knee so that the toe points into the open shoe, and lowers the leg so that the forefoot slides in. He now extends his wrist against the calf, pushing the foot and the shoe forward until the heel catches on the front edge of the footrest. If gravity does not slide the foot into the shoe, pressure on the knee will do so. Wheeling the chair against a wall will also push the shoe onto the foot.

Taking Shoes Off

Method 1. The patient holds his leg in position with one arm. He uses the heel of his other hand against the heel of the shoe to push it off (Fig. 6-96).

Method 2. The patient places his foot within reach, and pushes the heel of the shoe off with his thumb or dressing stick (Fig. 6-97).

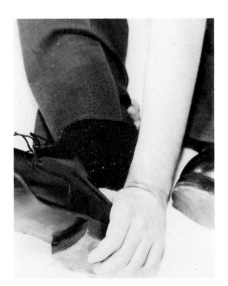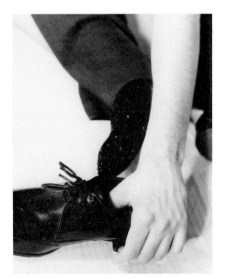

FIGURE 6-97

Method 3. (Fig. 6-98)   The patient lifts his leg and, by extending his wrist behind his calf, he pushes his lower leg forward, allowing his foot to drop in front of the footrest. He now lifts his knee, gently catching the heel of the shoe on the front of the footrest. His shoe will slide off as he replaces his foot on the footrest.

Method 4.   The patient lifts his leg under the knee and shakes his leg, causing the shoe to slide from his foot onto the footrest. Retrieving it will be easier from the footrest than from the floor.

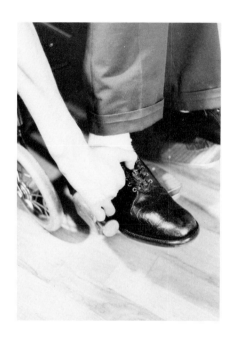
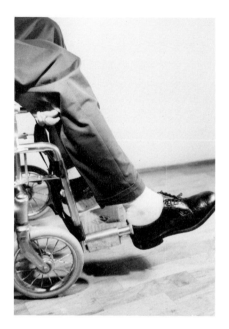
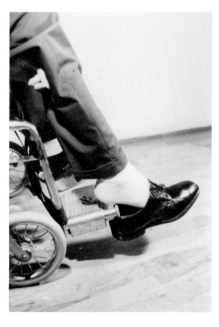
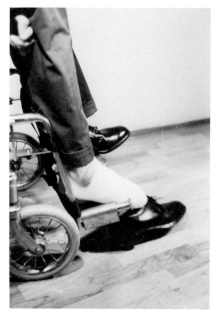

FIGURE 6-98

DRESSES AND SKIRTS

If dresses have fastenings, they should be at the side or the front. When the dress is fitted the patients should be seated, since length and skirt fullness may require adjustment in this position. Most patients prefer not to sit on a skirt owing to the difficulty of tucking it under and untucking it. For this reason full skirts or skirts with fullness at the back may be selected so that the skirt can be bunched behind and still appear smart in front. Some women prefer to have a split in the skirt at the back so that they do not sit on the skirt. This may be useful if the woman is transferring frequently to the toilet, or if occasional incontinence is a problem. Methods of putting on dresses are very similar to methods of putting on skirts or sweaters, and once she has mastered these she should be able to solve problems of putting on dresses and skirts. Skirts are put on over the head, and are fastened in the same manner as pant waistbands.

COATS AND PONCHOS

Jacket-length coats are more convenient to put on and wear. Roomy arm-holes in a slippery and light material are advantageous. Zippers that must be joined at the bottom are difficult to manage. If necessary, buttons or velcro should be substituted. Ponchos are easy to put on and require no fastening. A rain poncho is excellent protection for a patient seated in a chair.

TIES

Clip-on ties are easiest to manage for most patients. However, ties may be permanently knotted and the slip knot adjusted to put it on over the head. An open loop may be required at the inside of the small end of the tie to enable the patient to hold while pulling the tie knot up.

WATCHES

Watches should be self-winding or electric. The strap must be an expansion type or have a velcro D-ring fastening substituted for the buckler. When putting it on, the watch is worked over the hand using the thumb or fingers of the opposite hand. It is easiest to work the watch well down one side of the hand, so that it will stay in position when the hand is pressed onto some stable object, such as a thigh, while the strap is pushed over the other side of the hand. The thumb may be used to push the watch off, sliding the thumb from one side of the strap to the other. Friction on the pant leg or arm of the wheelchair may be used in conjunction with this.

Useful References And Aids

Functional and Self-Care Activities of Quadriplegia. Produced by Hall. J and Whittaker, M. $^{3}/_{4}''$ color video cassette. 35 minutes. GF Strong Rehabilitation Centre, 4255 Laurel Street, Vancouver, BC, V5Z 2G9, Canada, 1985.

Kernaleguen, A.: Clothing Designs for the Handicapped, University of Alberta Press, 1978. (Contains clothing adaptation ideas, and instructions for adapting patterns for a seated person).

Toward Independence: Male Quadriplegic Dressing. Color video, Dallas Rehabilitation Foundation, 1985.

Quadriplegic Functional Skills: Dressing. Color Film. 18 minutes. Producer, McLean, Elmer, Nugent. National Medical Audio Visual Center, Washington, DC 20409, or Atlanta, Georgia, 30333. 1974.

7

Bowel and Bladder Management

BOWEL TRAINING
  Timing
  Autonomic Dysreflexia
    (Hyperreflexia)
  Bowel Techniques
  Bowel Management

Suppositories
Bladder Management
Catheterizing
External Urine Collecting System
Menstrual Management

"Bowel training" is the program designed to reactivate the patient's regular bowel habits. "Bowel management" follows bowel training and explains the methods and equipment used to teach the patient to manage his own bowel regimen.

BOWEL TRAINING

TIMING

The patient must be toileted at the same time each day. If, after a reasonable length of time, the bowel movement shows a pattern of being more successful on alternate days, or every third day, the regimen should be changed to accommodate this pattern. Some patients find it desirable to evacuate their bowels in the evening. This may be due to practical reasons—pressure of time in the morning before work, previous habits—or because bowel initiation is easier in the evenings. If the patient is dependent on family or attendant for assistance in his bowel evacuations, it may be more convenient during the evenings. Later, during training, the patient may experience certain signs that indicate the bowel contents are starting to descend. These signs may be goose pimples, headache, sweating, muscular twitching, abdominal fullness, or indigestion.

AUTONOMIC DYSREFLEXIA (HYPERREFLEXIA)

It should be noted that the symptoms of autonomic dysreflexia may be somewhat similar, but are more severe and are described by patients as pounding headaches, flushing, and cold sweats. Because of the sharp rise in blood pressure, this dysreflexia is a medical emergency. A bowel or bladder procedure which may be the cause of the dysreflexia should be stopped immediately, and if the symptoms do not subside, the patient should be transferred to the bed in a seated position (to keep the blood pressure lower), and the bladder or bowel should be checked for distension. A physician may be required if the symptoms do not abate. Bowel or bladder distension cause most of the incidents; other causes may be trauma, strong skin stimulation, pregnancy, and labor. Patients must be counseled to take the condition seriously and to know how to remedy the cause, or when to call for medical assistance.

BOWEL TECHNIQUES

The patient must be able to tolerate sitting for at least half an hour before bowel training is started. Little is gained by starting earlier. A mild laxative may be necessary the evening before to ensure that the stools are of normal consistency, and a suppository may also be required to be inserted high in the rectum half an hour to an hour before toileting.

The patient transfers, or is transferred onto, a raised toilet seat or commode, and his feet are placed on a footstool to compensate for the additional height. A backrest adds to the security and comfort of the patient. Side bars may be necessary to give the patient complete security. Care must be taken when placing the patient on the toilet. It is especially important that the buttocks are not parted to cause tension on the skin of the natal cleft. On the other hand, the buttocks must not be compressed, thus inhibiting reflexes of evacuation. The patient must be comfortable if a bowel movement is to be achieved. The patient may initiate evacuation by pressing down on the abdomen, by holding a deep breath, by allowing the trunk to forward flex, or by raising the knees. Kneading the abdomen by hand or forearm along the level of the colon from right to left may assist.

The assistant's hand is gloved and a finger is well lubricated with a water soluble lubricant. A gentle massage with the finger on the skin around the anus will often be sufficient to relax the external anal sphincter. A finger may be inserted to further relax the sphincter if external massage is insufficient. The stool will then be expelled if it is of a soft consistency and is in the lower rectum. If the stool is too firm, it may have to be removed manually to prevent impaction. Plenty of lubricant must be used and extreme care taken to avoid damage to tissues. Two fingers may have to be used to break up the stool and gently work it out. If the stool is too firm, the laxative doses may be adjusted by the physician, and possibly fecal softeners added. The fluid intake may be increased and the diet adjusted to include more bulk and roughage to prevent recurrence.

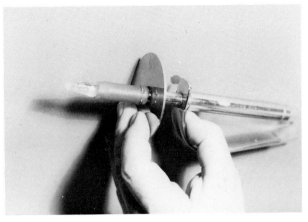 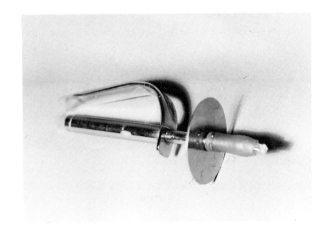

FIGURE 7-1 A   B

After evacuation the initial cleansing is done gently with toilet tissue. A protective pad or paper is placed on both wheelchair cushion and bed before the patient transfers. A pubic wash is done on the bed. The skin is now checked for abrasions or obvious pressure before drying and powdering.

BOWEL MANAGEMENT

When bowel regulation has been achieved and the initiation of evacuation methods has been established, the patient is ready to begin looking after his own bowel management. By this time the patient should have learned to transfer himself to commode or toilet seat, and to control his own laxative or diet regulation. Bowel movement may be initiated with no aids, by the regulation of diet or prescribed laxatives, or by kneading his abdomen and flexing his trunk forward. He may require suppositories or digital stimulation. As the management methods are developed, any equipment necessary to enable the patient to be independent must be provided.

SUPPOSITORIES

Method of Insertion

Patients with some finger function may learn to hold the suppository and insert it adequately.

Many patients will require a suppository inserter (Fig. 7-1). This type of flanged suppository inserter has been in use for over 28 years and has proved to be both safe and efficient. The flange controls the depth of insertion and the soft rubber tube is shaped and lubricated to prevent any damage to delicate tissues. The handle may be adapted so that it can be held firmly and at the correct angle.

An additional handle may be made, which can be attached to a standard suppository inserter and adjusted to establish the optimum angle for any patient who cannot manage the conventional angle (Fig. 7-2).

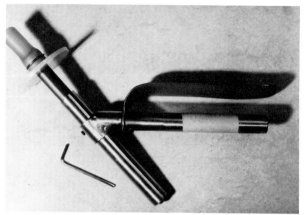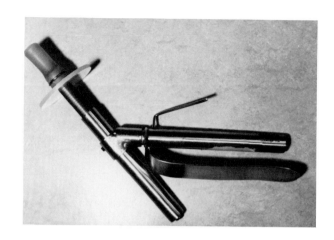

FIGURE 7-2

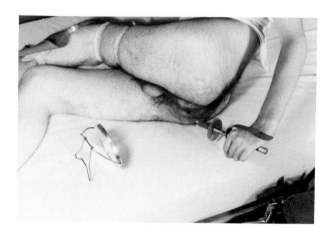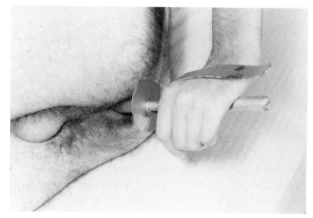

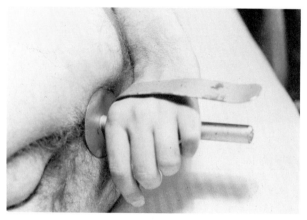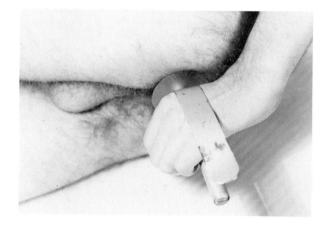

FIGURE 7-3

The appliance is inserted until the flange makes contact with the buttocks. Further pressure compresses the spring and moves the plunger down to eject the suppository (Fig. 7-3). A wrist-drive flexor-hinge or tenodesis-type splint is not recommended, as the wrist must be flexed in order to reach the anus. The flexor-hinge splint will close only when the wrist is extended.

It should be noted that generally men find it easier to use a suppository inserter because of their smaller buttocks.

Positions For Insertion

Position 1.   The patient lies on his bed with the dominant arm uppermost, the upper leg fully flexed at the hip and knee, and a mirror with a broad base placed on the bed. This position tends to turn the patient slightly onto his abdomen and makes it easier for him to reach.

Position 2.   The patient lies on his side on the bed with both knees flexed. This position parts the buttocks more than other positions, but makes the anus harder to reach.

Position 3.   The patient places his chair by the bed in side transfer position. He remains in the chair or commode chair, but rests his upper body in side lying on the bed, leaving his feet on the footrests or placing them on the bed. This position reduces the number of transfers required.

Position 4.   He may insert the suppository while in position on the commode chair or toilet, using a position as described below.

Positions for Insertion or Digital Stimulation on the Toilet

The patient positions himself on the toilet. He stabilizes himself with one arm, enabling him to reach his anus with the other using one of the following methods:

Position 1. (Fig. 7-4)   A table is placed by the side of the toilet. The height is adjusted so that the patient's elbow rests comfortably on the top. The patient leans

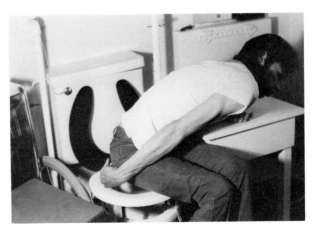

FIGURE 7-4

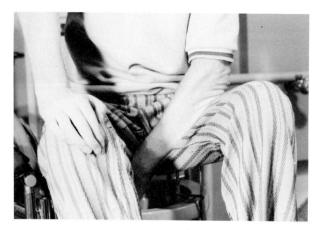

FIGURE 7-5

over this elbow, raising his buttock from the toilet seat on the opposite side. This permits digital stimulation without reaching under the toilet seat.

Position 2. (Fig. 7-5)   The patient flexes his trunk so that he can reach from the front through an open-front toilet seat. Depending upon the build and the ability of the patient, he may rest one forearm across his thighs, or he may rest his trunk upon his thighs. To use this method, he must be able to regain his upright position.

Position 3.   The patient hooks one forearm over a side bar at elbow height (Fig. 7-6A) or places his wrist in an overhead strap placed above his shoulder (Fig. 7-6B). He leans away from the bar or strap to reach under the side of the raised toilet seat.

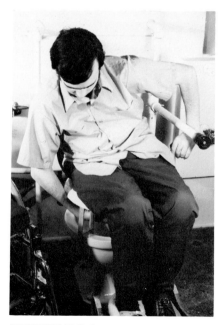

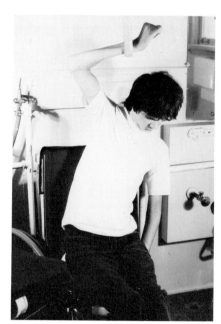

FIGURE 7-6 A   B

290

Position 4. (Fig. 7-7)   The patient places one wrist in an overhead strap and leans forward to reach through the front of an open front toilet seat. The overhead strap enables the patient to pull himself to an upright position.

Equipment for Digital Stimulation

Disposable gloves are donned and the finger to be used is lubricated. The patient may be able to use a gloved finger for digital stimulation, but where this is not possible, splints and aids may be used.

A simple splint may be used to hold the finger straight and the wrist and metacarpophalangeal joint in flexion; an ideal position for reaching the anus.

A length of $\frac{1}{8}$-inch (.32 cm) I.V. tubing (Fig. 7-8A) is looped around the base of the middle forefinger and is drawn over the palm to a wrist strap. The tension should be adequate to pull the finger forward so that it is held straight and away from the other fingers (Fig. 7-8B). Where there is difficulty in holding the other fingers back, a bar may be attached to the tubing behind the middle finger. The bar runs in front of the remaining fingers (Fig. 7-8C). The bar must be washable and adequately formed or padded to prevent pressure areas.

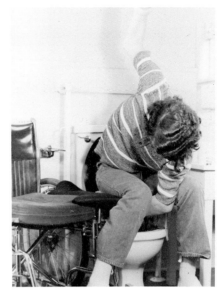

FIGURE 7-7

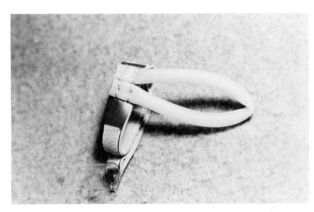

FIGURE 7-8 A

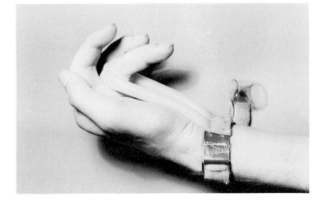

B

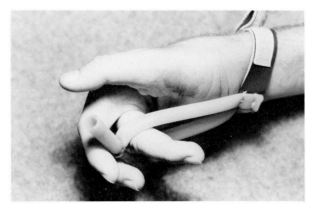

C

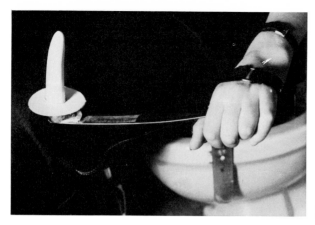

FIGURE 7-9

If a person cannot reach the anus with a gloved finger, a digital stimulator may be used (Fig. 7-9). A stimulator with some flexibility is felt to be safer than a rigid one. The surface of the stimulator must be smooth, and well lubricated with

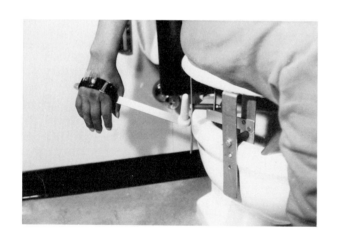

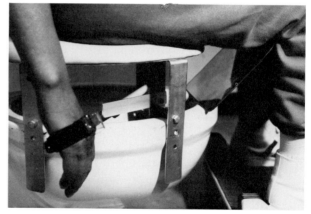

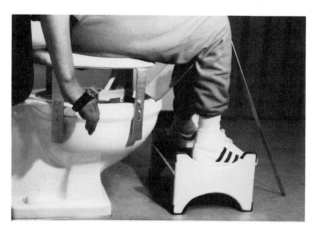

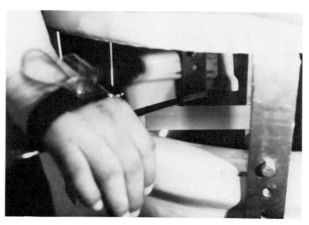

FIGURE 7-10

water soluable lubricant. Handles may be adapted, and the shaft may be curved or twisted to accommodate the hand position.

If a person requires more strength and has difficulty holding the stimulator in position, a lever bar may be attached to the toilet seat extensions (Fig. 7-10). The stimulator handle may be made of flat material which can be twisted slightly so that when it rests on the lever bar, the angle of the stimulator is correct. Slight pressure downward on the handle will raise the stimulator into position. A mirror must be used unless sensation has been spared. In this instance the mirror is placed between the knees with the mirror resting on the toilet bowl, and the bent aluminum handle resting on the floor.

Cleansing

The positions adopted for digital stimulation, described above, will also stabilize the patient for the first steps in cleansing.

The patient who has some ability to grasp may find that he needs more tissue to provide a firm grip. A large amount of toilet tissue may be wound around one hand. Wiping is done with the paper on the dorsum or radial side of the hand.

A toilet-tissue holder may be constructed (Fig. 7-11A). The handle must be adapted to attach to the patient's hand firmly enough to provide good control. The shaft is curved as required and the length is adjusted to the patient's needs. The holder at the tip may be made of two or three horizontal coils of wire. Coat hanger wire is suitable for experimentation and easily obtained, but stainless steel wire should be used in the permanent appliance. The two ends of the wire should finish at the handle so that there are no unprotected ends. Toilet tissue is inserted into the center of the coils and arranged so that it folds over the wires (Fig. 7-11B).

A dampened paper cloth is less abrasive than toilet tissue, and is often easier for a patient to manage. A stainless steel welding rod is formed to make a holder for a disposable paper cloth (Fig. 7-12). The damp cloth is tucked between the projections and wrapped around the holder several times. The soiled towel may be placed in a receptacle near the toilet, rather than flushing it down the toilet.

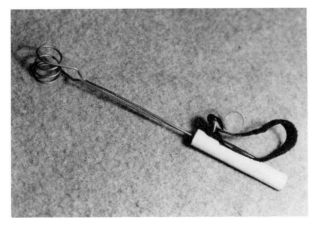
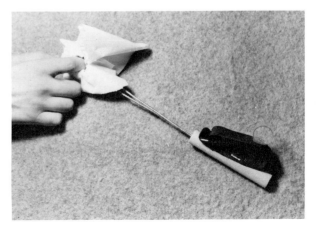

FIGURE 7-11 A   B

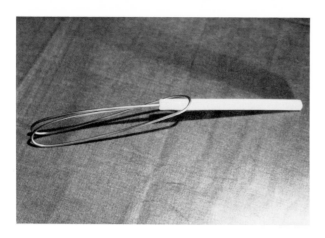

FIGURE 7-12

The patient transfers onto his wheelchair and then to bed, so that he can wash to ensure cleanliness.

Pubic Wash

Before transferring to the bed, the patient places a basin of water and his washing equipment in a convenient position by the bed. A stacking plastic storage unit makes a most useful washing basin because it does not tip easily and is easy to reach into (Fig. 7-13). A small plastic drain basket may be rivetted on the inside top edge so that the wash mitt may be squeezed out.

The patient must be careful to test the temperature of the water before placing the basin on his knees or lapboard to transport it. He then spreads a plastic or flannelette sheet or an absorbent pad on the bed. After transferring to the bed, the patient will roll onto his side and flex the upper leg. The patient reaches over his buttock to wash the posterior area thoroughly with a washing cloth or mitt. The anterior area may be washed conveniently when lying supine or sitting up. Since the patient is unable to wring out the wash mitt, he must verify that the pad or plastic is well placed to protect the bedding.

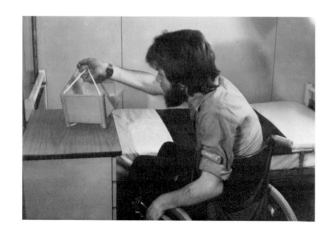

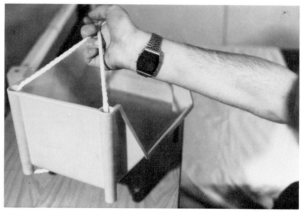

FIGURE 7-13

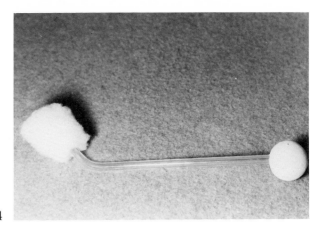

FIGURE 7-14

The patient dries the area and applies powder, using powder directly from the container, or using an adapted powder puff (Fig. 7-14). The puff may be made of artificial sheepskin sewn to a metal or plastic handle, which may be curved and adapted for an adequate grip.

BLADDER MANAGEMENT

Male and female patients may with training achieve spontaneous voiding; this is the optimum method of management.

A man may achieve spontaneous voiding without the necessity of independent toilet transfers. He may use a urinal or, if he knows that he will not be able to reach a toilet at the requisite time, he may apply a urine-collecting apparatus for the occasion.

Intermittent catheterization is a safe management method. Many men can manage intermittent catheterization as a permanent method of management, since it needs to be done only three to four times a day on the average. Women may find intermittent catheterization more difficult because transfers may be required. Women have further to reach and require more dexterity.

Urine-collecting apparatus may be used by the man who voids spontaneously.

A satisfactory and safe method of external urine collection for quadriplegic women has not been developed. At the moment these women are limited to the choice of a spontaneously voiding bladder with toilet transfers, intermittent catheterization, or to the use of an indwelling catheter.

Some women opt for the use of a permanent indwelling catheter because of the difficulty of doing frequent transfers, inability to manage clothing, the inconvenience of having to have access to a bed or toilet, and the general social and vocational inconvenience. The medical disadvantages of using an indwelling catheter must be clearly explained so that the woman can make an intelligent choice in her method of bladder management.

Some patients have an ileal conduit or a suprapubic catheter for medical reasons. Many of these patients learn to apply the urine-collecting system, provided that the outlet is conveniently placed and the patient is sufficiently dextrous. These procedures are not done frequently.

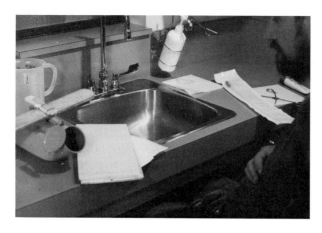

FIGURE 7-15

Advancing medical knowledge is changing procedures. These changes must be monitored.

Self Catheterization for Men Using "Clean" Technique

All equipment is prepositioned: a water soluble, sterile lubricant, a urinal, which may be modified so that it can stay positioned between the knees, a jug for measuring output, forceps, and a catheter are placed by a wash basin (Fig. 7-15).

Pants may require adaptation so the fly can be opened wide to permit easy access to the penis (Fig. 7-16). A long zipper, a flap with a velcro closure, or track pants that can be pulled down to hook over the knees are alternatives.

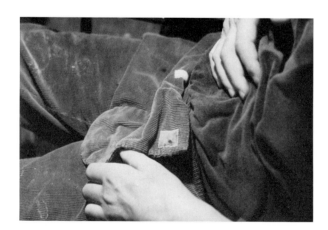 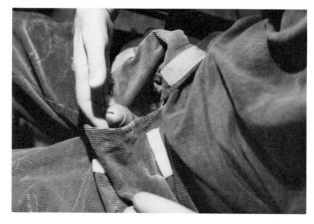

FIGURE 7-16

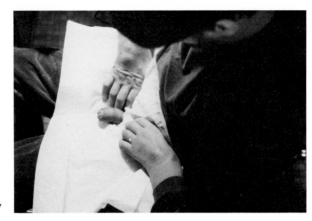

FIGURE 7-17

The patient washes and dries his penis and then washes and dries his hands. He places an incontinence pad or a clean towel on his lap under his penis. The patient illustrated prefers to tear a hole in the incontinence pad so he can place it on his lap with his penis protruding through (Fig. 7-17).

People using a catheter at home usually use a clean catheter, which has been washed in soap and water and stored clean and dry, that is, in a paper or cloth towel or a tobacco pouch for carrying.

Because of the danger of cross-infection in an institution, a sterile catheter is used.

The patient takes the sterile catheter package, and using his teeth and fingers, he opens the package at the opposite end to the tip. He pulls the package only partially open, taking care not to touch the catheter (Fig. 7-18).

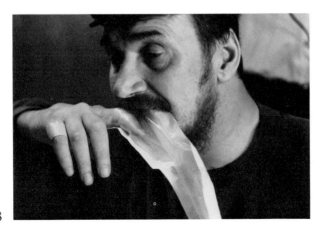 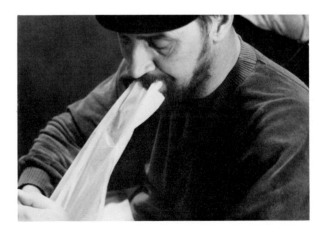

FIGURE 7-18

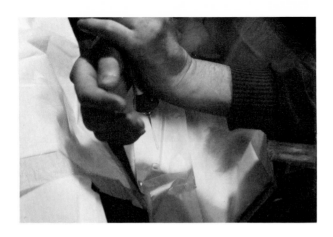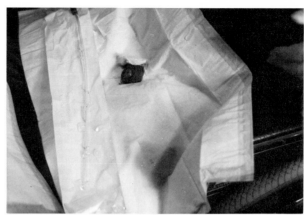

FIGURE 7-19

He places the untouched catheter on his knees, and squeezes lubricant onto about four inches (10.16 cm) of the tip of the catheter (Fig. 7-19).

He pulls himself up to the basin to wash his hands again, using great care that nothing touches the catheter or the package. He now places a clean pad on the sink edge and washes his hands thoroughly several times. If forceps are to be used, he washes them also, and holds them by a handle in his mouth to keep the tips clean. He now pushes away on the clean towel on the edge of the sink (Fig. 7-20).

He picks up the catheter and twists it to spread the lubricant before inserting the catheter (Fig. 7-21).

He may hold the catheter using one hand, or two hands, (including using the heels of both hands), or forceps. The catheter is inserted about 9 inches (23 cm), which places the tip near the internal sphincter.

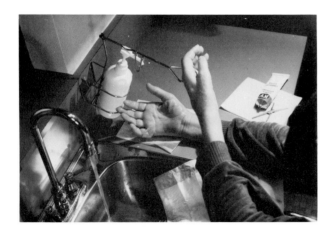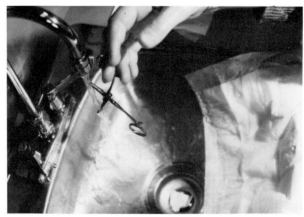

FIGURE 7-20

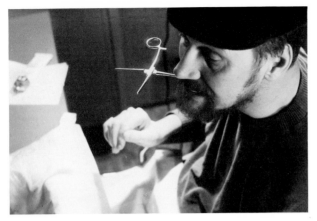

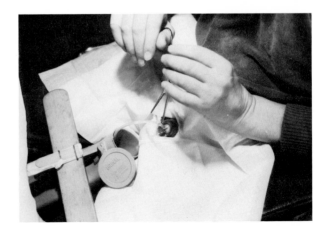

FIGURE 7-20 Continued

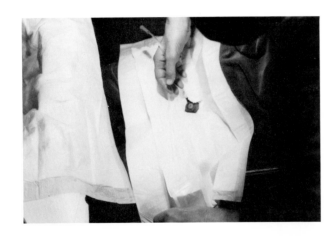

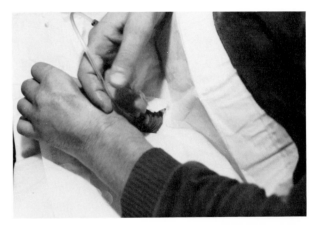

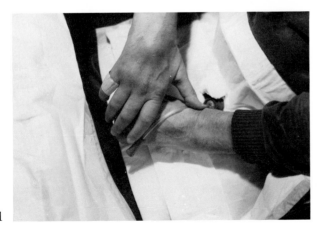

FIGURE 7-21

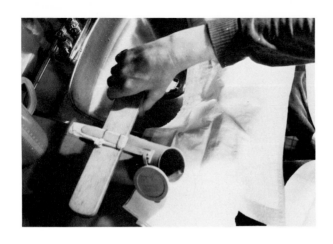

FIGURE 7-22

At this point the patient may reach for the urinal and position it, because his hands will not have to touch the part of the catheter close to his body (Fig. 7-22). Many patients will preposition the urinal at the beginning, before they wash their hands.

The free end of the catheter is now placed in the urinal. The patient now inserts the catheter fully. He may encounter a slight resistance as the tip of the catheter comes into contact with the internal sphincter. He must not force the catheter in, but may keep a gentle continuous pressure, which can be combined with a slight twist. Taking a deep breath in and then releasing it may cause the internal sphincter to relax.

When the urine has stopped flowing, the catheter is eased out about an inch (2.54 cm), because often a further small flow will occur.

After the flow ceases the urine remaining in the catheter must be prevented from running back because any sediment from the bladder is likely to be in the last trickle of urine. The catheter may be clamped off using forceps (Fig. 7-23), or it may be bent sharply; alternatively, the catheter can be withdrawn down into the urinal so that the urine is not allowed to run back. The catheter is removed completely and the urine is measured.

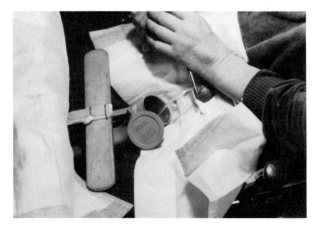

FIGURE 7-23

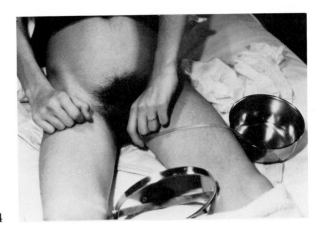

FIGURE 7-24

Self Catheterization for Women Using "Clean" Technique

It is more difficult for women to self catheterize than it is for men.

Positioning. A woman may transfer to the bed to do catheterization so that she can lean against the head gatch or head board for balance, and thus free both hands (Fig. 7-24).

She may slide forward to the edge of the wheelchair, and may either place one foot on the toilet (Fig. 7-25A) or outside the footrests (Fig. 7-25B). She must swing her footrests out of the way to allow a close approach, and even so may require an extra length of tubing on the end of the catheter to allow drainage into the toilet bowl.

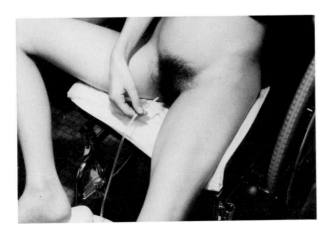

FIGURE 7-25 A

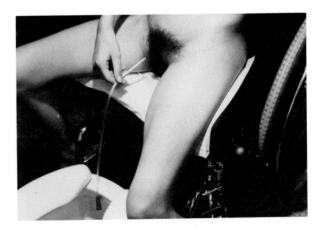

B

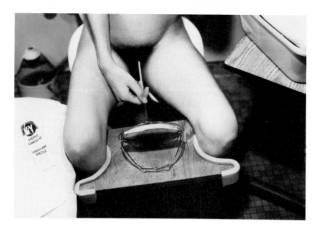

FIGURE 7-26

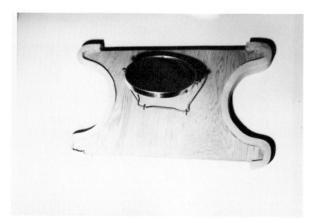

FIGURE 7-27 A

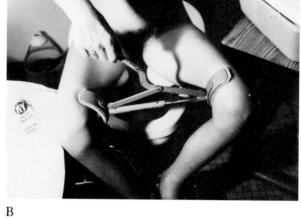

B

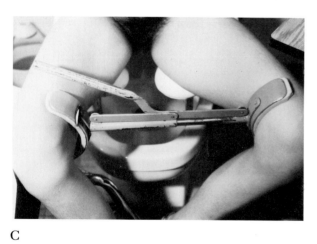

C

She may transfer onto the raised open front toilet seat (Fig. 7-26). In this case only a short catheter, such as a sound or female catheter, is required.

Mirrors. Mirrors are required by some women, particularly when learning catheterization. Some women find it useful also to use a flashlight at first, because the urethral opening is small and hard to see. The flashlight may be fastened to the base of the mirror. Adjustable mirrors may be placed on the bed (see Fig. 7-24), clipped onto the wheelchair or toilet, or fastened to a knee spreader (Fig. 7-27A).

Once a women has become accustomed to self catheterization, she should not require a mirror.

Knee Spreader. A person whose legs do not fall into abduction will find a knee spreader useful for positioning (see Fig. 7-27A). A person who has adductor spasticity may use a mechanical knee spreader (Fig. 7-27B). This spreader extends by pulling a lever down into a locked position (Fig. 7-27C).

CATHETERIZING

Because of the danger of cross infection in an institution, a sterile catheter is used, but once the person is at home she should use a clean catheter, washed in soap and water, and stored clean and dry in a paper or cloth towel, in a handy zipper purse.

All equipment is positioned ready for use, (hands are well washed) and the catheter is removed from its package; care must be taken not to touch the tip (Fig. 7-28).

Some women will lubricate the tip of the catheter with a water soluble sterile lubricant but many will not require this (Fig. 7-29).

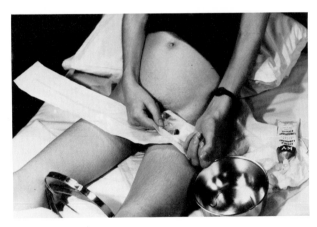

FIGURE 7-28

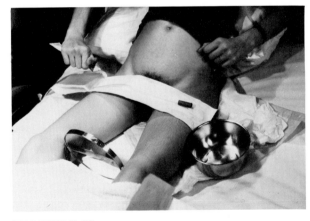

FIGURE 7-29

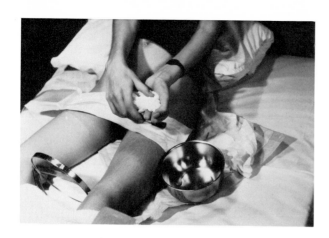 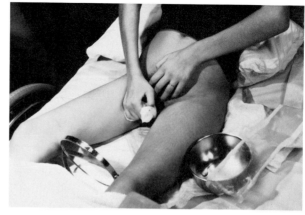

FIGURE 7-30

Hands are wiped with damp toweling or "Wet Ones", and the vulva is cleansed, wiping downwards to avoid contamination from fecal bacteria (Fig. 7-30).

The urethral opening is hard to reach and hard to see, even in a mirror. If the labia must be held apart, good dexterity is required. For these reasons, a woman will usually locate the urethral opening with a finger (Fig. 7-31). This is easier if the finger has some sensation. She can then slide the catheter by the finger into the urethral opening. After practice, many women can locate the urethral opening using the tip of a sound or female catheter. Sensory sparing will of course make the procedure much easier.

A labia spreader was developed, but though it worked, the whole process was too time consuming and therefore it was later rejected (Fig. 7-32).

The end of the catheter must be placed in the bowl before inserting the catheter because the urethra is short and the urine will flow almost immediately (Fig. 7-33).

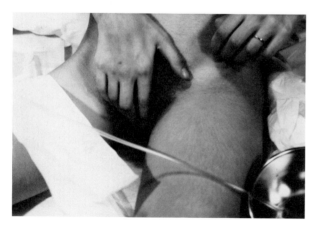

FIGURE 7-31

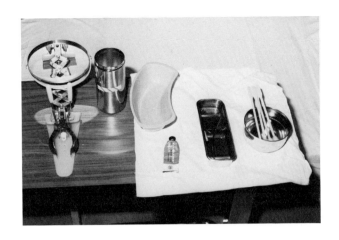

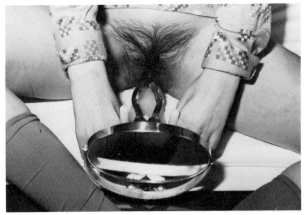

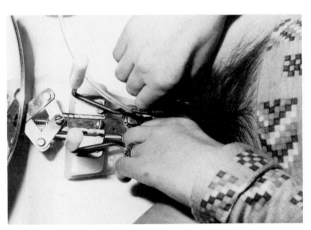

FIGURE 7-32

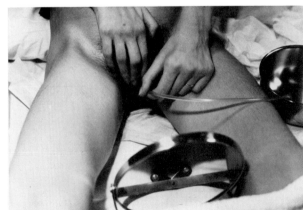

FIGURE 7-33

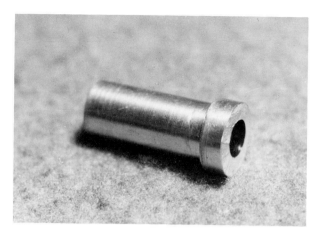

FIGURE 7-34

EXTERNAL URINE COLLECTING SYSTEM

It may be decided that external urine collection should be used rather than intermittent or indwelling catheterization. The urine collecting system consists of a condom attached to the penis, with a tube fastened to the other end of the condom leading to a collecting bag.

Assembly and Preparation of Urine-Collection System

When the method of urine collection has been established, it becomes desirable for the patient to perform the task of assembly and attachment himself. The equipment should be assembled and the smaller items kept on a tray so that they are accessible. Quadriplegic patients with adequate grip will manage the application using no aids. The flexor-hinge hand splint is a most useful aid for others who could not otherwise accomplish application of the drainage system. Many patients, who initially rejected the use of a hand splint, find its use so vital for this task that they perceive its use in other situations as well and accept it.

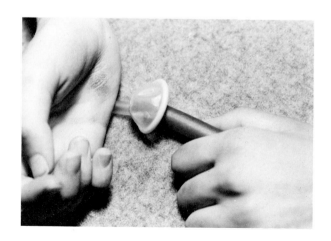
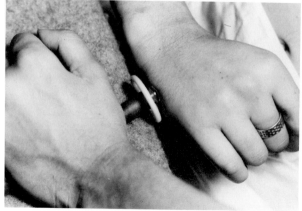

FIGURE 7-35

Joining Tubing and Condom

The tubing is made of a pure gum surgical tube ³/₈ × ³/₁₆ inches (1.00 × .50 cm). The plug (Fig. 7-34) is made of ¹/₂-inch (1.27 cm) (outside diameter) and ¹/₄-inch (.64 cm) (inside diameter) acrylic plastic tubing cut into 1-inch (2.54 cm) lengths. It is turned down on a lathe to ³/₈ of an inch (1.00 cm) (outside diameter) except for ¹/₈ of an inch (.50 cm) left at one end as a collar.

The following are methods used to insert the plug through the condom into the tubing and sink the plug. In all cases the condom must be punctured before application. A stick is generally used for this purpose.

Method 1. (Fig. 7-35) The patient uses tenodesis to hold the tubing and leans the condom against the end. The plastic plug is maneuvered into position against the condom and tube, using the heel of the hand and the table surface to tip it. Once the plug has been started into the tube the hands can be repositioned to enable more force to be applied to sink the plug home.

Method 2. (Fig. 7-36) The patient rests the condom over the end of the tube, using tenodesis to hold it in position, and starts the plug into the tube, hold-

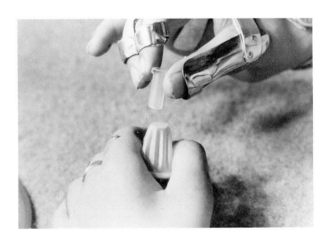

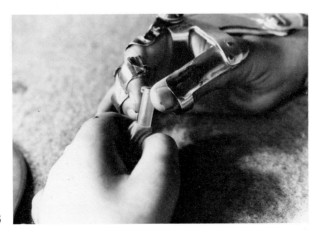

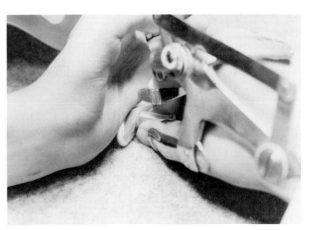

FIGURE 7-36

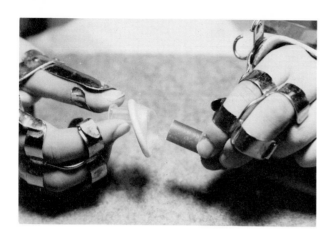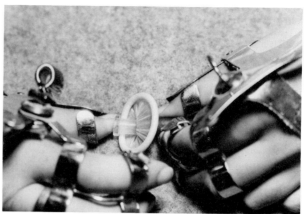

FIGURE 7-37

ing the plug with a flexor-hinge splint. Once it is started, he changes position so that he can drive it home. This may be done by holding the tube down with the side of his hand and using the thumb of the splinted hand to push the plug all the way down to the collar.

Method 3. (Fig. 7-37)   The patient uses two flexor-hinge splints to attach the condom to the tube in a normal fashion. He may complete pushing the plug into the tubing with one rigid thumb tip.

Method 4. (Fig. 7-38)   A simple clamp may be made of two pieces of wood, lined with foam and hinged at the end with leather. This requires little pressure to hold the tubing firmly while the plug is inserted.

Method 5. (Fig. 7-39)   A wooden pencil is held between the teeth and the sharpened end is inserted into the flanged end of the plastic plug. This holds the plug firmly, while enabling the patient to see what he is doing. He holds the urinal

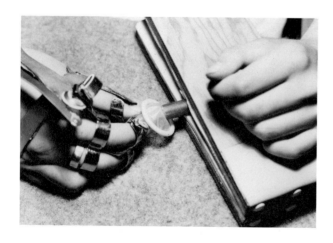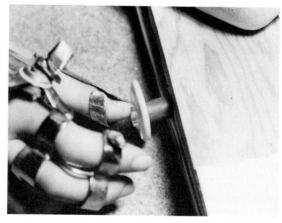

FIGURE 7-38

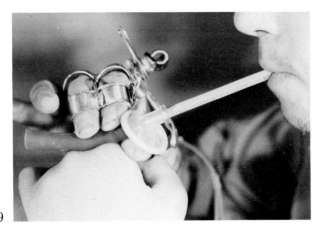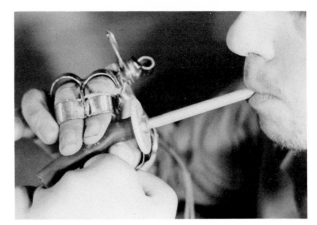

FIGURE 7-39

tubing either between the heels of his hands or, using his splint, maneuvers the condom until it rests over the tubing. The condom is placed so that it will unroll towards him. Using the pencil in his teeth, he inserts the plastic plug into the tubing through the condom. He checks to ensure that the condom is punctured.

Method 6. (Fig. 7-40)   A jig may be made to hold the plug securely for both assembly and disassembly of condom and tube. A length of two-by-two is sanded smooth, and a groove is cut down one side to fit the depth and diameter of the collar of the plug. A thin sheet of metal or plastic has a slot cut into it to fit the body of the plug. The slot is aligned over the groove and fastened down so that the plug can be dropped in and held in place by the collar. If a clamp is used to hold the tube, the plug height should be regulated to align with the tube. A hole may be drilled through the two-by-two, using the hollow plug in place as a guide, so that the condom can be punctured through it following assembly.

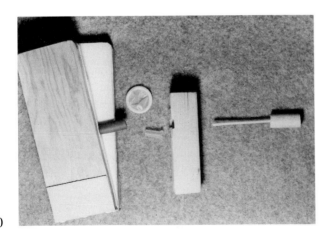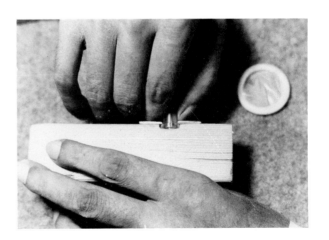

FIGURE 7-40

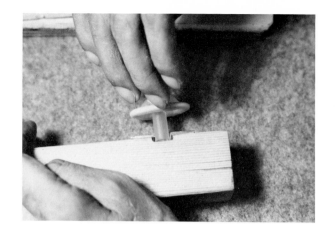
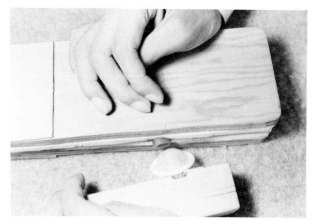
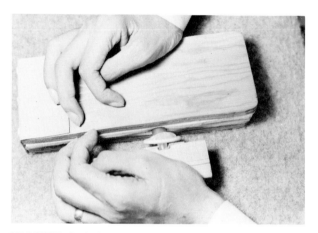
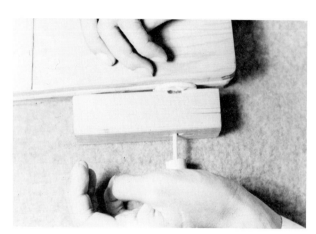

FIGURE 7-40 Continued

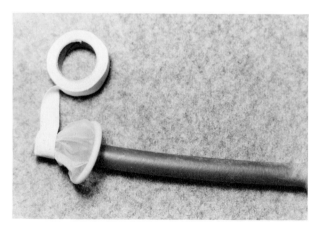
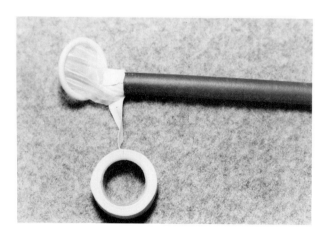

FIGURE 7-41

310

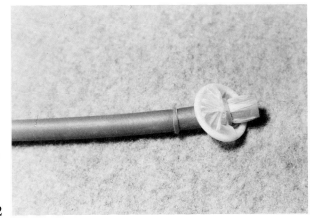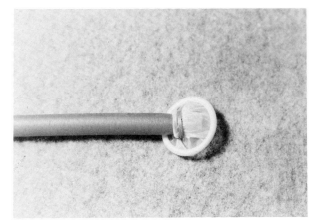

FIGURE 7-42

Method 7. (Fig. 7-41)   If a plastic plug is not available, the condom may be attached to the tubing with ¹/₂-inch (1.27 cm) adhesive tape. The condom is first pulled down over the tubing and taped. It is then pulled back over this tape and is taped again. This method requires considerable dexterity.

Method 8. (Fig. 7-42)   A condom may be attached by using two rubber bands cut off the tubing. One band is slipped about an inch (2.54 cm) down the tubing. The condom is pulled down over the tubing and the other ring is slipped over condom and tubing about ³/₄ of an inch (1.90 cm) down. The condom is now pulled back and the first ring is lifted over the second. This is the same principle as the tape method. It is unlikely that a quadriplegic patient will be able to manage this method himself.

Method 9. (Fig. 7-43)   A prepared commercially available external catheter may be used. This is very convenient, though more expensive.

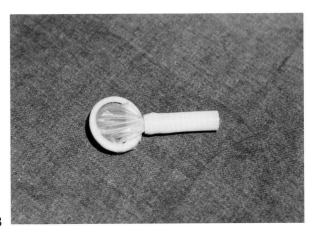

FIGURE 7-43

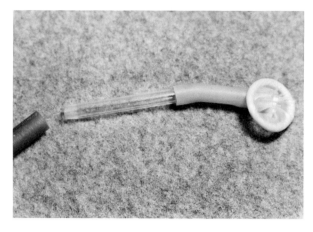

FIGURE 7-44

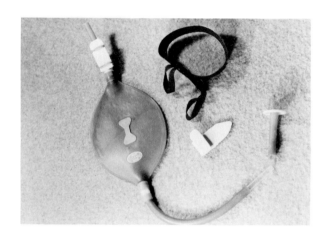

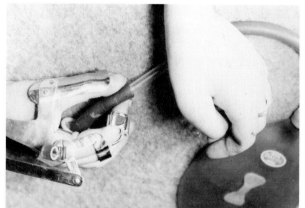

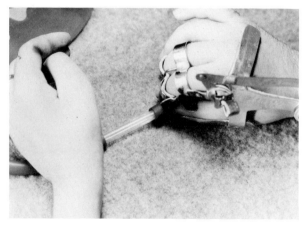

FIGURE 7-45

Securing Tubing and Urinal Bag

The urinal tubing extends approximately 6 inches (15.24 cm) to be slipped over a 3-inch (7.62 cm) plastic connector tube (Fig. 7-44). The connector is used to observe flow of urine and also to reconnect to the night drainage system if it is used. Once the system has been established, some patients prefer not to use a connector, as it creates additional assembly problems. The connectors are made of 3/8-inch (.96 cm) (outside diameter) and 1/4-inch (.64 cm) (inside diameter) acrylic plastic tubing. These are tapered at either end. Plastic connectors may also be purchased.

The urinal bag has a tube attached to the top and adjusted in length for the individual patient. The patient attaches this to the plastic connector (Fig. 7-45).

Urine Collecting Bags

A bag should be selected so that it has sufficient capacity to suit the individual's needs while remaining inconspicuous. If a very large bag is selected, it is hard to camouflage, and the weight of the bag when full may tend to pull on the collecting apparatus. Women who use an indwelling catheter often prefer to use a small collecting bag, and to wear it above the knee so that a skirt may be worn. Care must be taken that the flow is downwards.

Several methods may be used for attaching the urinal bag to the leg. For independent emptying, it is desirable to have a bag which can be lifted from the garter for easy emptying. The method must be varied according to the type of bag and the individual's needs.

Method 1. (Fig. 7-46)   The conventional rubber leg strap is removed, and a plastic clip is placed in the rubber slot of the bag.

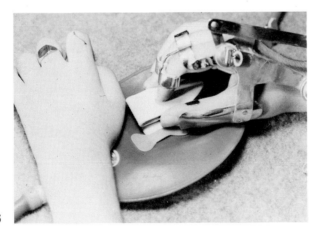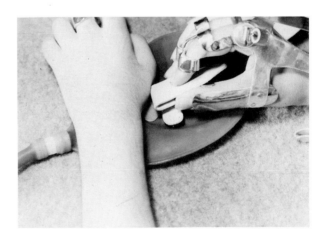

FIGURE 7-46

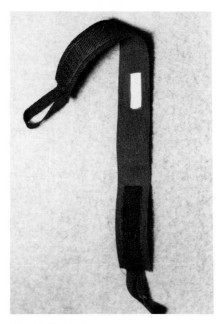
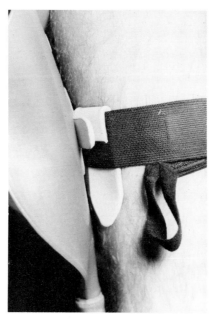

FIGURE 7-47 A   B

A strip of 1½-inch (3.81 cm) elastic with loops at either end and a velcro fastening forms a garter (Fig. 7-47A). This is wrapped around the lower leg just below the knee, and the plastic clip is slipped behind it (Fig. 7-47B). The clip is made of a thermoplastic material such as plexiglass. A jig will simplify manufacture of these. The clip is designed to fit into the slot on the urinal bag, and therefore must be made for a left or right leg so that the bag does not slip off the clip.

The same pattern of plastic clip may be bent to form a left or right clip (Fig. 7-48). The small projection is placed pointing to the left and bent back for a left clip, and facing right and bent back for a right clip, so that the bag does not fall off the clip when the patient's leg is extended.

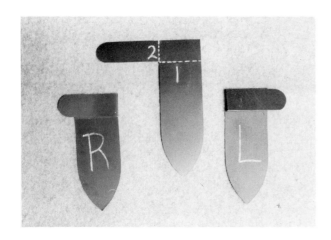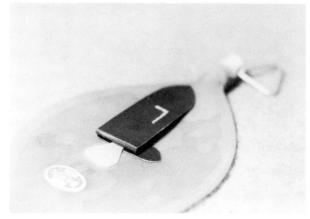

FIGURE 7-48

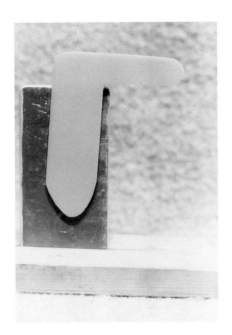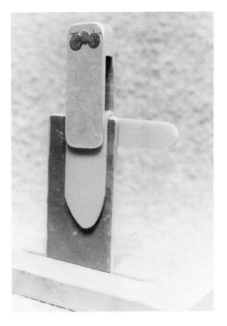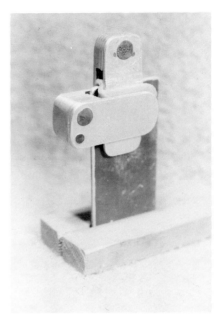

FIGURE 7-49

A three-piece jig may be made to be used to make the clips accurately and quickly. The heated material is held over the number one jig which is on a solid base. The number two jig is pressed down over the material forming the first bend. Number three jig is pushed over both jigs and the plastic projection to form the final bend (Fig. 7-49).

Usually a garter of the same style is used to position the tubing above the knee (Fig. 7-50). Sufficient tubing must be allowed so that the urinary apparatus will not be pulled when the patient changes leg position.

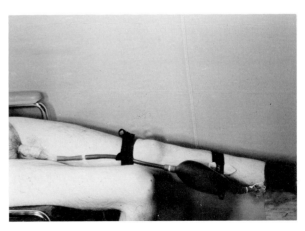

FIGURE 7-50

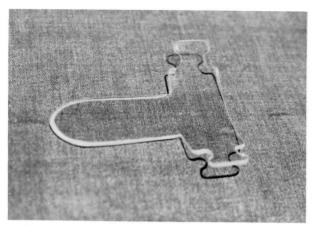

FIGURE 7-51 A

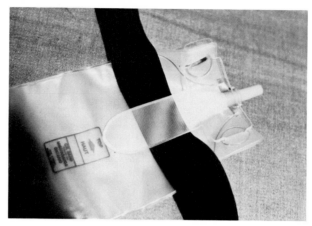

B

Method 2. (Fig. 7-51A)   A simple clip may be cut and curved to fit the leg, with projections to slip into the garter slots on a disposable bag. This clip may be slipped behind a garter to hold it in position.

Method 3. (Fig. 7-51B)   A variation of this clip can be made for the patient who cannot easily slip the clip into the garter. Velcro may be used on the cross bar and the garter front so that with the help of a holding loop, the patient can pull the bag free, and replace it by touching the velcro surfaces together. The leg bag cannot be allowed to become very heavy if velcro is used.

Clamps

Type 1.   A short length of urinal tubing is attached to the urinal bag outlet. A modified lever-type tubing cutoff is placed on this short tubing (Fig. 7-52).

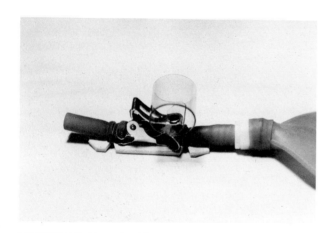

FIGURE 7-52.   A, Clamp closed

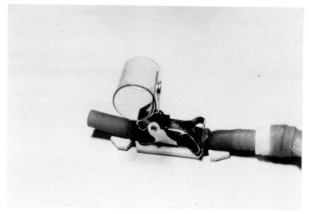

B, Clamp open

316

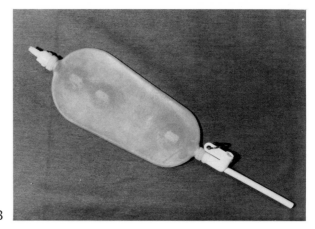

FIGURE 7-53

A stainless steel clamp can be obtained with a long lever arm; it may also have a thumb loop attached. A backing plate is frequently useful to stabilize the clip and increase the leverage for closing.

A ring is cut off the tubing and slipped over the end of the tubing to maintain the clamp in position.

Type 2. A Urocare type plastic clamp may be used, either on a Urocare bag, or adapted to a disposable bag. If a disposable bag is used, an extra short length of tubing is glued onto the external outlet as a packing to allow the urocare tubing to fit snugly. This clamp is favored by many quadriplegic people as it is neat and reliable (Fig. 7-53).

Type 3. A cutoff clamp can be made of solid stock, hinging the lever so that the tubing is shut off with a roller-cam action (Fig. 7-54). This clamp is extremely easy to manage and is reliable. It is not commercially available and must be custom made.

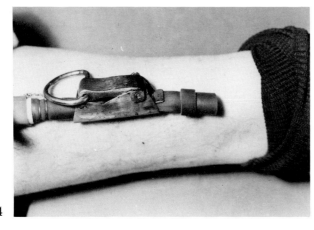 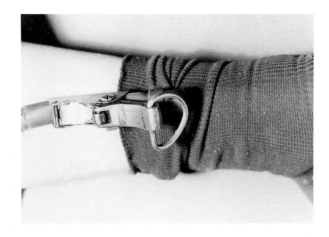

FIGURE 7-54

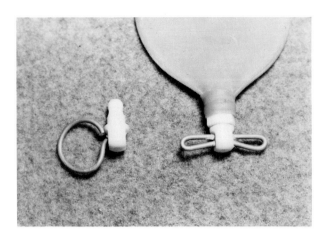

FIGURE 7-55

Type 4. Nonferrous wire is used to modify the cutoff plugs on the end of the urinal bag (Fig. 7-55). This is short and easy to camouflage and provides leverage to twist the plug.

A patient who requires a long tube to permit him to empty the collecting bag will require a way to camouflage it. A method that is easy to manage is shown in Figure 7-56. A velcro strap is fixed around the tube above the clamp so that when the end of the tube is folded up the small velcro strap holds it in place. The clamp is then tucked into the top of the sock if possible.

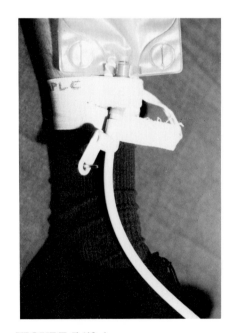
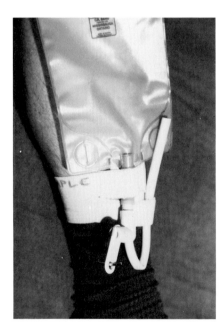

FIGURE 7-56 A   B

318

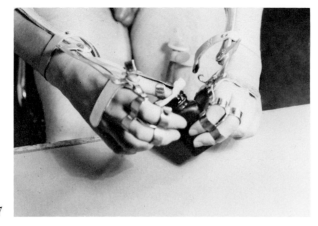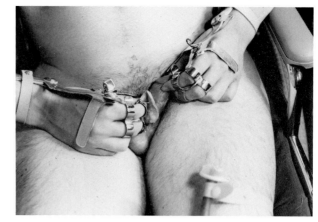

FIGURE 7-57

Application of Urine Collecting System

The patient assembles all his equipment and places it within easy reach. Some patients will prefer to sit up in bed so they can lean against pillows placed against the back of the bed. Other patients may find it more convenient to sit in the wheelchair with feet either on the footrests or on the bed. A patient may slide his buttocks forward on the wheelchair seat to improve his balance and free both arms.

The patient applies skin barrier to the shaft of the penis (Fig. 7-57). Skin barrier may be obtained as a wipe, a spray, or as a liquid in a can with its own brush attached to the lid.

Using Skin Cement. To prevent cement from spilling to unwanted areas a shield made of a square of vinyl with a hole to fit the shaft of the penis is useful (Fig. 7-58).

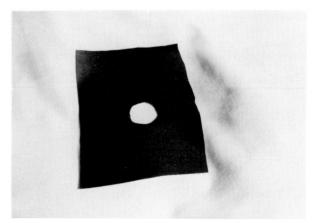

FIGURE 7-58

319

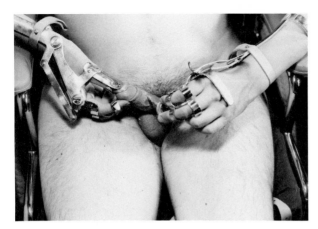

FIGURE 7-59

Finger tips or a swab may be used to apply the cement to the shaft of the penis (Fig. 7-59). Cement may be bought in a tin can with a brush fastened to the inside of the screw top lid. This is a very convenient utensil for brushing on the cement. If pubic hair interferes with cementing or application, the hair should be clipped.

When the cement is tacky the patient unrolls the condom for about half an inch (1.25 cm) to ensure that the plastic plug does not touch the head of the penis (Fig. 7-60A). He puts the condom over the head of the penis until the roll makes contact with the cement. Once the condom has made contact with the cement, it can be rolled on easily (Fig. 7-60B).

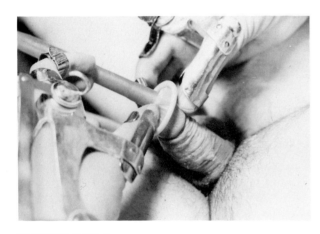

FIGURE 7-60 A

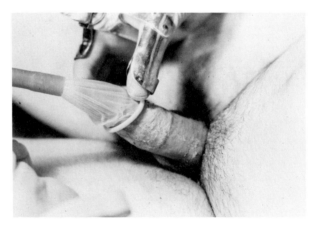

B

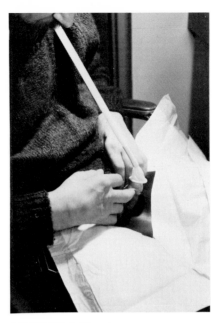

To enable a patient to use two hands to roll the condom onto the penis, a plastic stick may be held in the teeth, and the prepared condom may be held on the tapered end of the stick (Fig. 7-61). The length of the stick must be varied to suit the patient.

Using Double-Sided Adhesive Foam. The double-sided adhesive foam must be wrapped in a spiral around the shaft of the penis to prevent constriction. The condom will be rolled over the adhesive, and the collar snipped or removed (Fig. 7-62).

FIGURE 7-61

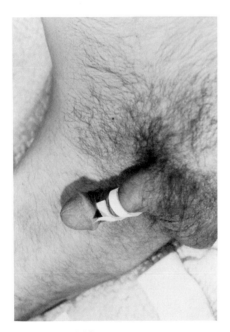
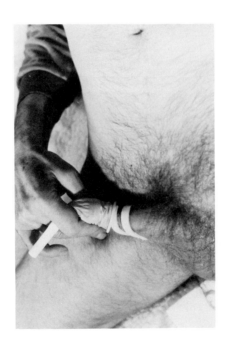
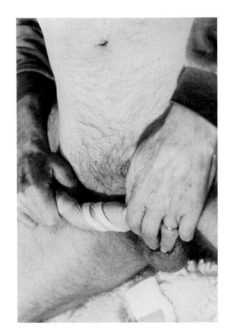

FIGURE 7-62

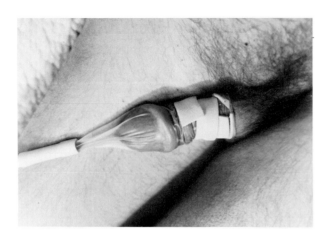

FIGURE 7-63

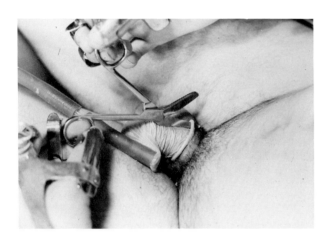
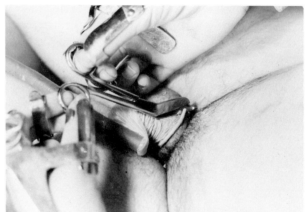

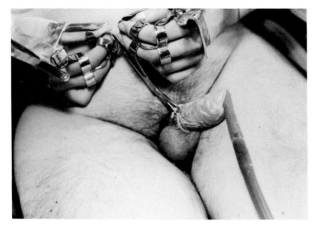

FIGURE 7-64

Using Single-Sided Adhesive Foam. (Fig. 7-63). The condom may be rolled onto the penis, and the one-sided adhesive foam may be spirally wrapped over it.

The patient pushes the blunt point of a pair of bandage scissors under the collar of the condom and cuts the collar by using the thumbs of both hands to close the scissors (Fig. 7-64). This prevents constriction of the penis. The scissors are pointed towards the patient's abdomen to ensure that he will not snip his skin. Some patients will remove the entire collar to eliminate any possible pressure area.

Draining the Urinal Bag

Even if the quadriplegic patient cannot attain complete independence in other areas of self-care, he may be able to empty his own urinal bag. Independence in this aspect of management is of great psychological benefit and enables him to remain alone for a greater length of time. These comments, and the methods of emptying apply to both men and women.

Method 1. (Fig. 7-65) The patient positions himself by the toilet and reaches down to unzip his pant leg or, if he does not use a zipper, he pulls the pant leg up, using the heels of his hands or a dressing stick. He lifts the bag by pulling

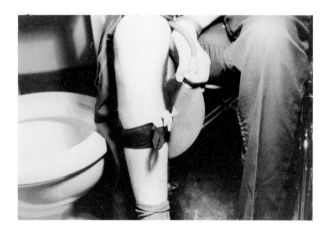
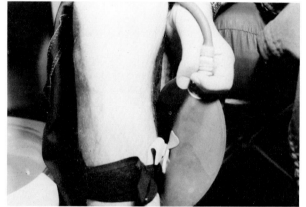
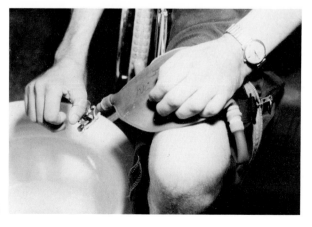

FIGURE 7-65

the clip out of the garter and rests the bag across his knee. He holds it down with one hand so that he can insert a thumb into the plastic loop and pull it open. He closes the clip by pressing down with the heel of his hand or with his thumb. The firm base on the clip prevents the tubing from tipping or buckling during closure.

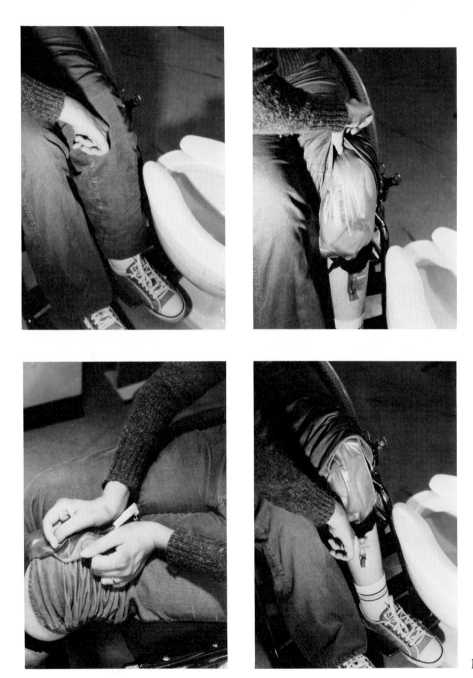

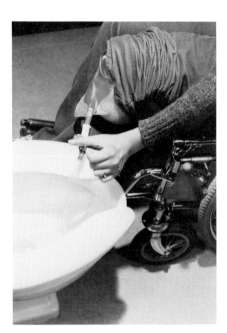

FIGURE 7-66

324

Method 2. (Fig. 7-66)   An alternative that is similar to Method 1 eliminates the need to use a clip to slip behind the garter on the lower leg. The top of the bag is fastened with a garter above the knee, and the garter on the lower leg has an extra velcro flap to fasten the lower end of the bag to the leg. Emptying requires only one hand or a dressing stick, but closing this clamp requires two hands unless a base plate is used. Generally, the urinal bag is worn on the side of the knee, usually on the inside, but occasionally on the outside if it makes emptying more convenient. Most people do not wear the bag directly over the knee, as in the illustration, because it shows more.

Method 3. (Fig. 7-67)   The patient lifts his leg onto the toilet seat and reaches down to unfasten the drainage clamp. He may unclip the bag from the garter if he must rest the bag on the edge of the toilet seat in order to open the clamp. This position is stable, and also prevents him from leaning so far forward that he may not be able to sit up again.

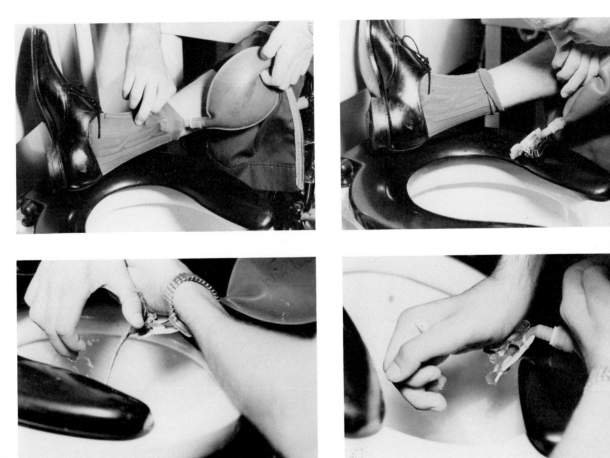

FIGURE 7-67

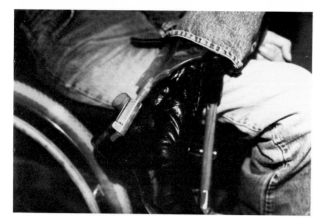

FIGURE 7-68 A

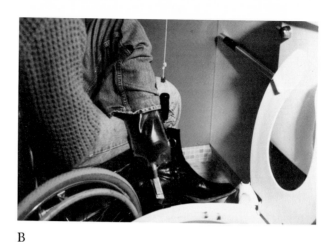

B

Method 4. (Fig. 7-68)   A patient who uses a post for transfers and positioning instead of an arm rest may find it useful also to hold his leg up within reach. This position is quite stable and enables the patient to use both hands freely.

Night Drainage

The patient places an absorbent pad under the connector when he is in bed. He disconnects the urinal bag tube and attaches the connector to a long tube that leads down to a receptacle such as a gallon plastic bleach bottle, which is left on the floor under the bed. A patient must be encouraged to change position every two hours even if he must use an alarm clock to rouse himself at first. He usually starts the night on one side, then turns to supine, and then to the other side. Each time he turns he must make certain that the urinal tube crosses his leg below the knee so that drainage is ensured (Fig. 7-69). If a turning bed is used the night drainage must be led to the foot of the bed.

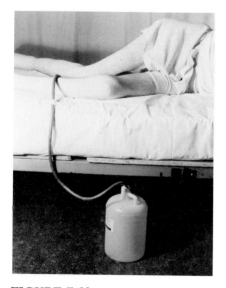

FIGURE 7-69

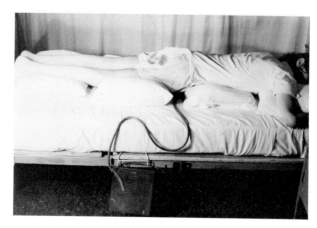

FIGURE 7-70

326

Sometimes a patient should lie prone because of pressure areas, or because a dependent patient requires turning less frequently in this position. When a male patient is prone, he may require elevation with pillows, leaving a space between genital area and bed (Fig. 7-70) so that he does not lie on his drainage tubing and so that involuntary erections will present no problem.

A patient's night connection may lead to a disposable plastic bag that hangs from a detachable hook on the bed (Fig. 7-71). Many people who travel take disposable bags with them, because they take up less room than a plastic bottle and can be discarded.

Removing and Disconnecting the Urine-Collection System

The clip of the urine-collection bag is slipped out of the lower garter and the garter above the knee is removed. The bag is placed on the bed or on a convenient surface below the level of the condom to ensure continued drainage. The condom is peeled off, using hand friction, and the whole assembly is dropped into a receptacle. Skin cement should be removed completely once a week, using a cement solvent or ether. Cement solvent will scald the skin if used too generously or if left on too long. The area should be thoroughly washed and powdered before reapplying the clean urine-drainage system.

All plastic connectors should be moved from side to side to work them out of the tubing. Pulling will merely clamp the tubing tighter. The assembly apparatus may also be used for taking apart. The tubing connected to the top or bottom of the urinal bag is removed only periodically for thorough cleaning. Only quadriplegic patients with good finger function will be able to perform this task.

Care of Urinal Apparatus

The urine-collecting apparatus should be completely disconnected and connectors checked for sediment. The interior of the bag and tubing must be rinsed well in cold water before soaking them in diluted antiseptic. The equipment can then be suspended to dry.

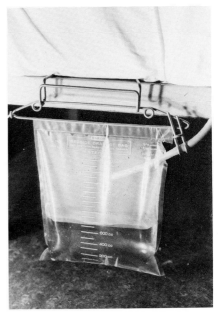

FIGURE 7-71

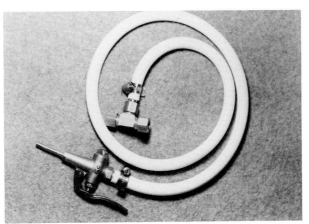

FIGURE 7-72

Two bags may be used, one every other day, to permit proper cleansing and disinfecting.

To facilitate rinsing, a flexible hose may be "T'd" into the cold water line of the toilet or sink with a nozzle with a long nose to insert into the urinal tubing at the end (Fig. 7-72). The lengthened nozzle will need to be specially made, but the lever-type release can be obtained commercially. This system is valuable, as the water pressure washes the urinal apparatus with little trouble to the patient. If this is not available, a syringe can be used instead.

MENSTRUAL MANAGEMENT

Management of the menstrual period will be a major problem for many quadriplegic women, especially those with a heavy flow, who need to change sanitary napkins or tampons frequently, or have limited time or access to bathroom facilities during work or recreation time.

Tampons

A woman who wishes to use a tampon must have fair grasp and wrist flexion in at least one hand. An open front, raised toilet seat enables the patient to reach to insert the tampon and to use two hands to eject the tampon, without losing balance (Fig. 7-73). Less effort is required to eject a tampon in a cardboard applicator, but strength of grip is required to pull on a cord which is not looped.

Some women can insert a tampon if they slide to the front of the wheelchair. Stretchy panties or a crotch flap will provide easy access (Fig. 7-74).

Some women who are learning bladder control may find that tampons create too much pressure on the bladder; they should use pads until the pattern is well established. The dependent patient and her helper may choose to manage by using tampons because it is easier to keep the perineum clean and it eliminates hazards of pressure from pads.

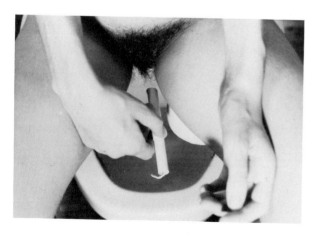

FIGURE 7-73

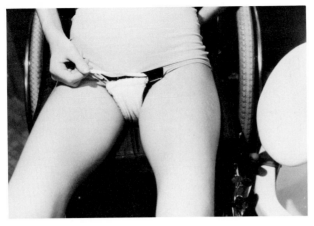

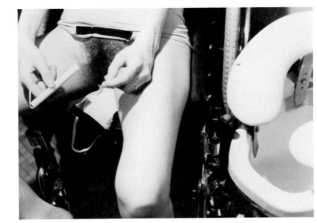

FIGURE 7-74 A   B

Sanitary Pads or Disposable Diapers

Sanitary pads can be obtained with a strip on the back which will cling to underpants and keep the pad in place. A pad may be placed in the crotch of the underpants before pulling them up. This will normally be accomplished in whatever position the patient uses for putting on her pants, and is generally done on the bed so that an incontinence pad can be used for cleanliness (Fig. 7-75).

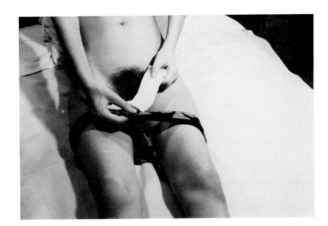

FIGURE 7-75

329

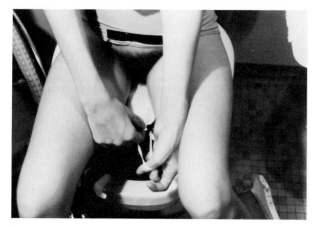 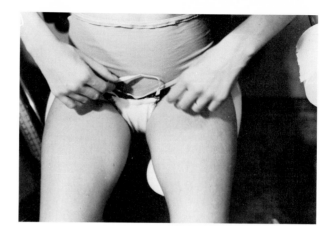

FIGURE 7-76 A   B

The front of the crotch of a pair of stretch underpants may be cut from leg opening to leg opening and a velcro closure and loop sewn in (Fig. 7-76). When the patient is seated on the toilet she can undo the crotch flap to replace her pad.

Even with a crotch flap, the pad cannot be placed far enough underneath by a woman seated in a wheelchair even if she slides to the front of the seat. Only a person who can lift up from the cushion can manage this.

Many women cannot tolerate sitting on a normal sanitary pad owing to a combination of the bulk of the material, dampness due to bypassing or frequency, and their particular skin tolerance and build. A combination of a disposable diaper and an incontinence pad is often used because it is less bulky and can be placed to cover a large area, distributing pressure and reducing risk of soiling.

Control Through Medical Means

The physician may prescribe birth control pills to be taken on a daily basis in an attempt to eliminate the menstrual period entirely. Menstrual periods may be such a problem to some women that they and their physician may consider surgery.

USEFUL REFERENCES AND AIDS

LLOYD, EE: Bowel stimulator for quadriplegic patients: A follow-up survey, Rehabilitation Nursing. Volume 8, May-June 1983.

MARTIN, N et al.: Comprehensive Rehabilitation Nursing. McGraw-Hill, 1981.

MCCARTHY, BP: Disabled Eve: Aids in Menstruation, Disabled Living Foundation, London, England, 1981.

Nursing Management in Neurogenic Bladders. Part I—45 colour slides with audio (normal and abnormal micturition), Part II–80 slides with audio (assessment, management and education, spinal cord). Purchase source: Educational and Training Center, Rehabilitation Institute of Chicago, 345 East Superior Street, Chicago, IL 60611.

Quadriplegic Functional Skills. Bowel and Bladder Techniques, 16 mm film, 14 minutes, 1974. Producer: McLean, Elmer, Rowee, Illinois. US Department of Health, Education and Welfare. National Medical Audio Visual Center, Station K, Atlanta, GA 30324. 1974.

Self-Catheterization, Using Clean Technique. Patient Instructional Package. Color slides, audio and guide book. Purchase source: Educational and Training Center, Rehabilitation Institute of Chicago, 345 East Superior Street, Chicago, IL 60611.

Strategies of Bowel and Bladder Management. Part I—67 color slides and audio, 15 minutes. Part II—29 color slides with audio and script, 10 minutes. Producer: Diane Talbot, Sister Kenny Abbot, North Western Hospital Inc. Publications Audio Visual Office, #314 -2727, Chicago Avenue, Minneapolis, MN. 55407. (Assessment, Planning, Methods of Management, Aids)

WILLIAMS, L, GARETZ, D: Independent leg bag emptying technique for cervical five quadriplegic clients. The American Journal of Occupational Therapy. Pages 40-42, Volume 35, No. 1. January 1981.

8

Holding and Manipulating

MAINTENANCE

Early in rehabilitation resting splints will probably be required to maintain web spaces, palmar arches, and functional finger and wrist positions for all patients (Fig. 8-1). Later, many activities help to maintain joint positioning; for

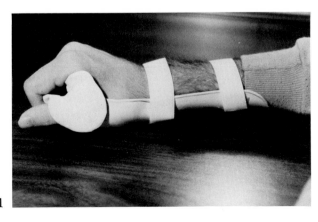 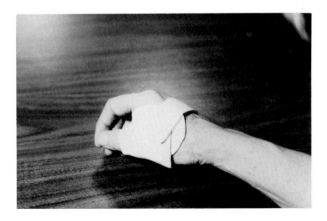

FIGURE 8-1

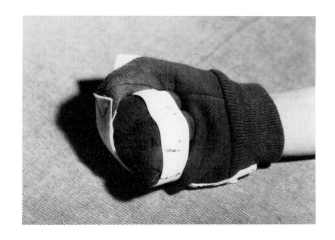

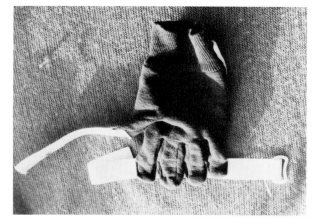

FIGURE 8-2

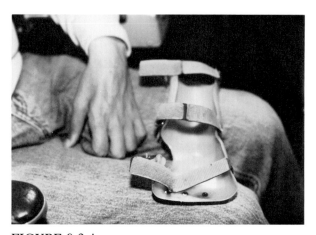

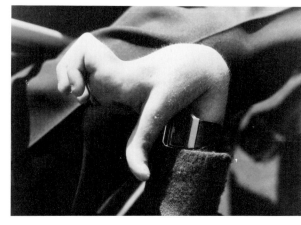

FIGURE 8-3 A

B

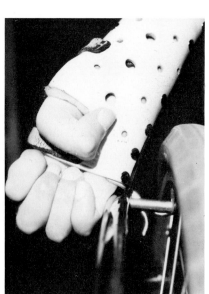

C

334

instance, pushing against the arm front uprights to move back in the wheelchair will help to maintain the thumb web space.

The person who is doing transfers, manual wheeling, and other activities of daily living must make sure that his fingers and thumbs do not become either over-stretched or too tight, but he is unlikely to have major problems with contractures. If he finds that his fingers are becoming too loose, a "boxing glove" may be used at night to try to allow the finger flexors to tighten. The thumb web space is maintained by letting the thumb rest over the fingers (Fig. 8-2).

When both hand and wrist lack power, the wrist may contract into flexion, especially if the wrist is allowed to hang over the edge of the wheelchair arm. The fingers will then be drawn into hyperextension at the metacarpophalangeal joints and flexion at the interphalangeal joints. The tendency can be seen in Figure 8-3A, and the result of such wrist contractures twenty years after injury can be seen in Figure 8-3B. Even if a functional wrist splint is used, care must be taken to prevent finger deformity (Fig. 8-3C). This is also an example of a deformity 35 years post injury, which could have been prevented by occasional stretching, and which now causes problems in washing and drying the fingers.

Good maintenance habits should be developed early. For instance, lying down with the elbows extended for at least part of the time will help to avoid elbow contractures if a person has no triceps. Placing a hand over a ball shape in a positioning trough on the wheelchair arm (Fig. 8-4) will help in a wrist lacking active extension.

Occasionally a person will develop a habit that enhances poor positioning, and this can occur so slowly that it is unnoticed. For instance, the person illustrated (Fig. 8-5) has sat for years with her cheek supported on her fist. The resulting hyperflexed metacarpophalangeal joints are not in fact a detriment to her function, but they illustrate the damage which may be caused by habit patterns. The patient should be made aware of good positioning to maintain appearance and function so that he or she can be responsible for this in the future.

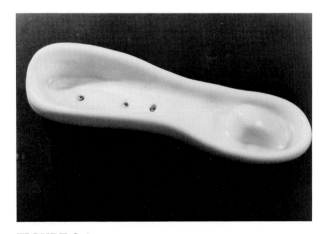

FIGURE 8-4

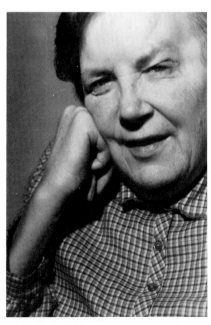

FIGURE 8-5

335

HAND FUNCTION

Before hand function can be examined, the patient must be comfortable and well balanced in the chair, and if he is to work at a table or counter top, the optimum height and depth of these must be established. Adjustable tables may be useful to estimate heights at first. Later a patient will usually be able to adapt himself to slightly different heights of surfaces.

Intrinsic Loss

The quadriplegic patient lacking only the intrinsic muscles of the hand should not need aids or splints. He will lack some dexterity and strength that could hinder him in some vocational and avocational pursuits, but should not interfere with his self-care.

Active Finger Extensors Only

A person who has active finger extension, but no finger flexion, often finds this movement useful, and will usually reject a flexor hinge splint, even though this might be expected to increase function.

Tenodesis—Lack of Finger Flexors and Extensors

A patient who lacks finger flexion may pick up, hold, and manipulate to a varying extent using tenodesis, the normal finger flexion caused by extension of the wrist (Fig. 8-6). (Tenodesis action can be demonstrated on a nonparalyzed, relaxed hand by moving the wrist through its range and noting how the fingers flex when the wrist is extended with the other hand.)

The finger flexors must have some tightness to make their grip functional. Care must be taken not to overstretch fingers for this reason, but range must be maintained in the thumb web space and the distal joint of the thumb.

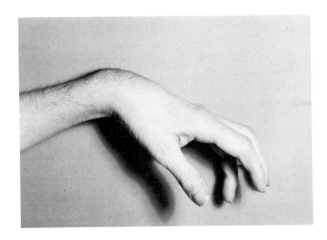 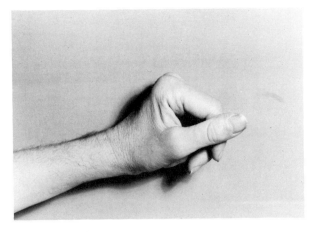

FIGURE 8-6

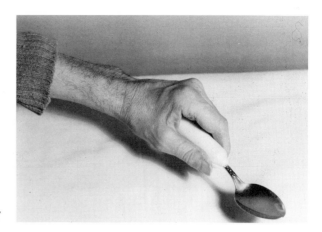

FIGURE 8-7

Weak Tenodesis

A patient may require padded handles (Fig. 8-7) to use his tenodesis effectively if his fingers are not sufficiently contracted or his grip is weak. Padding should be made of lightweight, nonslip material, and be either washable or removable. Plastizote, ground to shape, or rubbazote tubing are excellent padding materials. Another is foam-backed leather with velcro or press-stud fastenings to allow cutlery to be removed for washing. Stainless steel tubing may be brazed to cutlery to make a permanently built up handle which will last well.

"Weaving"

He may hold and use a thin-handled tool by weaving the handle into the fingers, that is, over the first, under the second, over the third, and under the fourth, or vice versa (Fig. 8-8). He may tighten the grip by using tenodesis, or finger extension.

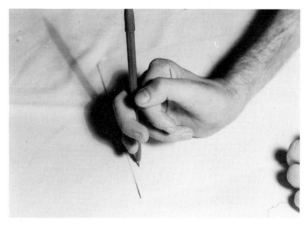

FIGURE 8-8

337

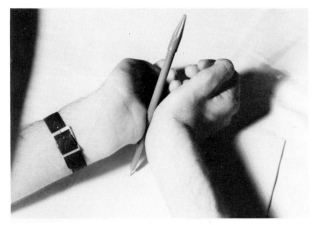

FIGURE 8-9

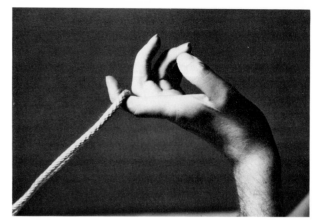

FIGURE 8-10

Two-Hand Hold

Many objects may be held between the heels of the hands. Legible writing is possible and may be useful if a small amount of writing, such as a signature, is required (Fig. 8-9). This method does, however, preclude using a telephone or holding the paper down simultaneously.

Use of Extreme Range

The patient may push or pull by placing his hand and arm into such a position that a digit can be put into its extreme of joint range, using ligaments rather than muscles (Fig. 8-10).

TYPES OF AIDS AND SPLINTS

Joint Positioning Splints for Function

Splints may be made to stabilize joints, such as the thumb joints, so that the thumb meets the finger tips when the wrist is extended (Fig. 8-11).

When the opponens splint is made, the palmar arch must be maintained, and the splint must not extend beyond the palmar crease, or the fingers will not be able to flex adequately at the metacarpophalangeal joints. These splints may be used for assessment for possible surgery, such as fusion of a joint. Patient, therapist, and surgeon can determine the practical value beforehand.

Palmar Pocket Strap

A patient may use a strap with a pocket in it to fit common tools such as a spoon, tooth brush, or pencil (Fig. 8-12A). This strap may be made with velcro and a D-ring, putting the pocket on the palmar side of the hand, with the narrower end of the pocket at the ulnar border. The strap is fastened around the hand

338

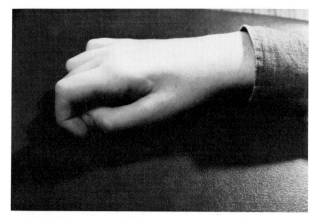

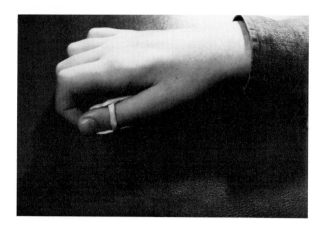

FIGURE 8-11A.   Plastic D.I.P. joint splint

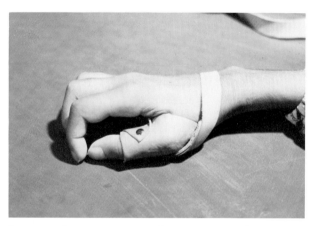

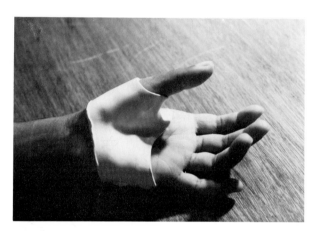

B.   Leather opponens and P.I.P. joint splint

C.   Plastic opponens splint

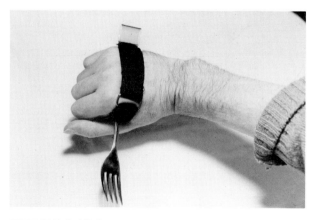

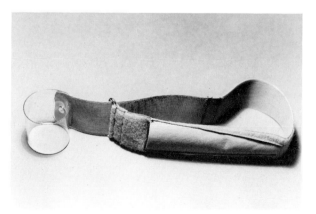

FIGURE 8-12 A

B

proximal to the metacarpophalangeal joints. This is both easy to put on and to secure.

The velcro D-ring pocket strap is made from approximately 8 inches (20.32 cm) of 1-inch (2.54 cm) wide pile velcro, with 4 inches (10 cm) of hook velcro sewn to the end facing the same direction. To form the pocket, a 3-inch (8 cm) length of pile velcro is sewn facing the pile velcro strap 1½ inches (4 cm) from the end of the pile velcro. The pocket is usually tapered, wide to grip tools at one end, and narrow to grip a pencil at the end where the hook velcro is sewn. Modifications may be made—a sewn base to the pocket or a 2-inch (5.08 cm) width of velcro sewn to the 1-inch (2.54 cm) strap to fit cooking utensils, etc. A square 1-inch (2.54 cm) D-ring is sewn to the free end of the pile velcro. The hook velcro is threaded through it, and an open loop of plastic is rapid-riveted to the back of the free end of the hook velcro (Fig. 8-12B). The plastic loop may be made of .040-gauge polished polyethylene chloride sheeting, 1 inch (2.54 cm) wide by 3 inches (7.62 cm) long.

U Handle

A U-shaped handle may be obtained with a swivel pocket which takes various utensils, such as spoons or writing clips (Fig. 8-13).

Loop Handle

Loop handles of plastic, leather and elastic, velcro and D-ring, metal, etc., may be permanently fixed to the tool. The loop should be placed proximal to the metacarpophalangeal joints, firmly enough to prevent the tool from sliding around the hand (Fig. 8-14). The rigid loop handle with an open end will be practical and easier to put on than a handle with a complete loop, particularly for those with very wasted hands, or those with large metacarpophalangeal joints. Velcro and D-ring fastenings are practical for the majority. Tools must be fixed to the loops so that they are in the optimum positions. This can be ascertained by temporary taping before the loop is permanently fixed.

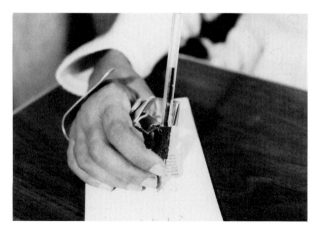

FIGURE 8-13

Wrist-Drive Flexor-Hinge Orthosis

A wrist-driven flexor-hinge orthosis may be useful to allow a firm grip. This is a plastic or metal splint that causes the first two fingers to meet the thumb when the wrist is extended (Fig. 8-15). The wrist extensors must be strong enough to take some resistance plus gravity. The patient must be capable of maintaining his hand in a pronated position while holding his wrist in extension. It is preferable to fit the dominant hand, even though it may be a little weaker.

An adjustable wrist position enables the patient to grip objects in the most comfortable position. For instance a glass requiring a wide grip can be held using the same wrist position as that used when holding a pencil, simply by changing the slot position on the wrist joint.

A spring pencil holder attached near the MCP joint of the splint provides a stable point for many tools, as well as a pen or pencil, and is a valuable addition (see Fig. 8-55).

The splint must be carefully fitted, both to prevent pressure areas, and to ensure that the thumb and fingers meet correctly. All joints must be aligned with the anatomic joints, or the splint will ride up and down on the arm, hand, or

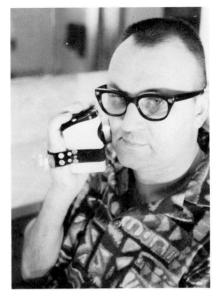

FIGURE 8-14

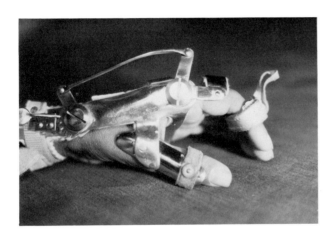
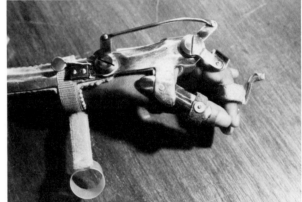

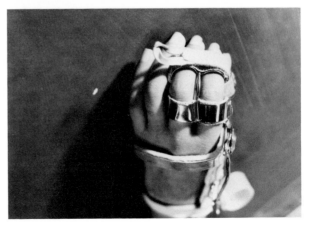

FIGURE 8-15

341

fingers. If the splint is correctly aligned, the fingers should remain in position under the finger rings as the splint is moved; if it is not correctly aligned, the rings may dig into the fingers as the splint operates, or the fingers may be twisted to one side.

Quite often, the wrist, as it is extended, will radially deviate because the wrist extensor muscles on the thumb side of the wrist are stronger than those on the little finger side. This radial deviation can make the wrist joint of the splint bind. If this occurs, the wrist strap can be left loose so that the wrist can move away from the splint. If the problem cannot be overcome simply, a polyaxial joint can be used, which will bind less (Fig. 8-16).

Leather thumb and finger straps on the gripping surfaces near the thumb and finger pads allow a better hold than if metal or hard plastic is used, which tend to skid on hard utensils.

It is most useful for a patient to have an opportunity to use a trial splint provided the fit is reasonable, before the custom built one is made. Very early fitting is not recommended because the hand changes shape considerably, early, and because the patient is not usually able to evaluate the potential use at an early stage. It is probable that the use of the splint enhances good alignment of the fingers and thumb, and also wrist strength which improves tenodesis. The appearance, time taken for putting on the splint, ability to wheel with it on, and concrete uses for it will influence splint use for a patient.

If, after practice, the splint takes more than about a minute for the patient to put on, it is unlikely to be used, unless it is to be used for a long period of time, or the person is very patient and determined.

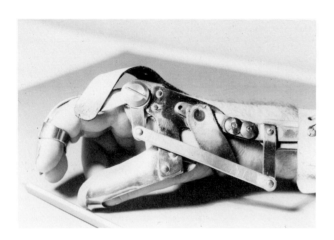 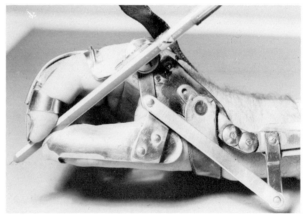

FIGURE 8-16

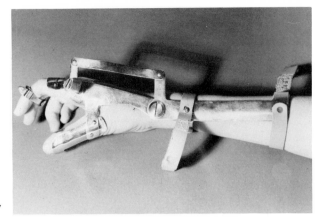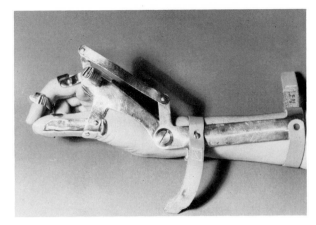

FIGURE 8-17

Generally, a patient will prefer a flexor-hinge splint if he has definite uses in mind for it, which he is unable to perform conveniently without. For example, some patients may find that they require a splint for applying a urine collecting apparatus, others may require them for work or leisure. Some activities performed with flexor-hinge splints include hobbies such as mosaic work, carpentry, and sewing. Work activities include writing, operating typewriters, telephones, and calculators. Everyday activities may include cooking, eating, and housework.

A person who finds a first splint useful for these activities may decide to have a second splint to enhance function.

Training a quadriplegic in the use of his splint includes counseling the patient in the advantages and disadvantages of the splint, in gradually working up wearing time, in checking for pressure points, and in practicing useful activities to increase strength, dexterity, and endurance.

External Power—CO_2 Muscle and Electrically-Driven Prehension Splint

When a patient cannot operate a splint with his own muscle power, external power may be selected. This power may be electrical or CO_2 muscle power (Fig. 8-17), and may be activated by mechanical pull of a valve or switch, by myoelectric-operated solenoid switches, or by contact-operated microswitches. The type of switch and the movement required to operate it must be selected so that the device can be operated in a near natural manner, unrestrictive to other functional movements. The device must not take an excessive amount of time to put on and must be acceptable and useful to the patient. Patients using external power will need to have the apparatus put on for them.

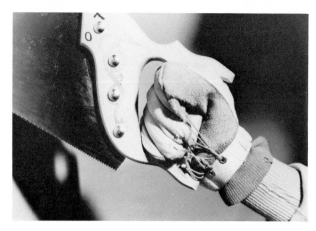

FIGURE 8-18

Glove Grip

A firm grip that will not release can be provided using a glove with the fingertips fastened to a strap. The fingers are then drawn down and the strap is fastened around the wrist (Fig. 8-18). If the strap is fastened with velcro it may be undone independently. This aid may be very useful for many sports activities, for gripping racquets, bats, and so forth. Nonslip type sports gloves and resins may be used to prevent slipping, and additional straps of webbing or elastic may enhance the grip.

Clamps

A patient may stabilize objects in clamps (Fig. 8-19) or vises (Fig. 8-20).

When a scissor-action tool such as a side cutter, pliers, or a leather punch is frequently used, a clamp may be permanently brazed under the lower lever arm so that it may be fastened to the working surface and one lever only operated (Fig. 8-21).

Rings

Small objects may be manipulated using forceps or pliers with an accuracy which may not be possible with the fingers (Fig. 8-22A). Forceps may be manipulated using two hands. They have the advantage that they can be locked and used for holding. Pliers can be adapted with two thumb rings, like the forceps, or they may be adapted for use with a wrist-driven flexor-hinge splint. A ring is brazed to the lower lever of the plier to fit around the thumb and elastic is fitted over the fingers and fastened to the top lever (Fig. 8-22B).

Wrist Support Splint

A commercially available wrist support splint with a swivel pocket is obtainable for the patient who has little or no wrist extension (Fig. 8-23).

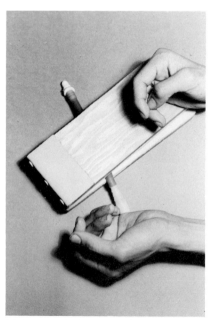

FIGURE 8-19. Leather-hinged wooden clamp, rubber lined for optimum grip

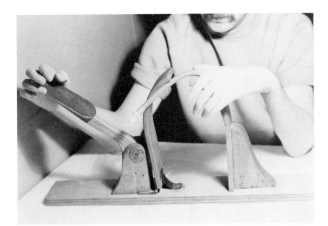 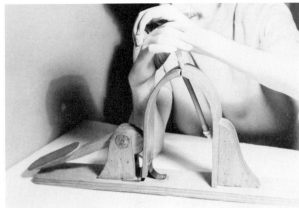

FIGURE 8-20.   Leather worker's vise leaves both hands free

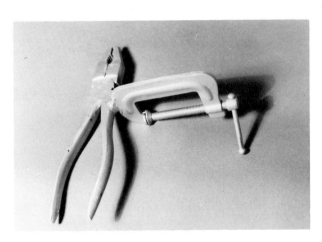 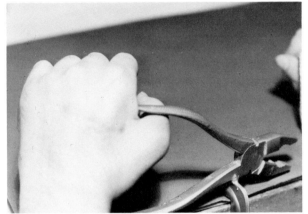

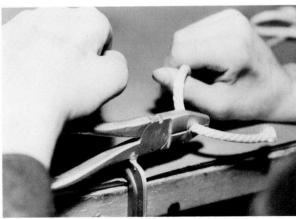

FIGURE 8-21

345

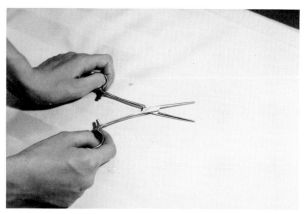

FIGURE 8-22 A

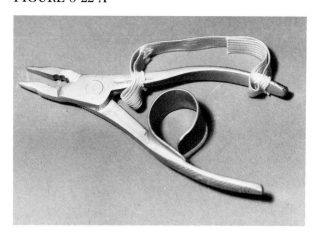

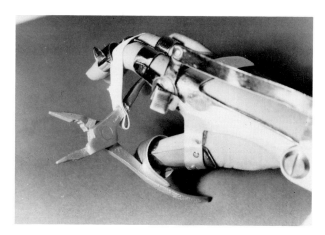

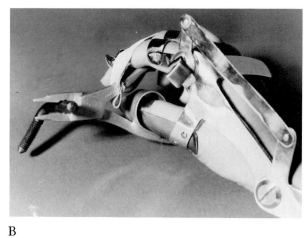

B

Molded Wrist Splint With Metal Pocket

   Fiberglass or plastic splints may be made which immobilize the flaccid wrist. These are fitted with metal sockets for holding the tools most commonly used by

346

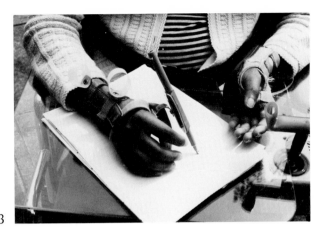

FIGURE 8-23

the patient, such as projections for propelling the wheelchair, typing sticks, or pens. This is used for patients with flail wrists, but with elbow flexion and shoulder control (Fig. 8-24).

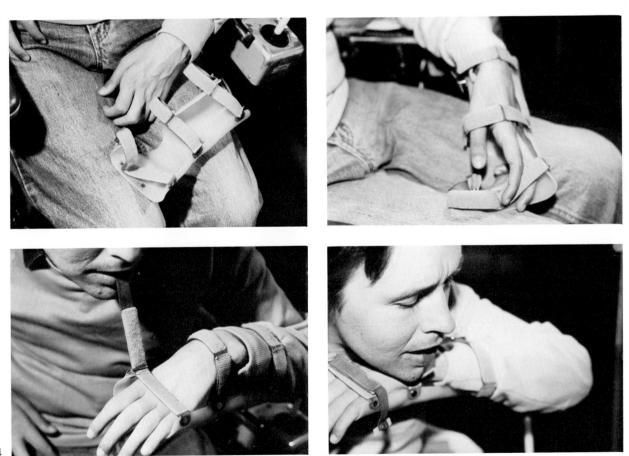

FIGURE 8-24

Many patients can put on their own splints, provided that the straps are fastened by velcro and D-ring or post and hole, and that the straps are left long enough for the patient to insert a hand. The strap should not be able to slip out of the D-ring; this may be done by blocking the end of the strap with a thumb loop. The splint may be fastened using the teeth or the other hand. The method used determines the direction of the strap fastening.

The tools used may be slipped into the socket by using teeth or hands or by fitting the splint onto pre-positioned tools.

This metal pocket has a leaf spring with a small ball on the tip which clicks into the hole in the utensil to hold it in place. A sharp pull on the utensil will allow the ball to slide out of the hole (Fig. 8-25).

Mobile Ball-Bearing Arm Support

The commercially available ball-bearing arm support may be useful for a patient with a high lesion but very little spasticity (Fig. 8-26). This arm support usually requires a supinator attachment. The support requires careful adjustment and training in its use (See "Adjusting a Mobile or Rocker Arm Support," Page

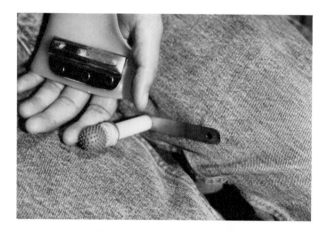

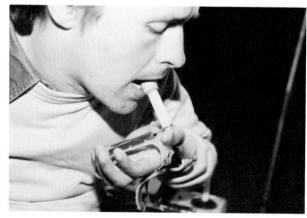

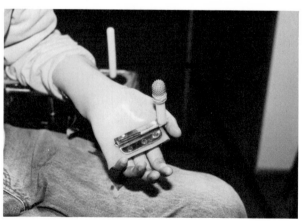

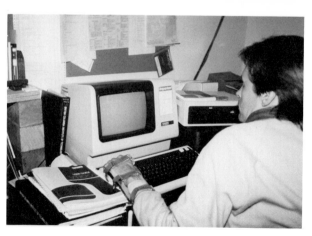

FIGURE 8-25

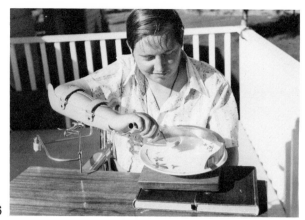

FIGURE 8-26

365). The arm trough may be replaced by molded plastic or fiberglass so that pressure areas are avoided and the arm is stabilized in the trough.

Rocker Arm Support

More commonly used is the rocker arm support suitable for quadriplegic patients who may have some degree of spasticity (Fig. 8-27). This may be clamped to the table or to the wheelchair arm. Usually a supinator attachment is necessary. The rocker arm support has a universal joint under the trough which may be more or less mechanically restricted in movement, depending on the degree of control of the patient. A rocker arm support may have a horizontal bar to permit some horizontal motion, the length again depending on the amount of control possible. This bar fits vertically into a tube on the clamp or wheelchair arm and then is bent at right angles.

An adjustable stop may be fitted to the vertical part of the bar. The height of the apparatus, length of the bar, and point of balance of the rocker require adjusting to the individual patient. (Details on adjustment procedures will be found

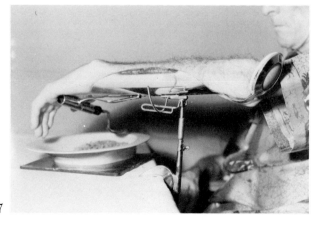

FIGURE 8-27

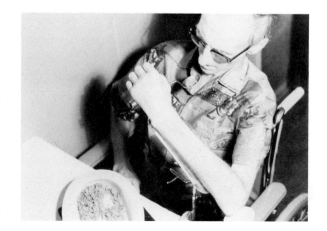

under "Adjusting a Mobile or Rocker Arm Support", Page 365). The metal trough may be replaced with a molded fiberglass or plastic trough.

Overhead Slings

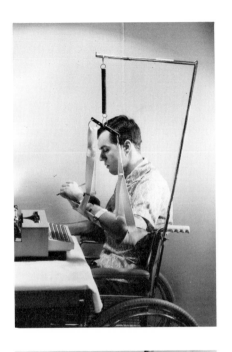

Overhead slings may be used as a means of training for later progression, or may be for permanent use. The sling support bar should be easily detachable from the wheelchair for transportation. The height of the bar can be varied to increase or decrease the pendulum action. The bar is raised for the patient with more control and vice versa. The suspension unit can be spring or webbing, again, the spring for the patient who can control it, but who can benefit from the feeling of liveliness and from the increased reach. The suspension can clip directly to an elbow sling and must be adjustable to the most useful height. This height is often decided by the spoon-to-mouth test.

Two slings may be used, one for the elbow and one for the forearm (Fig. 8-28). These have adjustable straps that clip to either end of a horizontal metal strip or rod above the two slings. This strip has holes drilled at approximately 2-inch (5 cm) intervals and the rod has a set-screw adjustment on a metal sleeve. The strap or spring from the overhead bar is clipped to one of the holes in the metal strip, thus creating a fulcrum and allowing the metal strip to pivot. The position of the fulcrum is adjusted so that the forearm can be held horizontally when relaxed. Further adjustments for optimum function can be made from this point. A patient who must use slings will usually require a splint to support his wrist. A slot may be incorporated to accept frequently used tools.

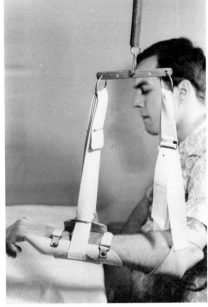
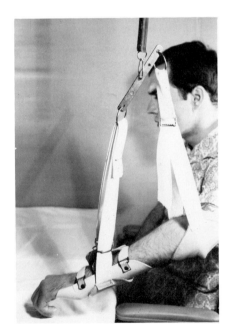

FIGURE 8-28

Mouthstick

A patient who lacks strength or control of shoulder and elbow movement may use a mouth or head controlled stick for page turning, painting, writing, typing, and so forth. He may use these aids for all activities, or only for those requiring fine control.

Mouthstick length is determined by the patient's eyesight, and by the power required. For instance, a person who is doing clay or soap carving using a mouthstick may require a short stick for better leverage (Fig. 8-29A), whereas someone typing or painting may wish to use a longer stick (Fig. 8-29B).

Most patients find that a fitted plate with a stick attached requires a great deal of head movement, and is not as useful as a stick which can be moved in the mouth; however, if a patient uses a mouthstick a great deal of the time, he may require a plate fitted over his teeth by a dentist in order to protect his teeth and maintain a good bite.

The portion of the mouthstick which is held by the teeth may be widened and

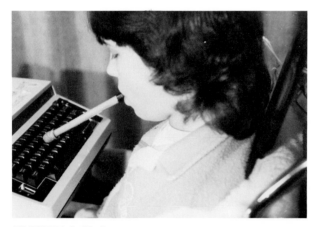
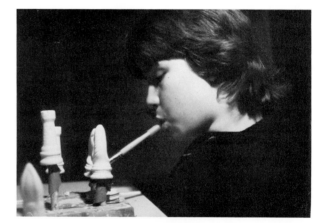

FIGURE 8-29 A

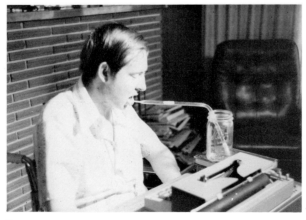
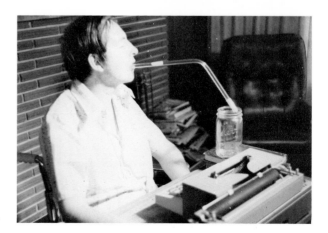

B

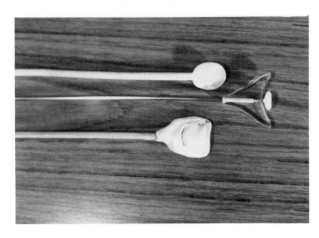

FIGURE 8-30

flattened for comfort and may be rubber covered (Fig. 8-30). A bamboo stick with a flattened end has been found to be useful by many people. This is made from a bamboo back scratcher with the "fingers" ground off. The bamboo stands up well to moisture, and has a pleasant taste and texture. Plastic mouthpieces may be molded for comfort and tooth protection. Toxicity may be a problem with some types of plastic. Dentists may be very helpful in advising about nontoxic plastics, as well as tooth protection.

The length and strength of the shaft of the mouthstick again depends upon the use. A long and thus more flexible stick may be used for card playing, or for page turning, where a less flexible stick may be required for typing or for operating elevator buttons. Generally a straight stick is easier to control; a bent one has a tendency to twist, but may be required for a comfortable head position compatible with eyesight. Only a limited number of light materials suitable for mouthsticks can be bent and still maintain strength. These materials may be aluminum tubing, or plastic rod or tubing. Commonly used materials for the shaft of the straight mouthstick are: bamboo, wood dowelling, plastic rod, plastic tubing, or aluminum tubing. The tip of the stick may be rubber or dycem covered, or may be made to slot into pre-positioned tools such as paint brush holders. If the mouthstick is long, particular care must be taken to keep the end of the stick light. Generally, pickup type sticks have not been found very useful, as the objects cannot be manipulated once lifted. For instance, it has been found easier for patients to use continuous-roll paper, rather than feed in individual sheets to a typewriter with a pickup stick. The patient should be able to rest a mouthstick in a holder so that it can be retrieved easily.

Pre-Positioned Apparatus

Apparatus may be mounted in a stable and convenient position and operated by head movement. Such apparatus may be an electric razor, toothbrush, comb, or electric switches (Fig. 8-31).

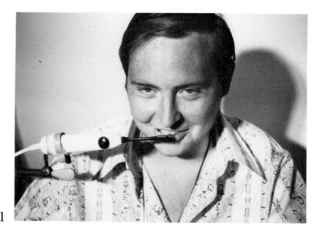

FIGURE 8-31

Environmental Controls

Patients may require controls to switch electrical equipment on and off, or to control a rheostat, required for graduated switches such as a dimmer switch.

These controls range from extremely simple to very sophisticated, depending on need and availability. For instance, one patient may require only a call bell, which can be constructed easily from components bought from a hardware store: batteries, pressure switch, electric cord, and bell. Another person may need to control such items as a television, radio, air conditioner, door lock, dictaphone, telephone, computer terminal, or recreational equipment, and may require these controls both when he is resting in bed and when he is operating from a wheelchair (Fig. 8-32).

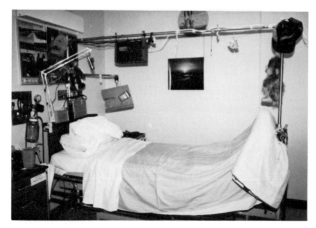 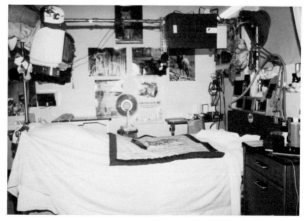

FIGURE 8-32.   Beds set up with environmental controls for television and radio. The control is more visible on the bed on the left (A), and the apparatus controlled is more visible on the right (B).

Assessment

When assessing the needs for environmental controls there are five major questions to be considered:

1. Do the patient and his assistants wish to use environmental controls? Some people prefer the human contact; others wish to control their environment and enjoy a different quality of human contact.
2. What equipment will the patient wish to control?
3. Is the equipment controlled by on/off switches, or is a rheostat control required also?
4. Is the equipment to be controlled from one area or several, that is, bed, school, desk?
5. What switch (interface) can the patient operate in the different positions required?

Examples of interfaces are: pressure, breath, myoelectric, moisture activated, voice, and eye controlled switches (Fig. 8-33).

Many "environmental controls" are already used by the general public, for example, remote television controls, garage door openers operated by radio, and so forth. If these controls can be utilized by disabled people also, it is usually cheaper, and equipment is easier to replace or repair than special or custom built equipment for the disabled. As robots and remote controlled arms become more commonplace and reliable, these will be a great boon to the disabled.

Animal Assistance

Animals may be trained to do certain chores. Monkeys are very dexterous and can be taught to substitute for some lost hand function. Dogs may also be trained to be useful. The dog illustrated will pick up objects such as letters and pass them to his mistress. He is also very good at vacuuming any food spills (Fig. 8-34).

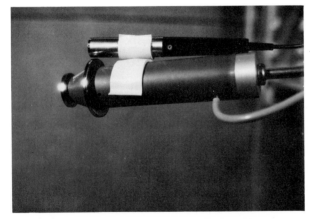
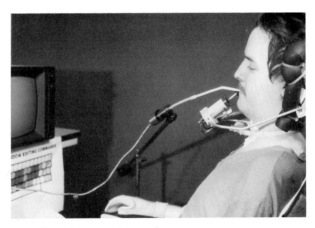

FIGURE 8-33.   A. A touch control interface   B. A breath control interface

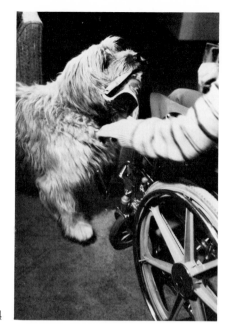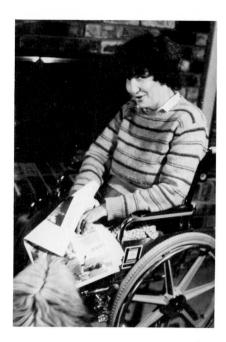

FIGURE 8-34

HOLDING METHODS APPLIED TO SPECIFIC TOOLS

Toilette

Tooth Care

Toothpaste. Toothpaste should be stored within reach, with the cap screwed down just enough to hold. It may be picked up by tenodesis, or between the heels of both hands. The cap may be removed by using the teeth and tongue, and the amount of toothpaste desired sucked from the tube or squeezed onto the teeth. The cap may be replaced with a minimal twist by both head and hands. The toothpaste can be squeezed onto the toothbrush bristles by using the heels of the

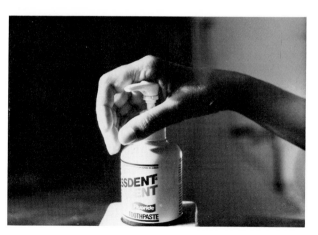

FIGURE 8-35

355

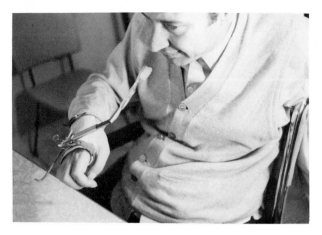

FIGURE 8-36

hands, by using a flexor-hinge splint to squeeze the paste out, or by using the teeth while holding the bottom of the tube in the mouth. A press-cap-type toothpaste may be used (Fig. 8-35).

Toothbrush. The toothbrush may be picked up by using tenodesis, the flexor hinge splint, or a pocket splint (Fig. 8-36). An electric toothbrush is managed in the same manner. It should be possible to swivel the toothbrush so that the inside and outside of the teeth can be cleaned. The toothbrush should point towards the back of the mouth so that a turn of the head will allow the teeth on both sides of the mouth to be cleaned. The toothbrush handle may be bent, or the holder angled, to allow all the teeth to be reached.

With an ordinary toothbrush, a combination of hand and head movement is used for brushing. If up-and-down brushing is difficult, side-to-side brushing is substituted. To save swiveling the toothbrush twice, the outside of one side and the inside of another is cleaned, then the toothbrush is swiveled using the tongue and teeth. Teeth may be further cleaned by eating raw carrot, or similar food, if toothbrushing is inadequate. Frequent visits to the dentist will help to preserve the teeth, the equivalent of the quadriplegic patient's third hand.

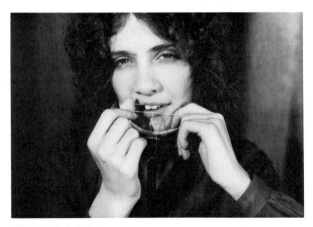

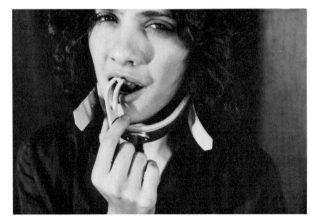

FIGURE 8-37 A   B

Dental Floss. Suitable lengths of loops of dental floss may be knotted by an assistant and stored for later use. These loops are easier to handle than lengths of floss. The floss may be wrapped around the thumb to prevent slipping (Fig. 8-37A).

A floss holder may be used. This can be held by tenodesis, or it can be held in a suitable splint (Fig. 8-37B).

Dentures. Dentures can be ejected with the tongue into the cupped hands or into a container of denture cleaner. The dentures may be cleaned by using a nail brush fastened to the sink with suction cups. They may be held by tenodesis or between the heels of the hand to replace them in the mouth. Arms may be stabilized by resting the elbows on a solid surface.

Care of the Hair. Short hair is easiest to manage for both men and women. Pins, rollers, and similar items, are very difficult to manage, and visits to a hairdresser or help at home must be available for longer or more complicated hair styles. Because the patient may have a problem with excessive sweating, hair may have to be shampooed frequently.

Brush. A military-style brush, or a shampoo brush, may be adapted by fastening a length of elastic to either side of the brush with screws and washers. The elastic must fit snugly over the hand. D-ring and velcro can be substituted for elastic. A brush with a handle may have an elastic loop, a D-ring and velcro, a metal or plastic "U" handle, or a padded handle (Fig. 8-38). For mechanical advantage, the hand should be placed close to, or over the back of the brush, rather than on the handle where the leverage will work against the patient. If the patient is unable to reach parts of his head, he could rest an elbow on a table or dresser and flex his neck and upper trunk until his hand reaches his head; this is a method of obtaining increased shoulder flexion. A flexor-hinge splint may be used to hold the handle of a hairbrush.

Comb. A rat-tailed comb may be held in a wrist-drive flexor-hinge splint, in a pocket splint, a rigid splint, a wall-mounted bracket, or by using a padded handle (Fig. 8-39). The rat-tailed comb may be twisted, bent, or lengthened to allow all parts of the head to be reached.

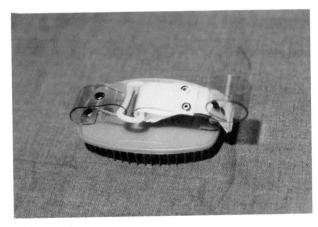

FIGURE 8-38

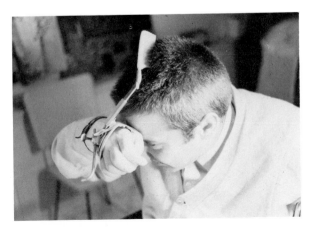

FIGURE 8-39

Electric Razor. A strong tenodesis can be used to hold an electric razor, vibration will cause the razor to slide out of a weak grip. A flexor-hinge splint may be used to hold most makes of razor, weight being the limiting factor. During training a long elastic may be taped to the razor and hung around the neck as a safety measure. A plastic handle may be bent to fit the hand and fastened to the razor with strong glue. The handle must be positioned so that the beard can be completely shaved, including the difficult areas under the corners of the jaw.

Velcro and D-ring, as in a pocket splint, may be taped to the razor to establish the correct angle before permanently riveting the velcro D-ring to a detachable leather razor jacket (Fig. 8-40).

The razor may be attached to a bar which may be slipped into a slot in a rigid cock-up splint (Fig. 8-41). The angle of the razor should be adjusted so that all the face can be shaved. The razor may be fixed to a swing away bar projecting from the wall (Fig. 8-42). The patient can move his wheelchair around so that he can reach both sides of his face. The plug on an electric cord may be enlarged for easier handling by jamming an empty spool (such as an adhesive tape spool) per-

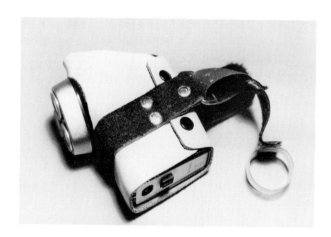

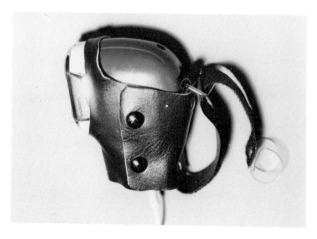

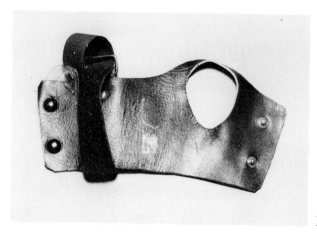

FIGURE 8-40

358

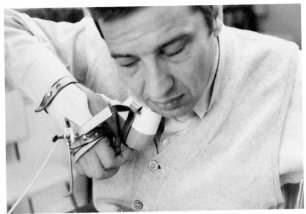

FIGURE 8-41

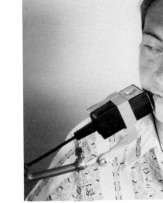

FIGURE 8-42

manently over the plug. A metal spool should be insulated for safety. It may be eaiser to adapt the plug than to adapt the razor switch which is often small or inset. The use of cordless razors may be an advantage, but weight, shape, and cost must be taken into consideration. A switch may be wired into the cord, and the razor left permanently plugged in.

Safety Razor. Occasionally a safety razor is preferred to an electric razor. The razor may be held in a flexor-hinge splint, or by padding the handles. Since there are so many makes of safety razor with as many different methods of inserting and extracting blades, this problem must be worked out individually.

Contact Lenses. The quadriplegic patient's ability to place contact lenses depends partly upon the previous ease of insertion and the method used before the onset of disability, as well as on the present hand function of the individual. This patient can remove his lenses by pulling on the skin at the side of his eye so that when he blinks the contact lens drops onto a clean towel (Fig. 8-43). This individual with his excellent tenodesis pinch is also able to wash and care for his lenses.

To replace the lens, he picks it up from the towel using a finger dampened

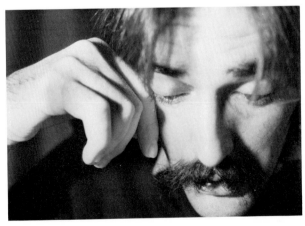

FIGURE 8-43

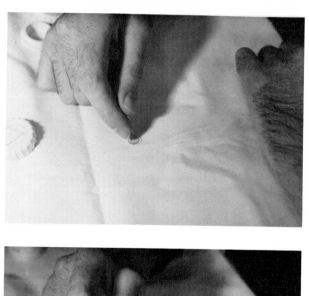

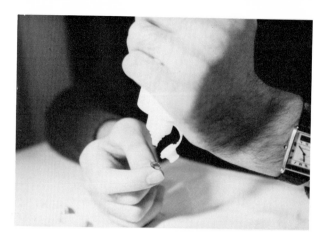

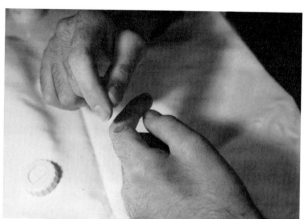

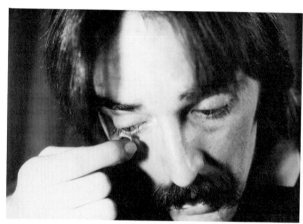

FIGURE 8-44

with saline solution. He then puts more saline onto the lens from a bottle which drips slowly when held inverted. He places the lens on the knuckle of his other hand so that he can adjust the position of his lens on the forefinger exactly for easy insertion (Fig. 8-44).

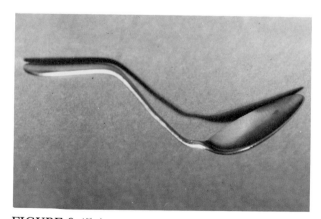

FIGURE 8-45 A

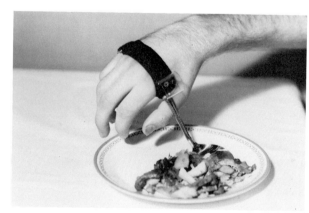

B

360

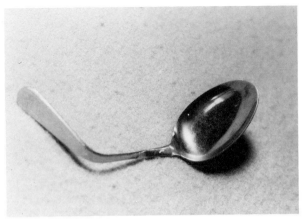

FIGURE 8-46

MEAL MANAGEMENT

Plates. Plates may be fitted with plate guards, or a Mannoy plate may be used if the patient has difficulty pushing the food onto a fork or spoon. A nonslip pad will stabilize the plate. Soup bowls may be more functional than dinner plates for some patients because their rounded shape fits the spoon bowl and permits more food to be picked up.

Spoons and Forks. Some patients manage an unadapted spoon but many spoons must have two bends of about 120°, giving a step effect. One bend should be by the bowl and the other about 2 inches (5 cm) up the handle, thus the rest of the handle and the bowl will be approximately parallel (Fig. 8-45A). The spoon can now be used in a deep bowl and the fingers will be kept out of the way (Fig. 8-45B).

A spoon may require not only a double bend, but also a twist so that the spoon tip will point towards the mouth. Patients with inadequate range may require a lengthened handle (Fig. 8-46).

A length of stainless steel or plastic may be fixed to a spoon and then bent back to form a loop which is fitted proximal to the metacarpophalangeal joints

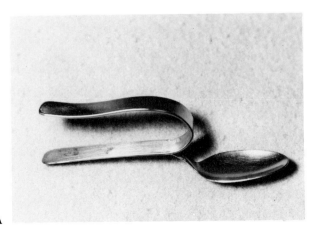

FIGURE 8-47 A

361

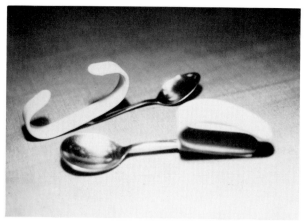

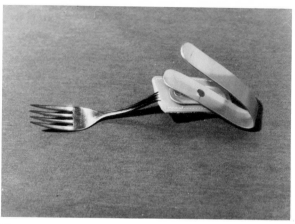

FIGURE 8-47 B   C

(Fig. 8-47A). This spoon handle is easy to apply. Commercially available cutlery adaptations may be obtained and fitted (Fig. 8-47 B & C).

Spoons or forks may be held by threading the handle through the fingers, or by the use of a pocket splint, a padded handle, or a flexor-hinge splint. A double finger ring may be used to stabilize fingers, so that a handle can be held between them. A rigid cock-up splint may have a slot on the palm to receive the modified handle. This spoon may be a swivel-handled spoon or fork with stops and two bends in order to keep the bowl or tines level (Fig. 8-48 and 8-49).

Knives. Cutting can be a difficult and lengthy procedure for some quadriplegic patients. In these cases it is preferable to have meat cut beforehand so that the patient can eat a hot meal. The patient may hold a sharp knife between the heels of both hands and use direct pressure, rather than a sawing action. Greater pressure and some rocking action can be achieved by using the knife tip, although the area cut is less.

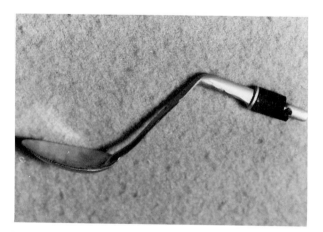

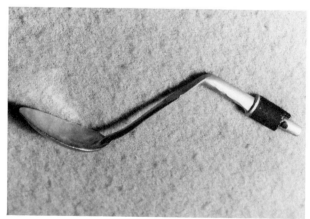

FIGURE 8-48.   Swivel spoon with stops. Black sleeve fits into a metal tube on the splint which protrudes from under the palm of the hand.

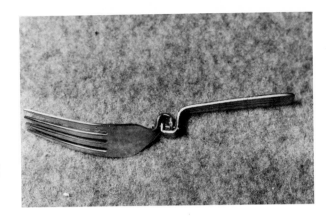

FIGURE 8-49.   Simply constructed swivel fork made by cutting and bending the fork handle, drilling a hole through the bent ends, and inserting a cotter pin as an axle.

Commercially obtainable knives may be fitted to the patient's hand (Fig. 8-50A). A rigid metal or plastic handle may be attached to the knife near the blade and bent back over the dorsum of the hand (Fig. 8-50B). The other end is not

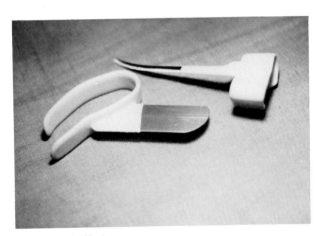

FIGURE 8-50 A

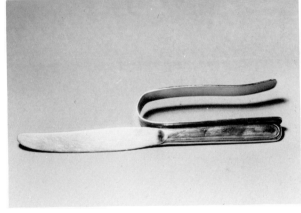

B

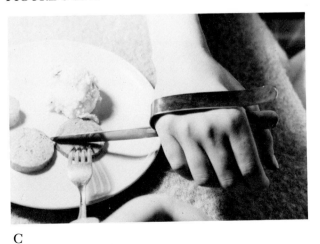

C

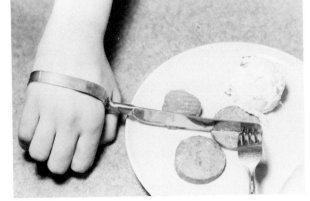

D

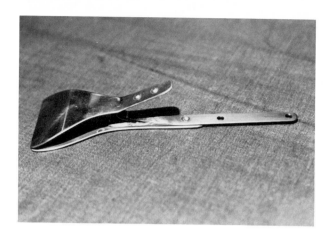
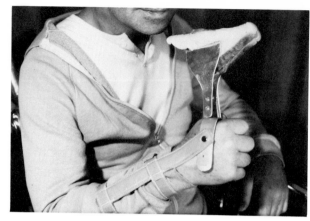

FIGURE 8-51

attached to the knife handle, but left open for easy insertion of the hand. The knife blade may require some bending for better function. The knife must be firmly held to enable the patient to apply adequate pressure. The knife may be held conventionally so that the blade points toward midline (Fig. 8-50C) or, if more pressure is required, the knife may be reversed so that supinators which are generally stronger may be used effectively (Fig. 8-50D).

Sandwich Holders. These will be required only for those who cannot manage a tenodesis grip. The sandwich holder may be held in a pocket splint, a rigid wrist splint, or in a stand within reach. The sandwich is moved in the spring holder by pulling the sandwich out a little before biting off a piece, leaving the sandwich in position for the next bite (Fig. 8-51).

This handle requires a twist so that the sandwich is held straight at mouth level (Fig. 8-52). Other patients may lift the elbow more easily and will not require the twist.

Glasses and Cups. Many quadriplegic patients have finger flexors adequately contracted to use tenodesis for holding a cold glass. The glass is pushed into the

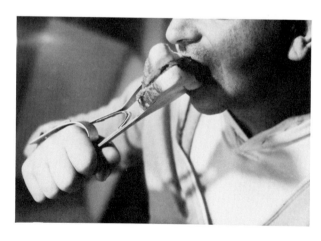

FIGURE 8-52

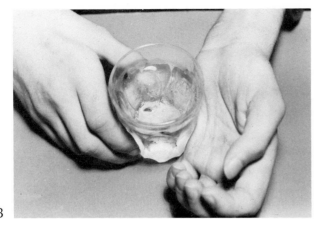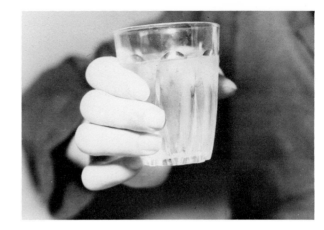

FIGURE 8-53

hand with the other hand (Fig. 8-53). A wrist-driven flexor-hinge hand splint may be used to pick up a small glass, provided the drive bar is above the hand. A plastic straw may be used for hot or cold liquids. Some people require a long straw or a raised cup stand.

Mugs and some cups may be managed by pushing the thumb into the handle, so that with the wrist extended, the lower part of the mug rests against the dorsum of the flexed fingers. Care must be taken that hot cups do not cause burns on anesthetic fingers. The heels of both hands may be pressed against the opposite sides of the glass and the glass raised to the mouth. Resting the elbows on the table while raising the glass adds to stability.

Quadriplegic patients have been known to pick up a glass in their teeth and drink, but this method is not recommended because of the possibility of breaking teeth or glass.

Adjusting a Mobile Arm Support or Rocker Arm Support

The patient is seated in his normal position in the wheelchair. The trough, elbow, and hand piece are adjusted for length and comfort and a tentative point of balance is found (Fig. 8-54A). The final point of balance is dependent on the height and position of the trough. The height of the support is adjusted so that when the elbow is down it clears the table or chair arm. The hand should be about level with the nose (Fig. 8-54B).

The double angles of the spoon should be as shallow as possible so that the hand does not have to be raised high, but should be long enough so that the lever arm is sufficient to maintain the spoon bowl in a horizontal plane (Fig. 8-54C). Much depends on the efficiency of the swivel, which must not bind. Once the length of the drop in the spoon is established, the spoon-to-mouth test will be used to establish final positioning (See Fig. 8-54B). If either the up or down movements should be difficult, the balance may be adjusted to compensate.

The rocker support may have two points permanently marked on the vertical adjustment: one for eating, which often requires considerably more height than other activities, such as typing.

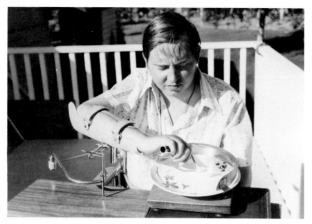

FIGURE 8-54 A

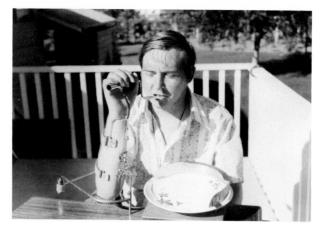

B

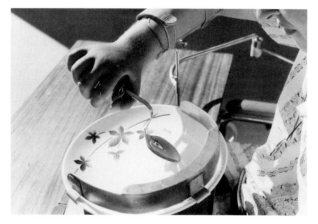

C

The table or plate height is adjusted so that the spoon reaches the plate. Sometimes the plate must be raised on a block so that the elbow can clear the table. The plate may require a plate guard, or a Mannoy plate made by Melaware may be used. A nonslip pad may be required to stabilize the plate. A turntable may also be required to compensate for limited movement if the patient is unable to reach parts of the plate. Finally, the stop on the swivel spoon is fixed so that the spoon remains stable while picking up food, but is able to swivel freely as the spoon travels towards the mouth.

Water, or dried peas or beans may be spooned when working out mechanics so that the levels can be easily seen and little mess made. During eating training a patient should be given privacy until he becomes proficient. The type of food chosen for training is important. Foods that tend to stick to the spoon, such as purees or stews, are preferable to dry food or thin soups.

WRITING

The table surface must be at a comfortable height and the wheelchair must be wheeled well under it so that the elbows can rest on the table. Paper may be stabilized on a nonslip mat, or by using magnets or weights, and the paper angle may have to be changed for the new writing pattern.

Tenodesis may be adequate to hold a pen in the normal manner. The top of the pencil rests in the thumb web, and the tip under the pads of any of the first three fingers. The elbow is usually raised to compensate for the extended wrist, and the hand is not completely pronated.

The pencil may be held by threading it through the fingers: over the first, under the second, over the third, or vice-versa. This is not usually a very firm hold, but may be useful for writing a small amount, for instance a signature. This is a particularly useful grip for those with active finger extension but no flexion. A pen may be held between the heels of both hands pressed together. This precludes the use of a telephone or holding down a paper at the same time. In addition, it is hard to see around the hands to watch the pen tip; therefore, the pen tip must usually be tipped towards the writer. This method is useful mainly for writing a signature when equipment is not at hand.

If writing is shaky, the patient should try to write faster, to speed and control writing. Shakiness may not be reduced, but will not be as obvious in the writing. (Practice and writing exercises are usually helpful). A nylon-tipped pen may be easier to use than a ballpoint pen, as less pressure is required and the angle can be shallower.

If a patient is found to require a writing splint, assessment of the optimum hand angles, pen angles, and methods of holding the fingers and pen may be worked out using adhesive tape. It should be remembered that the pencil or pen will be held more firmly with tape, but there will be a good indication of which fingers or thumb should be incorporated in a splint.

A pocket splint may be useful for writing, particularly when control of pronation and supination is good. The pencil is pushed through the pocket so that the point projects about an inch (2.54 cm) below the ulnar border of the hand. The pencil must be held firmly in the pocket.

A flexor-hinge splint is very useful for writing, particularly with the addition of a hook or spring loop to hold the eraser end of the pencil near the metacarpophalangeal joint (Fig. 8-55). The position is determined by temporarily taping the

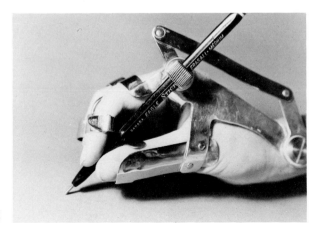

FIGURE 8-55

367

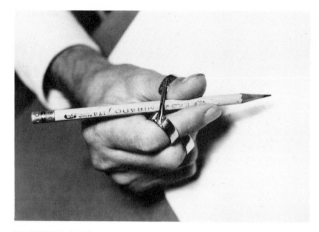 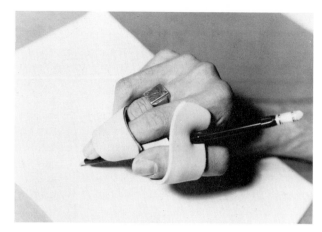

FIGURE 8-56

pencil in position for writing, then marking the correct placement for the spring clip.

A writing splint made of plastic or metal to hold the pencil between the thumb pad and finger may be constructed (Fig. 8-56). All the interphalangeal joints may need to be stabilized in this splint, thus creating a solid triangle, the finger forming one side, the thumb another, and the thumb web the third.

A great variety of plastic or metal splints may be constructed so that hand and pen are held comfortably (Fig. 8-57B, C, D). If the writing aid is to be permanent it must be made so that it will last, and be unobtrusive.

The "Z" splint (Fig. 8-57A) has been particularly popular with many people for a number of years. Amputee elastics may be used to fasten the pen to the splint.

A person requiring a wrist splint will find it easier to type unless only a small amount of writing is required (Fig. 8-58).

If a quadriplegic patient requires aids such as ball-bearing supports, rocker supports, overhead slings, or a mouthstick, he will find it more practical to type.

TYPING

Most patients require an electric rather than a manual typewriter. Care should be taken when selecting the typewriter to see that margin setting and carriage return buttons are within reach, and that the paper can be inserted independently. The paper may be rolled into an electric typewriter using the carriage return button once the paper is placed in position. The typewriter may be selected or adapted to take a continuous roll of paper to eliminate frequency of loading.

The typewriter should be placed at a comfortable height and distance to reduce fatigue. One finger of each hand may be used if the fingers are in a suitable position and the other fingers do not hit the keys inadvertently. Methods used by the patient for holding his pencil can be used with the pencil reversed so that the eraser hits the keys.

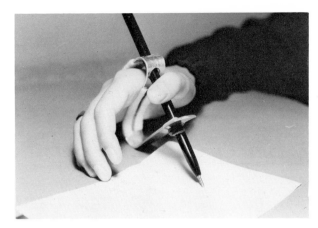

FIGURE 8-57 A

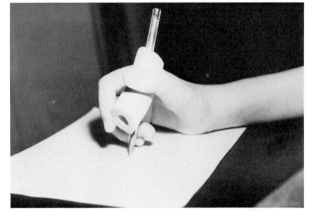

B

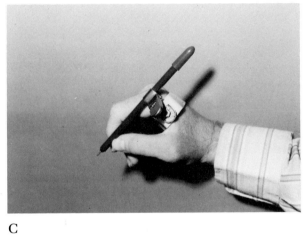

C

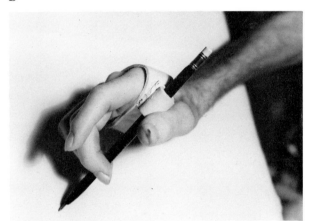

D

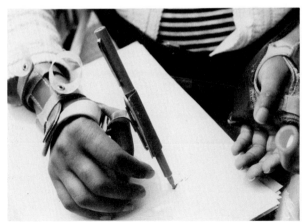

FIGURE 8-58

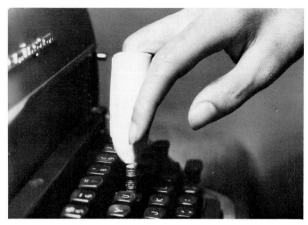

FIGURE 8-59

A plastic finger cot may be made with a typing stick projecting from the tip (Fig. 8-59). Arm slings or ball-bearing feeders may be used with a detachable typing stick firmly fitted to the handpiece. Typing sticks should be rubber tipped so that they do not slip on the keys or damage them, and they should be fixed at an angle and length to allow the patient to see the keys as he hits them. The typing stick should be short, if possible, to reduce the length of the lever arm. Typing sticks may be constructed from pencils with erasers at the tip or, if the sticks require a curve, a metal rod such as welding rod may be used with detachable slip-on erasers plugged to fit over the tips.

A mouthstick may be used (Fig. 8-60) but care must taken that the teeth are not damaged by excessive use with poor fitting. A dental plate incorporating the mouthstick may be fitted over the teeth by a dentist to prevent this damage. The mouthstick should be made just long enough so that the patient can look with comfort at the keys he is touching, and his head should be held in a comfortable position.

An interface system may be used to operate a computer by a patient with minimal or no head movement (Fig. 8-61). Some systems use morse code, via sip and puff or touch access, as the input to operate the computer, which may in turn

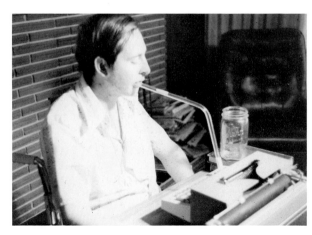

FIGURE 8-60

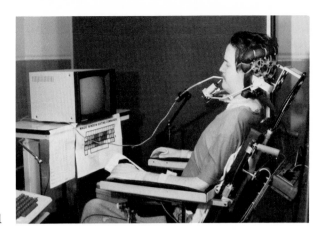

FIGURE 8-61

operate a typewriter, or be programmed to produce voice. These systems are changing and developing rapidly, and innovations must be monitored.

Methods similar to the above may be used to operate many business machines, computers, word processors, and similar devices.

TELEPHONING

Dialing. The receiver may be placed on a convenient surface while dialing. Dialing is facilitated by using immovable telephones, telephones placed on a nonslip surface, and telephones with deep dial holes and light return springs.

A rigid finger may be used for dialing. When a high number is dialed, the right hand must be pronated. As the number is rotated around the dial the shoulder is rotated and the hand supinated so that the finger remains in the same position relative to the dial. This is reversed for the left hand.

A pencil reversed in a pocket splint may be used with or without a flexorhinge splint worn simultaneously to hold the receiver. Dialing may be accomplished using a reversed pencil in the pencil holder of a flexor-hinge splint.

A portable telephone that can remain with a person in the wheelchair is a convenience, and also can be useful in any emergency (Fig. 8-62).

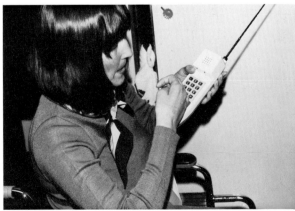

FIGURE 8-62

371

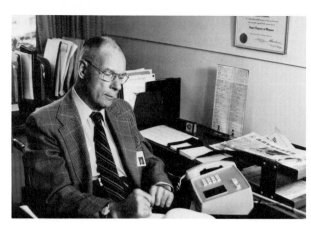

FIGURE 8-63

Pushbutton dialing (see above) or a speaker phone may be used (Fig. 8-63).

Numbers can be fed into a memory bank in a telephone, for later selection with a push on a single button. The phones may for handset use or "hands off" two way amplifier (Fig. 8-64).

Picking Up the Receiver. Picking up the receiver is easier if the receiver is light weight. The receiver may be pushed off the rest on the table while the number is dialed, or, less commonly, may be held in position while dialing. The receiver may be picked up using tenodesis, the heels of both hands, or a flexor-hinge splint, or it may be held permanently in position on a stand.

A simple, economical stand may be made for the patient who cannot hold a receiver. A lamp stand with a flexible arm may be used with broom handle clips fastened to the top to hold the receiver (Fig. 8-65A). The flexibility makes it easy to position the receiver for the individual.

Because the receiver is permanently off the telephone rest, another means must be used to depress the contact buttons. A wooden base can be made for the telephone with a 3-inch-square (7.62 cm) projection in line with the buttons. A corner brace is used to fasten a length of solid wood ½ inch by ½ inch (1.27 cm), and a hole is drilled in it, level with the contact button. Another length of wood is drilled so that one contact button is held down when the two pieces are attached at right angles using a bolt as an axle (Fig. 8-65B). Washers are used as spacers to reduce friction. An elastic is hooked around two screw eyes, positioned so that when the movable lever is vertical the elastic moves behind the fulcrum (Fig. 8-65C). A stop is necessary at the base to prevent the arm from moving past the vertical.

Holding the Receiver. After placing the receiver in position, it may be held as it was picked up. It may be held by shoulder shrug, as in holding a violin. Many types of receiver rests or speaker telephones are available, but solving telephone problems will depend to some extent on the types available in different localities.

CUTTING WITH SCISSORS

This method (Fig. 8-66A) may be useful for the quadriplegic patient, not only for hobby purposes, but also for trimming pubic hair and cutting the ring of a

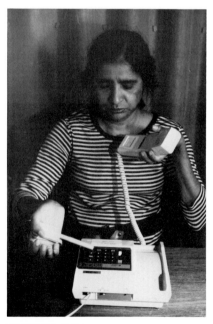

FIGURE 8-64

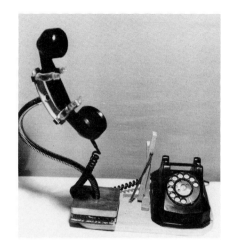

FIGURE 8-65 A

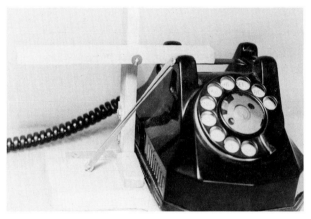

B

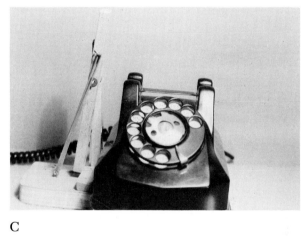

C

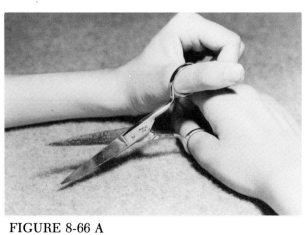

FIGURE 8-66 A

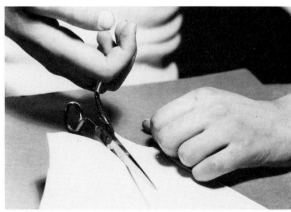

B

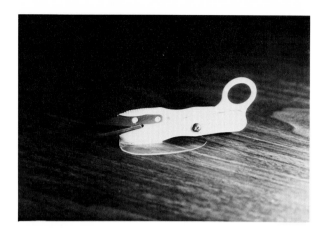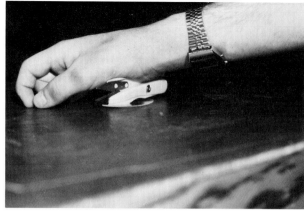

FIGURE 8-67

condom. Pressure down onto the table closes the scissors, while gravity will open them (Fig. 8-66B). The scissors must be chosen carefully so that they will open easily and still cut without requiring any twisting force.

Dressmaker snips may be adapted by gluing a flat plate underneath. These scissors have a spring return to make them very easy to operate with pressure only (Fig. 8-67).

Electric scissors may be adapted by using an elastic band around the scissors strong enough to depress and hold the switch. A thumb loop tied around the elastic band enables it to be pulled onto or off the switch (Fig. 8-68).

SMOKING

A table lighter may be used, or a pocket lighter may be stabilized by fitting it into a wooden base (Fig. 8-69). Grip may be aided by slipping elastic bands around the lighter or gluing sandpaper to it. The lighter should not require continuous pressure to maintain a flame. Electric lighters can be more easily operated than mechanically operated lighters.

Cigarette holders are recommended to prevent burns on anesthetic hands, or

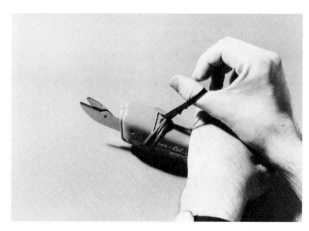

FIGURE 8-68

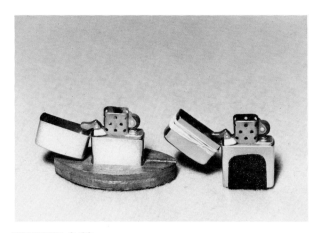

FIGURE 8-69

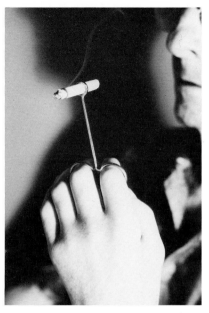

FIGURE 8-70

hands that cannot easily drop a cigarette that is burning them. The cigarette holder must be tested for easy insertion of the cigarette. A cigarette holder attached to the ashtray with a length of flexible tubing to the mouthpiece may be utilized safely by the dependent patient, but people who can manage conventional holders generally prefer to use them.

An ejector type may be held between the teeth while the body of the holder is pushed in, using the sides of both hands in order to eject the butt. The cigarette holder may be picked up using the teeth or by hand using tenodesis. The holder may be placed in the pencil holder of the flexor-hinge splint, provided the angle does not allow the fingers to be burnt, or it may be held in the normal manner in a flexor-hinge splint. The normal adduction of the fingers when the fingers are flexed by tenodesis is often adequate for the cigarette holder to be held between the fingers. The holder may also be held between the heels of the hands.

If a patient prefers not to use a conventional cigarette holder, he may use a ring which fits around the cigarette and attaches with an extension to finger rings (Fig. 8-70) or a handle to be held by tenodesis.

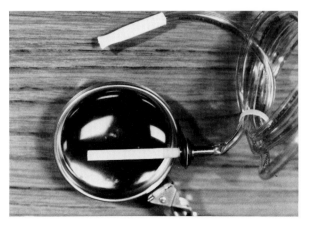

FIGURE 8-71

For some patients a stand must be used for the cigarette holder with an ashtray placed under the cigarette (Fig. 8-71). The patient reaches the holder by using head and neck movements and need not use his hands.

USEFUL REFERENCES AND AIDS

AINSLEY, J ET AL: Reconstructive hand surgery for quadriplegic persons. The American Journal of Occupational Therapy. Vol. 39, no. 11, November 1985. (Describes surgeries, therapy, functional gains, and patient satisfaction.)

BASFORD, JR AND ALLEN, EM: Adaptive equipment for C6 quadriplegia: An approach to effective, simple, and inexpensive devices. Archives of Physical Medicine and Rehabilitation. Vol. 66, Dec. 1985. (A reminder that patients are frequently excellent problem solvers and should be encouraged to develop aids which will be tailored to their own needs).

KOZOLE, KP ET AL: Modular mouthstick system. The Journal of Prosthetic Dentistry, vol. 53, no. 6, June 1985. (Molded mouthstick useful for long term use.)

MALICK, MH AND MEYER, CMH: Manual on management of the quadriplegic upper extremity. Harmarville Rehabilitation Centre, Guys Run Road, Pittsburgh, Pennsylvania 15238. 1978. (Highly recommended—detailed, with clear illustrations and text.)

SEPLOWITZ, C: Technology and occupational therapy in the rehabilitation of the bedridden quadriplegic. The American Journal of Occupational Therapy. Vol. 38, no. 11, November 1984. (Case study showing the improvement in quality of life possible through equipment, motivation, and adequate assistance for a severely disabled person.)

Upper Extremity Orthotic Systems for Patients with Quadriplegia. Slide-tape, 130 slides. Producer, Chapparo, C. Rehabilitation Institute of Chicago, 345 E. Superior St., Chicago, IL. 60611. 1981.

VANDERHEIDEN, G: Computers Can Play a Dual Role for Disabled Individuals. BYTE Publications Inc., Sept. 1982.

9

Sexual Management*

George Szasz, M.D.

Most quadriplegics who were already married or involved in a sexual relationship at the time of their injury report some kind of change in the frequency, nature, or enjoyment of their sexual practices. Other quadriplegics, who were not in a relationship, or who were too young at the time of their injury to have developed a sexual lifestyle, may be wondering what their sexual capabilities might be.

* This chapter was prepared with the assistance of Joan Stradiotti, B.S.N., R.N., and Wendy Turner, B.Sc.O.T., Sexual Health Clinicians.

It is not surprising therefore, that soon after the injury, it is common for quadriplegics to have urgent questions about sexual functioning: Will I be able to satisfy my partner? Will I be able to have sexual satisfaction? Will I be able to have children?

Later on the questions tend to become complaints or requests for help: I cannot satisfy my partner! I cannot get satisfaction! Could we have children? What can be done to recapture what used to be, or what promised to be, an important part of life?

Behind these concerns are unformulated ideas about the impact of the neurologic impairment on erection, ejaculation, or orgasmic capabilities. There may be worries about restrictions in movement and about the resulting lack of spontaneity. There may be concerns over the possible loss of urinary or bowel control in intimate situations. In addition, many quadriplegics sense negative social attitudes toward sexual practices involving disabled persons, and may become handicapped by their own judgment of having become sexually inadequate or unattractive.

In spite of these changes, there is a growing body of evidence provided by quadriplegics which gives rise to optimism for realistic sexual adjustment, even in the face of severe neurologic impairment and a multitude of physical disabilities. In line with this mood, there is increased demand by quadriplegics, their partners and families, and their attending professional personnel for more information and practical suggestions in the management of sexual practices. This chapter is, therefore, intending to accomplish two objectives: first, to provide a better understanding of sexual responsiveness in quadriplegia, and second, to provide guidelines toward the physical management of common sexual practices.

UNDERSTANDING SEXUAL RESPONSIVENESS

Quadriplegics engage in a variety of sexual practices and may experience a wide range of sexual responses. The degree of sexual responsiveness is highly individual, but it is influenced by physiologic impairments, physical disabilities, and personal and social handicaps.

PHYSIOLOGIC IMPAIRMENTS

Sex physiology has to do with reproductive functions discussed later in this chapter and the so-called "sexual response". This chain of events may include genital reactions (sexual sensations, erection of the penis, ejaculation, orgasmic reaction of the female genitalia); extragenital responses (perspiration, skin flush, heart palpitations, increased rate of breathing, body movements, etc.) and mental experiences (feelings of arousal, orgasmic sensations, state of mind after orgasm, etc.) An injury to the spinal cord may alter any of these responses.

CHANGES IN GENITAL REACTIONS

In the quadriplegic man with a complete lesion, accustomed genital sensations of touch or caress are lost. In spite of this, however, erection of the penis may occur quite reliably in response to any physical stimulus applied to it. This reaction is reflex in nature. The stimuli eliciting such a reaction may not be sexually intended. For example, tight trousers may press on the penis and cause an erection

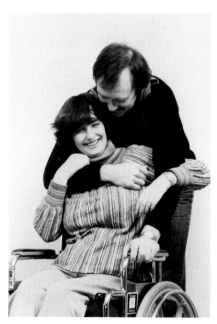

FIGURE 9-1

378

response to occur. Similarly, applying the condom or washing the penis may cause a reflex erection. The penis may become elongated and swollen within a matter of seconds. With further stimuli, the penis may become firm, although the tip often remains unengorged. The reflex erection may last from a few seconds to several minutes. Repeated squeezing of the penis usually brings about renewed engorgement of the organ. The capability for reflex erection does not alter noticeably with age or with the time elapsed after the injury. The reflex may be impeded by many factors, however; for example, the erection may not occur at all because of the side effects of certain medications or the complications of some types of urological surgery. Muscle spasms affecting the legs or abdomen may also interfere with the maintenance of reflex erections. Once the penis is inside the vagina, the reflex erection may be also lost because of insufficient stimulation.

Accustomed genital sensation is also lost in quadriplegic women with complete lesion. Stimulation of the genitalia, however, may bring about swelling of the lips and clitoral tissues. The vagina is usually moist, even without physical stimulation, and the preinjury tone of the vaginal muscles is retained. Spasms do not close the vaginal opening. The quadriplegic woman, therefore, is able to accommodate the penis in the act of intercourse.

The genital responsiveness of the incompletely spinal cord injured person is also variable. As reflex erections in men are usually the product of a complete high lesion, these erections tend to be quite unreliable in some incompletely injured men. In incomplete injuries with some nerve fibres still functioning, active and prolonged penile stimulation may lead to a degree of sexual arousal, and even orgasmic response, with or without ejaculation. In women with incomplete high cord injuries, the potential for genital responsiveness is also varied and often unpredictable.

The effects of ill health, the possible side effects of certain medications, (sedatives, muscle relaxants, antihypertensive agents) and nonmedical drugs (for example, alcohol) and the complications of genitourinary or other surgical procedures, may limit the quadriplegic's sexual response potential. Some of these limiting factors can be identified in the course of a medical assessment and assistance may be provided to remedy some of the limitations.

CHANGES IN EXTRAGENITAL RESPONSES

Quadriplegics, like nondisabled persons, may experience a variety of body reactions to sexual situations. For example, in response to caressing of the face, or other parts of the body with intact sensation, the quadriplegic's heart rate and respiratory rate may increase and the blood pressure may become elevated. The face and the neck may become flushed. Muscular spasms may occur in the abdomen and the legs. Similar reactions may also occur when, for example, the quadriplegic witnesses the partner's enjoyment of sexual stimulation.

Vibratory stimulation of the tip of the penis may produce rhythmic muscular contractions in the abdominal muscles, in the thighs and the lower legs. Some men have reported internal sensations reminiscent of orgasmic feelings in response to such stimulation. A few quadriplegics have reported seminal flow and even ejaculation with viable sperm in response to vibratory stimulation of the tip of the penis.

Active stimulation of the quadriplegic woman's clitoral area may also result in spasmodic contractions of her abdominal, hip and thigh muscles. Some women have indicated that these responses reminded them of orgasm-like sensations.

Vigorous genital stimulation may result in bowel or bladder discharge in quadriplegic men and women. Headaches are not unusual following all these body responses. In some instances, the headaches are manifestations of a milder form of autonomic hyperreflexia.

CHANGES IN MENTAL EXPERIENCES

A few quadriplegics have reported orgasmic experiences occurring during sleep. Others reported only the buildup, but not the release of tensions associated with the sexual responses. Other quadriplegics have described "referred" sensations in some sexual situations. For example, they may have experienced tingling in the chest area, itchiness of the scalp, stuffiness of the nose, all in response to caresses on otherwise "numb" areas. Sensations may also occur in the bladder, or the groin area. Pleasurable sensations may be experienced following the caress of the nape of the neck, the ear, eyelids or other, previously unexplored body areas. Some quadriplegics experience pain when stimulation is applied to skin areas bordering on the level of the lesion.

Many quadriplegics say that they learned to associate some of these new sensations with a variety of sexual practices. Eliciting these responses may, therefore, add to a couple's sexual satisfaction.

PHYSICAL DISABILITIES

The sexual significance of physical changes in quadriplegia relate primarily to the limitations in functional living skills and secondarily to the effects of chronic spasticity, body deformities, and chronic pain.

Limitations in functional living skills such as eating, dressing, grooming, bathing, and attending to bowel and bladder needs may significantly interfere with personal independence and spontaneity of actions in partnership situations. Most of these limitations can be transcended by physical management techniques and by love and affection.

Chronic spasticity may be associated with contractures and further loss of functional ability. Similarly, chronic pain or irritating tingling or burning sensations might lead to a cycle of loss of sexual motivation, moodiness, and emotional depression. Appropriate diagnosis of the problems followed by counseling, medications, and surgical treatment of pain or deformity may increase the quadriplegic's sexual interest level.

PERSONAL AND SOCIAL HANDICAPS

For many quadriplegics, resolution of their sexual concerns helps in establishing or re-establishing their feelings of self worth.

Quadriplegics with fond memories of a satisfying sexual lifestyle tend to have a strong motivation to re-establish their former practices. Those who in their preinjury sexual practices have been able to utilize the acts of intercourse, manual, oral, or mechanical stimulation as desirable options, seem to hold more flexible attitudes about the appropriateness of various sexual activities. For these persons, experimentation with different acts, different body positions, or altered sensations may now become an extension of their former approach to sex practices; or if their preinjury sexual experiences have been limited, they may now be motivated to explore the available options.

Quadriplegics who recall their past satisfaction in terms of "performance" may face certain difficulties. For example, some quadriplegic men may have difficulty visualizing how they could possibly be satisfactory sexual partners, without being able to actively thrust with their penis in the former accustomed manner. A quadriplegic woman may not be able to see how she could continue to be a satisfying partner without being able to voluntarily position herself to accommodate for her partner, or without being able to respond in her accustomed manner. Some quadriplegic women may even feel used; a quadriplegic man may feel inadequate, particularly if his erections are unreliable.

The partner may have concerns too. For example, thinking that the quadriplegic could not possibly have a rewarding sexual experience, a partner may feel selfish. The partner's sexual interest may diminish because of a degree of loss of spontaneity. Becoming a "nurse" to the quadriplegic may also diminish sexual motivation. Most quadriplegics and their partners seem to welcome information about their situation and the available choices. Some quadriplegics and their partners may need help to talk out concerns; others may need practical suggestions. Still others require professional help because they may experience helplessness and depression over their sexual losses. An important aspect of professional help should be a physical as well as a psychologic assessment of the individual's and the couple's sexual situation. In such an assessment, consideration may need to be given to the degree of sexual reponsiveness; functional ability in activities of daily living; bowel and bladder control and menstrual and genital hygiene as these play a role in sexual practices; fertility and birth control situation; the degree of sexual motivation, personal and social abilities to form and maintain partnerships; and self esteem.

Arising out of such an assessment, the professional will be able to clarify the partner's sexual-physiological functioning potential; correct possible limiting side effects of medications or surgical treatment; offer information about the relevant choices in sexual practices; suggest physical management techniques or use principles of sex therapy to assist the couple in discovering their sexual responsiveness potential. The professional will also recognize symptoms of depression, search for its cause, and offer appropriate management.

GUIDELINES TO THE MANAGEMENT OF SEXUAL PRACTICES

Sexual practices may be looked upon as including (1) preparation for sex activities; (2) engaging in activities (including various ways of touching, holding, manipulating, and moving one's own body and often a partner's body); and (3) disengaging from the activities. Consideration may have to be given also to assistive devices, and to family planning or birth control management.

PREPARATION FOR SEX ACTIVITIES

The quadriplegic may have to plan for and rehearse most of the activities that others may take for granted. Preparations may include bladder and bowel check, disconnecting urinary and drainage devices, oral hygiene, moving to a bed or other suitable place, transfers, positioning, and undressing.

The skills of independent management of each of these activities have been described in earlier chapters. However, many persons prefer a degree of continuity in sexual activities. A partner therefore may elect to help to disrobe the quadriplegic partner; may lift the partner into bed; or may elect to conduct their activity with the partner remaining in the wheelchair. New partners may first need guidance to the seeming complexities of wheelchair management, undressing, and catheter or hygiene routines. A recent partner may be surprised to learn about the skills required and energy expenditures needed for activities most people would take for granted. Most couples find it useful to keep towels, perhaps a dish, close by, in case of urinary or bowel accidents or to clean off perspiration or genital fluids.

PLACE SELECTION

Preparations may have to be made to find an appropriate place for sex activities. Privacy is an important consideration, particularly in group living situations. Almost all people want to be sheltered from the eyes and ears of others in intimate situations. However, the concept of privacy may have to be enlarged to include an attendant if two disabled persons want to get together. The attendant may be required for assistance in disrobing, transferring to bed, disconnecting urinary devices, or positioning.

Adequate space is another consideration in selecting a place for sex activities. If a bedroom is used, space should be made available for wheelchair movement, and for transfer to bed.

Some quadriplegics may prefer a water bed, for it may add to the rhythmic movement of some sex acts. When a hard surface or cramped quarters (such as the seat of a car) is preferred, the quadriplegic may wish to use supportng pillows and may want to change positions every few minutes to avoid pressures or abrasions to the skin.

BOWEL AND BLADDER HYGIENE AND PREPARATION

The quadriplegic may wish to plan ahead, and reduce fluid intake in the two or three hours preceding contemplated sex activities. When fluid intake is restricted, and the bladder is emptied just before the sexual act, urinary accidents are unlikely to occur. Quadriplegic men using a condom with urinary drainage bag may disconnect their apparatus. Some men might use a fresh condom to catch small amounts of leakage during the sexual play.

Quadriplegic women with indwelling catheters may disconnect the catheter and then tape the catheter end to the lower abdomen or the groin area (Fig. 9-2). Leakage can be avoided if a plug is used to close the open end. Alternately, the catheter end may be folded back on itself, and a clip, or rubber band might be

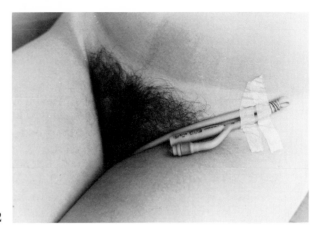

FIGURE 9-2

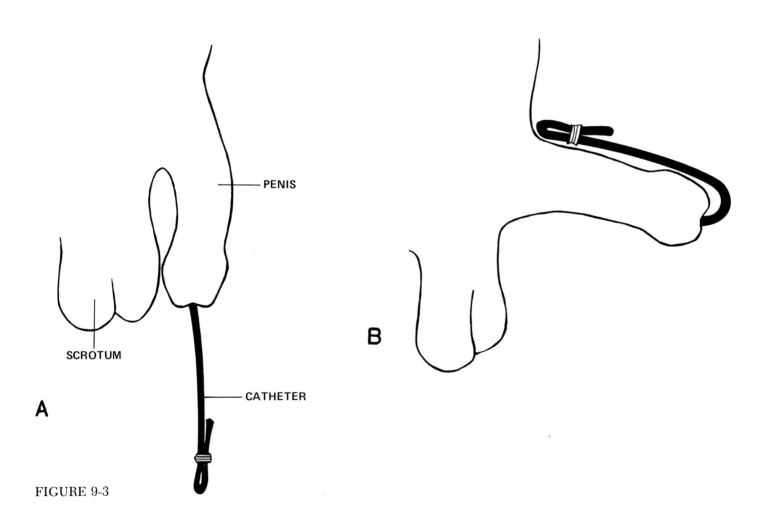

PENIS

SCROTUM

CATHETER

A

B

FIGURE 9-3

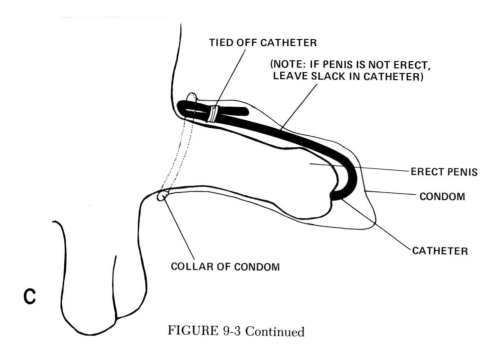

TIED OFF CATHETER

(NOTE: IF PENIS IS NOT ERECT,
LEAVE SLACK IN CATHETER)

ERECT PENIS

CONDOM

CATHETER

COLLAR OF CONDOM

C

FIGURE 9-3 Continued

used to shut it off tightly. Rarely, a quadriplegic man may use an indwelling cathe-ter. He may disconnect the catheter, fold the end of the catheter on itself and tie the folded end with a tape to prevent leakage (Fig. 9-3A). After producing a reflex erection, the free portion of the catheter may be laid back on the erect penis (Fig. 9-35B). Finally, a condom can be pulled over the erect penis and the catheter (Fig. 9-3C). Lubricant on the condom may facilitate easier entry into the vagina. A person requiring intermittent catheterization may wish to be catheterized before engaging in any sex activity.

STOMAS—HYGIENE AND PREPARATION

Some quadriplegics with high spinal cord lesions may have a tracheostomy, with or without a breathing apparatus. In preparation for sex activities, the quad-riplegic may have to learn what positioning might be best for easy breathing and for the continuous ventilating action of the respirator.

Ileostomies, colostomies, and urinary bags should not present undue compli-cations to sexual practices. Preparation may include emptying the bags and assur-ing that the adhesive holding the appliances binds well. Some persons may wish to wear an apron-like garment to cover the bags.

ENGAGING IN SEX ACTIVITIES

Sex activities generally include manual and oral stimulation of various body parts, and intercourse. The activities may take place in a heterosexual or a homo-sexual partnership.

MANUAL STIMULATION

The quadriplegic may wish to use the fingers, hands, arms, nose, lips, ears, or hair to rhythmically caress the partner. Some of these activities may be best accomplished if the able-bodied partner is positioned within reach, or if the partner moves against, for example, the immobile hand. Other activities may be managed with the movements that a quadriplegic has learned to use to manipulate various objects. For example, the penis may be held between the heels of the quadriplegic's hand. Principles of tenodesis could be adapted to facilitate breast or genital stimulation. The back of the hand, or the side of the hand may prove to be softer than the fingers in caressing the face, the breasts, or other desired areas. The partner may wish to hold and guide the quadriplegic's hand to provide appropriate stimulation. Aids and splints may be employed in several ways. For example, caressing may be accomplished using a hand splint with a pocket in it to fit in sheepskin or other soft covering material. A soft glove pulled on the hand may be a satisfactory alternative.

Caressing the spinal cord injured person may require a good deal of guidance. The quadriplegic may need to tell his partner which areas are still sensitive to touch and which areas might be hypersensitive or even painful to caressing. The nondisabled partner may need to prepare for longer periods of stimulation. For example, the male quadriplegic with incomplete lesion and some orgasmic response potential, may require strong, rapid, and long-lasting (e.g., 30–40 minutes) stimulation to the penis. This technique may cause skin abrasions.

The method devised for caressing, or the time spent on touching each other is perhaps not as important as knowing what the partner requires at that particular time. Directions to each other, therefore, may lead to exploration of a wide variety of high quality experiences.

ORAL GENITAL SEX ACTS

These acts may require body positioning by the able-bodied partner. Adequate hygienic preparation would reduce concerns over the degree of cleanliness of urinary or bowel openings. When the act is applied to the quadriplegic, urinary flow may occur in spite of normally adequate bladder management. Spasms in the adductor muscles of the hips and thighs may temporarily trap the head of the partner. If stopping the activity for a few moments does not reduce the spasm, then gentle, steady pressure on, for example, the knee, may reduce the muscle tension. Sometimes medication may be required to prevent the tendency to spasms. However, as it will be pointed out in the discussion of intercourse techniques, some quadriplegics may enjoy the rhythmical contraction of the hip and leg muscles in response to active genital stimulation.

Gagging or choking or not getting enough breath may be a problem to the quadriplegic engaged in the oral sex act. Such events may occur when, for example, a woman partner places her genitalia in contact with the quadriplegic's face, or when a male partner puts his penis to the quadriplegic partner's mouth. Experimentation with these acts and becoming proficient in giving clear signals to the partner to move off, are ways to manage these situations.

For many persons, sexual intercourse provides both emotional closeness and physical pleasure. Physical management of the suitable positions may require assistance by the partner or application of the techniques of self-positioning in bed. The various methods of turning, moving down the bed, and the use of an overhead bar for bed mobility can be well applied here.

Sitting on top of the quadriplegic male may provide for the comfort, mobility and stimulation required by the female partner. In addition, such position provides for the face-to-face view of each other which may offer additional stimulation (Fig. 9-4).

Some quadriplegic women prefer to lie on their back with their legs separated. Pillow support under the knees may help to maintain the position. Leg spasms may be utilized for holding the partner. In this "man-on-the-top position", the quadriplegic woman may have to pay attention to her freedom of breathing and may need to warn her partner to avoid pressing on her chest (Fig. 9-5). Other women may wish to lie on their side, with one or both knees pulled up, somewhat along the lines of the technique used in lifting legs into bed. The male partner would enter from behind. This position might be of special value when spasms are bothersome (Fig. 9-6).

Intercourse in the wheelchair may be an alternative to lying down. The quadriplegic man would want to ease forward in the chair, so that his partner may be able to straddle him in a "facing toward him" (Fig. 9-7) or "facing away

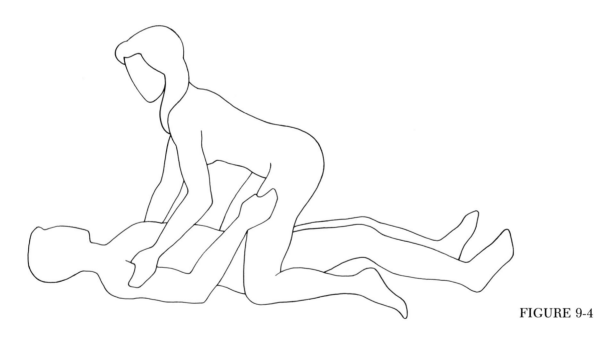

FIGURE 9-4

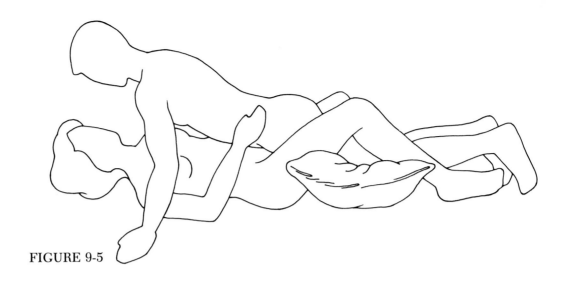

FIGURE 9-5

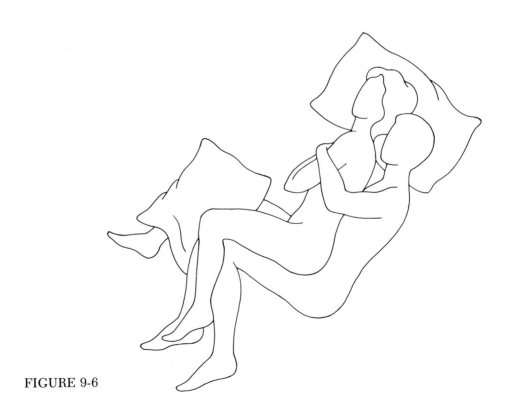

FIGURE 9-6

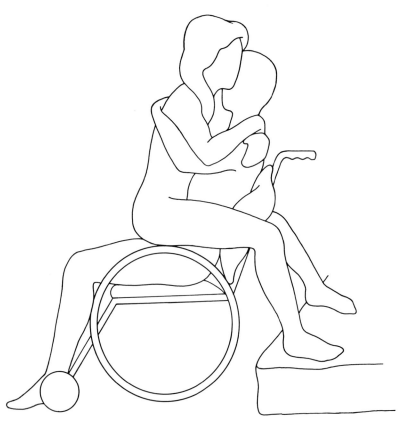

FIGURE 9-7

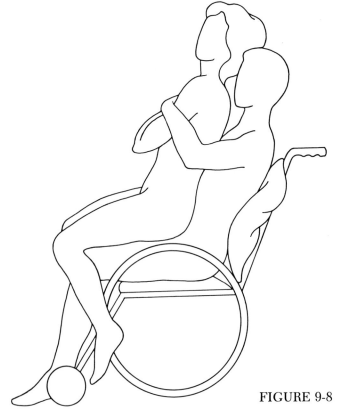

FIGURE 9-8

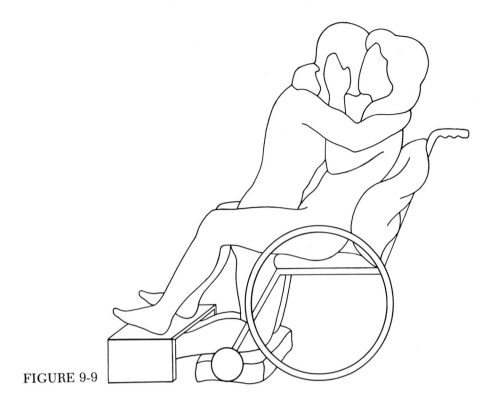

FIGURE 9-9

from him" (Fig. 9-8) position. Similarly, the quadriplegic woman may wish to slip forward in the chair; the partner then might kneel between her legs. In this position the woman's feet require some support (Fig. 9-9).

The mechanics of intercouse require thrusting the penis in the vagina in a rhythmical manner. The quadriplegic man lying on top of his partner may contribute to this action by using his skills to roll from side to side (Fig. 9-10). Lying

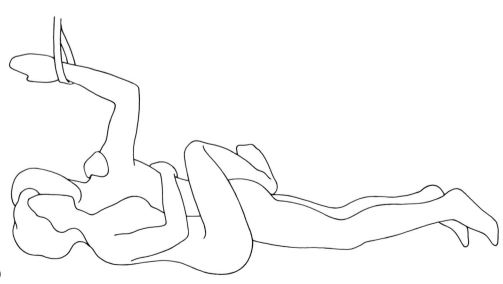

FIGURE 9-10

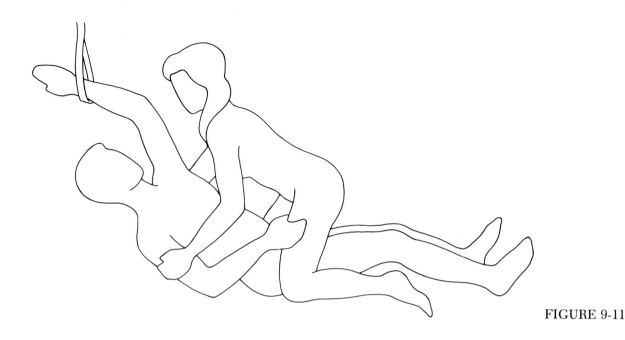

FIGURE 9-11

on his back, he may wish to use his overhead strap to produce a bouncing motion in rhythm with his partner's movements (Fig. 9-11).

Lubricating jelly applied to the penis may reduce chafing the vaginal opening and the vaginal wall.

Spasms occurring during intercourse may add to the rhythmical movement, but in quadriplegic men, the spasm may also cause a temporary loss of erection, and sometimes, loss of bladder control. In quadriplegic women severe leg spasm may make intercourse difficult. Gentle, steady pressure on the legs may release the spasms. Occasionally, medication may be required to control extreme sensitivity to touch.

The soft penis of the quadriplegic can be "stuffed" into the vagina. This technique is easier to accomplish with the quadriplegic on top, and the partner's legs drawn up. The partner moves her seat so that she can guide the well-lubricated soft penis into her vaginal opening. Then, she may wish to contract her vaginal opening in a rhythmical manner and gently move her hips to expose herself to the desired stimulation.

DISENGAGING FROM SEX ACTIVITIES

The technical aspects of disengaging may include bathing or washing the genitalia, getting dressed, and transferring back into the chair. Preparations for disengaging may take as much energy and organization as the preparation for the activity.

The period after sex activity may be characterized by elated feelings and strong energy. Some couples may find that they have become quite tired physically. Some find that they can go only so far, and then have to rest or stop their sex

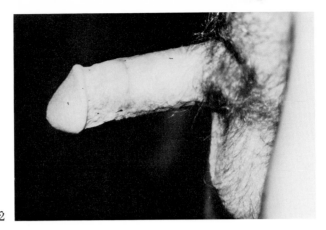

FIGURE 9-12

activities. Yet other couples may feel frustrated and angry because they could not achieve their objectives.

The "psychologic" aspect of disengaging is clearly of importance. This period may be of value to "debrief" each others about the preparations, positions, preferred ways of stimulation, nature of the responses, newly discovered potentials and plans for next time.

ASSISTIVE DEVICES

Some couples may wish to enhance their sexual experiences by technical means. These may be classed as penis enhancers, and as stimulation enhancers.

Penis Enhancers

The penis can be made reliably firm (Fig. 9-12) with one of the several types of internal prosthetic devices. Basically, these devices are firm rods (Fig. 9-13) or

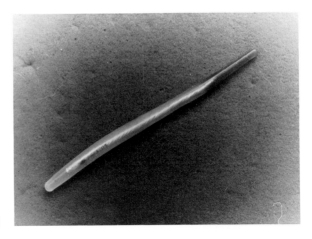

FIGURE 9-13

fluid-filled cylinder-like structures which are inserted into the erectile tissue of the penis in a surgical procedure. Some devices need to be pumped up when erection is desired. The pump is located inside the scrotum (Fig. 9-14A & B). Strong finger power is required to activate the pump, so that the quadriplegic may require assistance from the partner to bring about the mechanical erection. Similarly, manual dexterity and strength is required to press the release button on the pump device in the scrotum. This act may also require the partner's participation.

A side benefit of prosthetic devices is that the rods or the casings for the cylinders provide for a degree of firmness of the penis even in the resting state. Some quadriplegics find it easier to apply their condom drainage device over this semifirm penis.

The major problem with these devices is that the firm materials inside the penis may cause extensive pressure sores, infections, and scarring of the internal tissues of the penis. While such complications do not interfere with the urinary functioning of the penis, the extensive scarring of the erectile tissues may preclude the further use of internal prosthetic devices.

Penile rings and dildoes are some external methods to assist with erection. The idea behind using rings is that these may capture blood in the penis, and

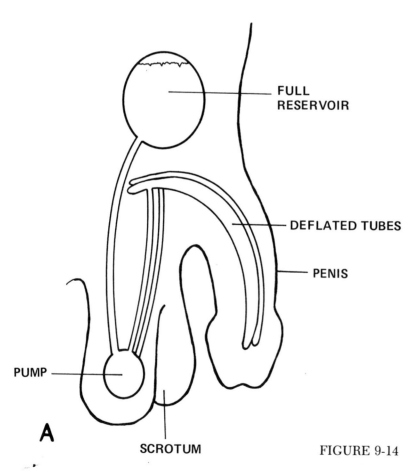

FULL RESERVOIR

DEFLATED TUBES

PENIS

PUMP

A

SCROTUM

FIGURE 9-14

392

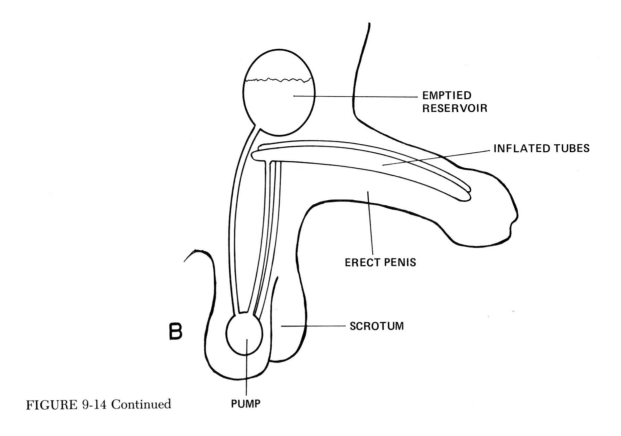

EMPTIED RESERVOIR

INFLATED TUBES

ERECT PENIS

SCROTUM

B

PUMP

FIGURE 9-14 Continued

therefore promote and maintain erection. The rings come in several forms: some are ordinary rubber bands, other are made of flexible plastic, yet others are more rigid. Any of the rings may be effective at times, if applied to the base of a partially swollen penis. Placing the ring on the penis requires a degree of manual dexterity which may not be available to the quadriplegic person. The ring should be just tight enough to block the exit of the blood from the penis, but not so tight that it stops blood getting into the penis. The risks of using rings are poorly documented, but there are medical concerns over causing skin damage to the penis, damage to the erectile tissue inside the penis, and even bruising of the urinary passage in the penis.

Dildoes are rubbery or hard casings, which fit over the soft or semierect penis. The casings may be held on with suction devices (Fig. 9-15A), adhesives, or straps (Fig. 9-15B). The purpose in using dildoes is to provide for the partner stimulation inside the vagina.

Some couples may enjoy using these implements; others may find them strange, even repulsive. None of these methods is specifically constructed for spinal cord-injured persons. They are available for any couple interested in exploring these alternatives.

There is a new medicinal approach to inducing a reliable and longer lasting erection of the penis. This method requires the injection of certain medications (mostly papaverine and phentolamine mesylate) into the spongy tissue of the pe-

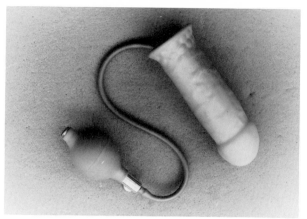
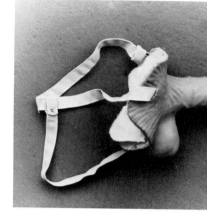

FIGURE 9-15 A   B

nis. The injection may induce an erection within 10–15 seconds that may last for an hour or more, depending on the dosage used. This method may be of value to quadriplegics whose reflex erection is incomplete, uncertain, or short lasting. Self-administration of the medication may not be possible for persons with quadriplegia, but a partner may learn the technique. One short-term complication is that the erection may last longer than desired. There is no information to date on long-term complications.

Stimulation Enhancers

Some of the stimulation applied to the body may be enhanced by vibrators. These are battery or electrically driven appliances that may be used by either partner, for several purposes. An able-bodied partner may enjoy the sensation of vibration on the body as well as on the genitalia. To provide this stimulation, the quadriplegic may need to use a splint to assure a good grasp on the vibrating appliance. The quadriplegic may enjoy the vibration sensation on the neurologically intact areas of the body. Application of the vibrator to the tip of the penis (Fig. 9-16) or the clitoral area may produce abdominal and leg spasms. The spasms may become rhythmical, and in some instances may be accompanied by internal feelings of tension, even though the genitalia may be insensitive to touch. In quadriplegics, prolonged application of the vibrator to the genitalia may also cause extragenital responses, including elevation of pulse and respiratory rates, and elevation of blood pressure. Some quadriplegics may experience headaches in such situations. The vibrator may cause skin abrasions or burns on the skin.

FERTILITY AND BIRTH CONTROL IN QUADRIPLEGICS

In many quadriplegic men reproductive capability is impeded by impairments related to sperm formation, seminal fluid secretion, and ejaculation.
Recent research findings with electrical stimulation of the nerves through the rectum, or with vibratory stimulation of the tip of the penis, have raised hope that

394

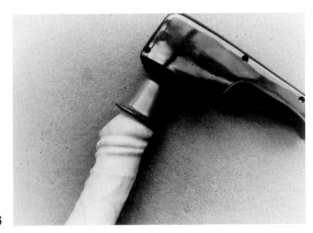

FIGURE 9-16

a flow of sperm-laden seminal fluid may be induced in men with quadriplegia. The fluid so obtained might then be used for artificial insemination of the partner. These techniques are still in an experimental phase.

Spinal cord-injured women of childbearing age usually retain their fertility and are able to carry their pregnancy to term. Close medical supervision is usually required to ensure a healthy pregnancy. Obstetric advice will be needed to decide whether vaginal delivery or caesarean section will be in the best interest of the mother and the infant. Chapter 10 deals with some aspects of management of the infant by the quadriplegic mother or father.

Professional advice may be required for the selection of the safest and most protective birth control method. The best methods may not be the most practical ones for the quadriplegic. It might be of value, therefore, to consider recommending technical methods in two categories: the "you do it" methods and the "done to you" methods. In the first category belong those methods which require hand manipulation to ease of access to the genitalia. Examples of these methods for women include the diaphragm, foam, cervical cap, and the birth control pill. (The latter has to be removed from its case or bottle, placed in the mouth, and water may be needed to swallow it. Some or all of these activities may be impossible for a number of quadriplegics). For men, the condom and the withdrawal method are the "you do it" methods. Both require coordination and motor power. The main "done to you" method for men is vasectomy. For women, this method includes the intrauterine device (inserted or "done to you" by a health care professional), tubal ligation, and removal of the uterus.

When an unprotected quadriplegic woman wants to avoid pregnancy, yet has had intercourse with an unprotected man, she may wish to consult health professional advisors for assistance. The "morning after" pill may be of value within the first two or three days after the sexual incident. In some countries abortion may be considered if pregnancy threatens the life or health of the quadriplegic woman.

Sexual adjustment is possible even in the face of severe neurologic impairment, opening the door to deeply satisfying physical and emotional relationships.

USEFUL REFERENCES AND AIDS

BECKER, EF: Female Sexuality Following Spinal Cord Injury. Accent Special Publications, Cheever Publishing, Inc., Bloomington, IN, 1978. (A question-answer resource for spinal cord injured women.)

BREGMAN, S: Sexuality and the Spinal Cord Injured Woman: Guidelines Concerning Feminity, Social and Sexual Adjustment. Designed for physically disabled women and health professionals who work with them Minneapolis, MN, Sister Kenny Institute, 1975. (Spinal cord injured women tell of sexual possibilities.)

MOONEY, T COLE, T, CHILGREN, R: Sexual Options for Paraplegics and Quadriplegics. Little, Brown and Company, Boston, 1975. (Easily readable and practical information, and explicit pictures.)

RABIN, BJ: The Sensuous Wheeler: Sexual Adjustment of the Spinal Cord. Injured Multimedia Resource Center, San Francisco, 1980. (Review of areas of sexual adjustment and counseling guidelines. Includes some illustrations.)

SZASZ, G, MILLER, S, AND ANDERSON, L: Guidelines to birth control counseling of physically handicapped. Canadian Medical Association Journal 120:1353-1358, 1979. (A series of suggested steps for counseling physically disabled men and women.)

SZASZ, G: Sexual health care, in Zejdlic, C; Management of Spinal Cord Injury Wadsworth, Inc., Belmont, California, 1983. (A comprehensive review of the principles of sexual health care for nurses working in the acute spinal cord injury treatment area.)

10

Parenthood

PLANNING

The expectant quadriplegic mother must plan carefully for her own, and her baby's care. A major factor in her planning must of course be the baby's health and safety, and her own physical ability. New mothers who are not quadriplegics can be quite apprehensive about looking after a new baby. The expectant quadriplegic mother will be even more apprehensive, and must plan methods of management to help to reduce her fears and to select a realistic plan of care for herself and her baby.

The average mother may do much of her planning later in pregnancy, but the disabled mother would be wise to practice baby care and work out problems early in her pregnancy before she becomes less able to maneuver, to approach tables and cribs closely. She may also have to plan for extra care for herself if her weight and bulk make it hard or impossible to care for herself independently. If she is normally dependent, new methods of transfer may be required; for example, if she must lean her trunk forward as part of the normal transfer, or if the extra weight is too much for her attendant.

HOME HELP

Part of the parents' assessment of possible methods of management may be to consider whether the mother or father should look after the child, and whether this should be complete or partial care. Perhaps other members of the family should provide some care, or another person should be hired; if so, the parents must decide how much control they wish to retain. It is all too easy for the nervous new mother to hand the baby over to more capable hands, only to discover to her distress that the baby turns to this person and not to her. (Fig. 10-1).

If the parents elect to have a home helper as the main caregiver, they must be prepared to accept that the baby will bond to this caregiver. The parents must therefore choose this person carefully, and should make it clear if they wish to be in control of the baby care methods. They may have to accept the baby's bonding to another and prepare to take charge later in the child's life. This can be very upsetting, even if it has been foreseen and accepted.

It may be helpful to note that this stage lasts usually until the baby is about 18 months old, after which parents usually become all-important to the toddler.

PRENATAL CLASSES

Prenatal classes may be avoided by some disabled expectant parents, perhaps because of difficulty of access, because transfer to a floor mat requires help, because the person does not wish to stand out among the crowd, or because of fear of bowel or bladder accidents.

The knowledge gained at prenatal classes by the first time mother is very valuable and allays many fears. It would be wise, if possible, to shop around for an accessible class and an instructor who is understanding.

The prospective quadriplegic mother will probably have to educate the instructor about her disability, as indeed she has to educate many people, but she and her partner usually gain a great deal from their participation in childbirth and baby care education. If the disabled mother cannot participate in a class,

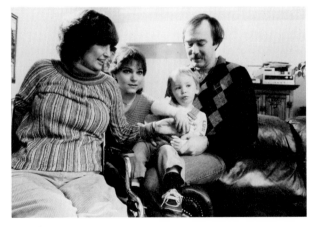

FIGURE 10-1

arrangements may be made for a prenatal educator to visit the home, or to supply educational material.

If a rehabilitation center is accessible, it can be helpful to have a short admission or outpatient attendance, so that baby care methods may be explored, and the expectant mother can work with babies under careful supervision to learn what is realistic for care giving later.

HOSPITAL CARE

Before the birth of the baby, the expectant mother should plan as far as possible for her own care during her stay in the hospital, including time to discuss her physical needs, transfer requirements, and turning and toileting, so that hospital personnel have an opportunity to learn the special care required by the disabled mother. This should assist both staff and the expectant mother to be more relaxed and familiar with procedures.

The mother should discuss the birth process thoroughly with her doctor; she should know of possible complications, such as autonomic dysreflexia, and what procedures may be required to minimize risks. The probability of vaginal delivery and the complications that might require caesarean section should also be discussed beforehand, together with types of anaethesia that may be needed. Some women are concerned about episiotomies because of fear of possible complications. Contamination of the wound owing to incontinence of bowel and bladder, the possibility of slow healing, and pressure on the wound when sitting may be concerns to be discussed with the doctor.

EMOTIONS

Even if the expectant mother has adapted to her disability, and has planned a pregnancy, a new wave of frustration with the disability can occur as she finds herself unable to look after her baby as much as she had hoped, or as the baby needs her and she cannot meet its needs. This frustration may be complicated by the emotional ups and downs experienced by most new mothers, and will be very hard to cope with if there is post partum depression.

The expectant mother who has not had time to adapt to her disability, who became quadriplegic during pregnancy, will need a great deal of support to cope with her frustrations and feelings, in addition to the stress any new mother experiences. She will also need a great deal of help in assessing her situation. Since she has had so little experience of living in a wheelchair, realistic planning may not be possible for her.

It is important that any new mother have someone to confide in, in addition to her partner, for support and reassurance. It is most important for a new disabled mother to establish this relationship early to help cope with her exceptional frustrations and apprehensions.

Although some physical limitations and frustrations are unavoidable, a disabled parent, mother or father, can be as good or as poor a parent as any nondisabled person. Most parents agree that understanding, guidance, love, and a sense of humor are more important than the physical ability to care for a child. Physical

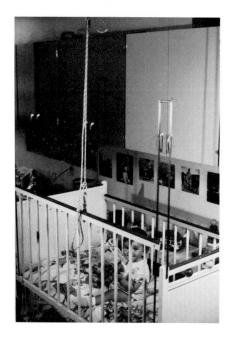

requirements must be met, especially during the first two years, but they can be met by careful planning, inventiveness, and adaptability.

METHODS OF MANAGEMENT

LAYOUT

The layout of the nursery should be planned so that working surfaces are at a convenient level and are accessible for the disabled parent. They must also be made safe for the baby. A small baby will be safe on a padded table top with no edge, but as the child grows a safety barrier will be required to prevent falls.

Supplies such as baby powder should be stored within reach, and if necessary, adapted for handling.

CRIB

The crib may be adjusted to wheelchair height, and a gate may be made to slide up and out of the way. In the crib illustrated (Fig. 10-2), bars have been

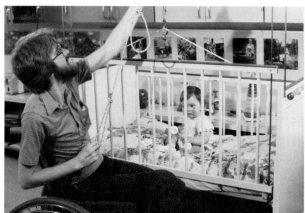

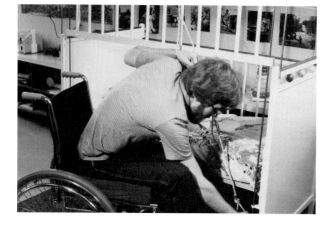

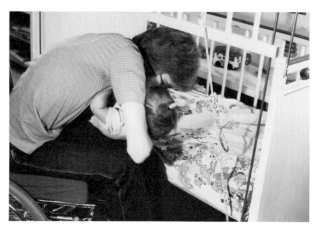

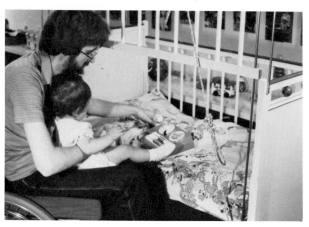

FIGURE 10-2

400

added at the corners as a sliding guide. An overhead pulley and rope are used for lifting and lowering the gate. Loops are placed in convenient positions in the rope, and the rope looped over a hook to hold the gate in the open position. With some sparing in his trunk, this father can reach forward to fasten the rope; others will fasten the rope to a hook at the base of the gate.

A slide up gate is more practical than a swing-out gate because it takes up less room, and it allows the wheelchair to be positioned before the gate is opened.

FEEDING

A mother may breast feed her baby in bed or in her wheelchair. In bed she will probably need help to position the baby and to change position so that the baby can be moved to the other breast.

The baby may need to be held in a 'cuddle sack' (Fig. 10-3) for safe bottle or breast feeding in the wheelchair. A cuddle sack which has worked well is made like an open sleeping bag to lie flat so that the baby can be slid onto it. The bottom corners are then zipped up diagonally, and the top of the sack is closed with velcro. The head piece remains under the baby's head for support.

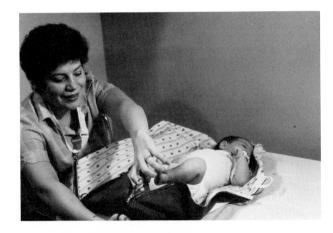
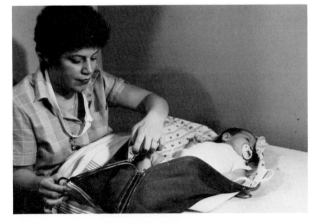
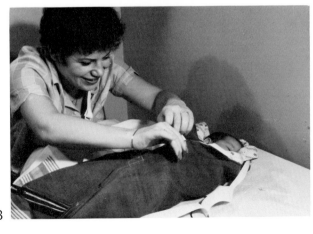
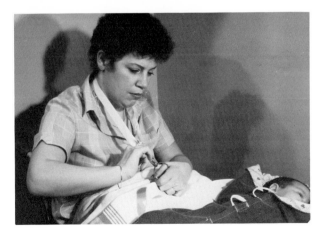

FIGURE 10-3

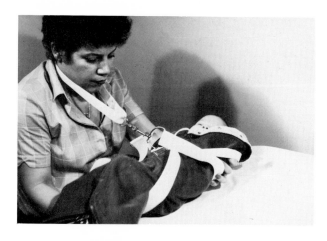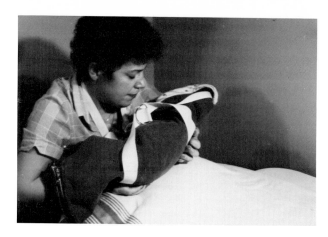

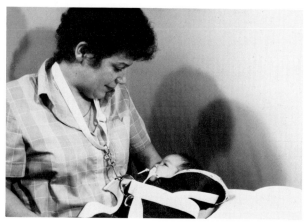

FIGURE 10-3 Continued

An adjustable neck loop of webbing for the mother is made to clip onto webbing straps sewn to the cuddle sack so that complete safety is assured.

As the baby grows older, a cuddle seat may be useful (Fig. 10-4). The adjustment clip may require lengthening to permit the mother to manage it. She may not be able to lift the baby in or out, but can feed or play with her very safely.

A disabled mother may have the satisfaction of feeding her child, even if she cannot lift him into his high chair (Fig. 10-5).

DIAPERING

Disposable diapers are not easy to handle, but are convenient to use because they save laundering. If the protective paper cannot be pulled off the sticky tab, adhesive tape may be substituted.

The mother in the illustration has adapted cloth diapers and practiced diapering a baby before the birth of her own baby (Fig. 10-6).

The diapers are rectangular, with velcro straps with loops sewn below the waist at the top. At the other end of the diaper, the hook velcro has been sewn so

402

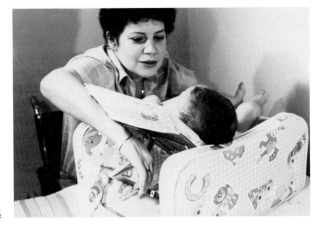
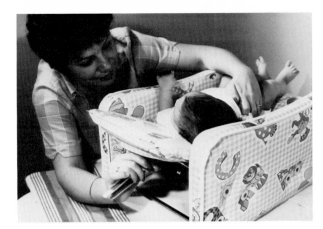

FIGURE 10-4

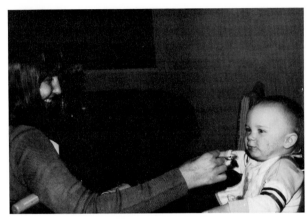
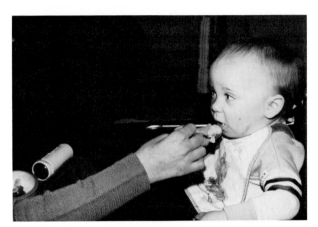

FIGURE 10-5

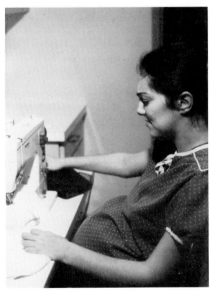

FIGURE 10-6

that when the diaper is positioned, the velcro straps will fasten. The diapers are about 12 inches (30.48 cm) by 18 inches (45.72 cm), and have five layers quilted together in the centre, leaving about an inch (2.54 cm) around the sides to reduce the bulk (Fig. 10-7).

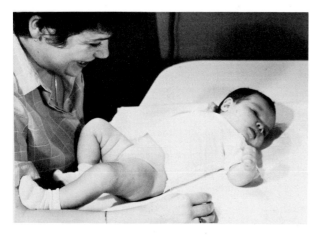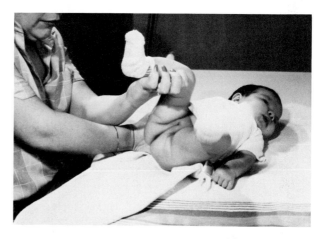

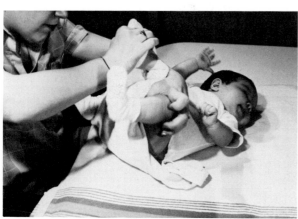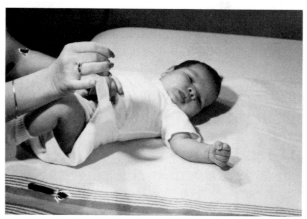

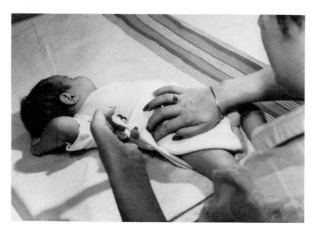

FIGURE 10-7

404

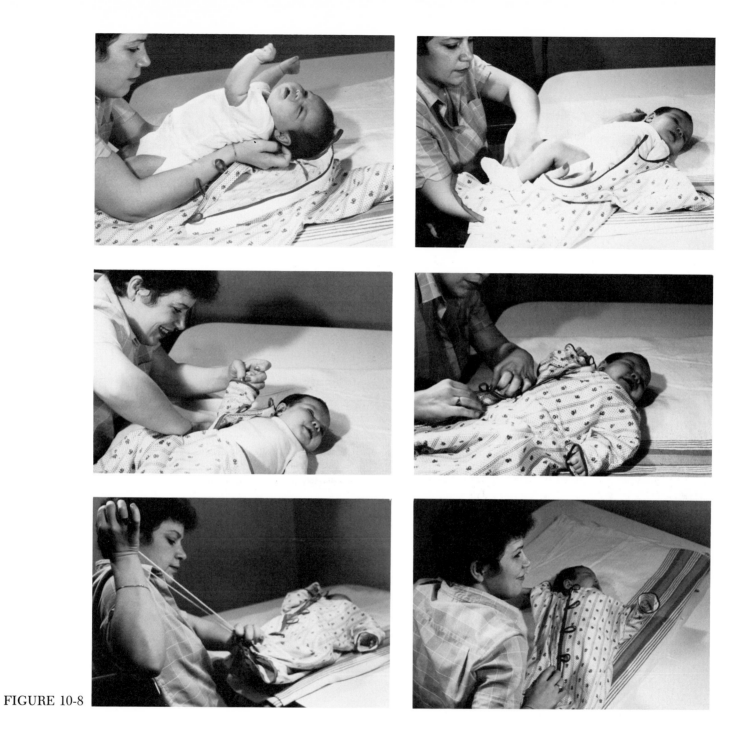

FIGURE 10-8

The nightdress has been adapted using wide openings, raglan sleeves, a drawstring bottom closure, and velcro and loop fastenings (Fig. 10-8). Clothing adaptions shown in Chapter 6 may also serve for children's clothing. The style of clothing selected is important. For instance, loose raglan sleeves are easy for both parent and child. Wide openings and large fastenings enable some disabled parents to dress the child more easily, and as the child grows and becomes more adept, these styles also allow the child to become independent earlier.

BATHING

Babies are difficult to handle when wet and slippery. A net stretcher with handles to lift a baby in and out of the baby bath may be possible, but this has not been tested, and may not be safe. It may be preferable for the disabled parent to wash the baby on the changing table, and to have an able-bodied person supervise the baby bath.

COOPERATION

This baby learned very early to cooperate with her father so that she could be lifted up or lowered (Fig. 10-9). If she did not feel like cooperating, her father could not keep her on his knees, nor could he pick her up (Fig. 10-10). This was extremely frustrating for him and is an example of child behavior that the disabled parent may have to face. Similar behavior is to remain out of reach. This is where patience and a sense of humor are needed!

SAFETY

Toddlers are at a particularly vulnerable stage, where they may dash impulsively into danger. Children at this stage should be restrained because the disabled

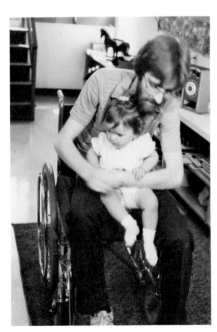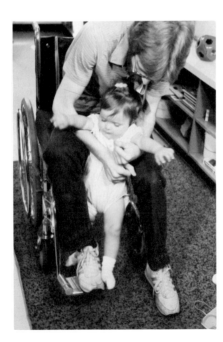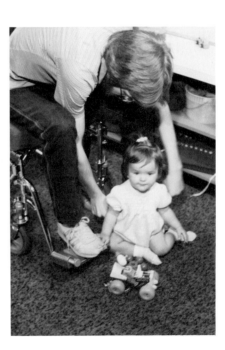

FIGURE 10-9

parent is not mobile enough to protect them in a normal fashion. Playpens and other restraints such as harnesses and leashes are accepted as a matter of course, just as children accept safety restraints in a car (Fig. 10-11).

As children grow older they normally become more responsive and controllable. A prearranged telephone network can be invaluable for the disabled parent's peace of mind and the child's safety. It is impossible to foresee every danger that a child may encounter; a seemingly impregnable fence may be a challenge to the toddler. Arrangements should be made for a call from a portable telephone to quickly bring a neighbor to the scene in any crisis.

Placing safety gates (Fig. 10-12), using safety plugs for electric outlets, and storing potentially dangerous substances such as cleaning fluids out of reach are normal procedures when a baby or a toddler is in the house. Unfortunately, these safety measures usually are inconvenient for the disabled person. Any measure to make a safety gate easy to open for a disabled parent makes it easy for a toddler. Again, preplanning, home help, and a sense of humor may be required.

PLAY

A child soon learns to climb onto mommy's knee for a cuddle, and then a story (Fig. 10-13). At this stage the disabled parent can participate actively in the child's care. Playtime, story time, and exploring are fun times and valuable for child and parent (Fig. 10-14). Frustration is reduced, and there is great satisfaction and enjoyment of the role of parenthood.

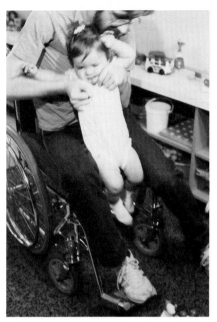

FIGURE 10-10

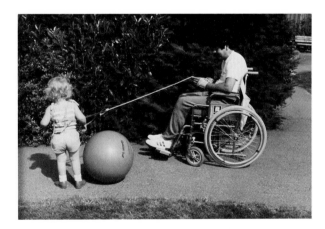

FIGURE 10-11

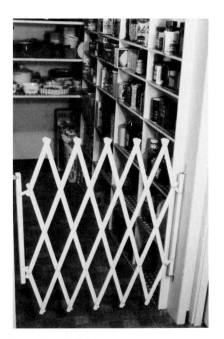

FIGURE 10-12

407

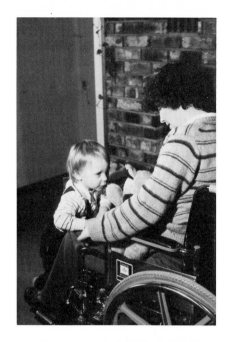
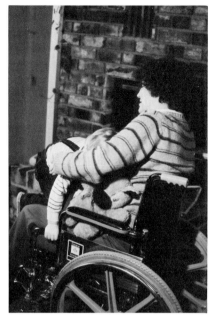
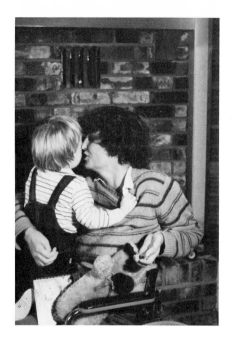

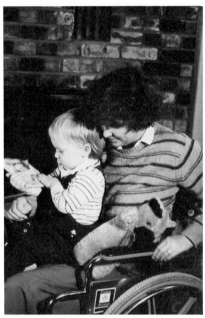

FIGURE 10-13

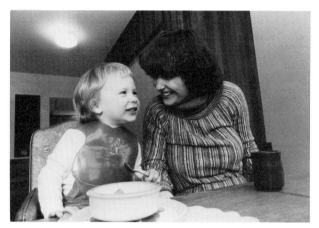

FIGURE 10-14

408

USEFUL REFERENCES AND AIDS

BOETTKE, EM: Suggestions for Physically Handicapped Mothers on Clothing for Preschool Children. School of Home Economics, University of Connecticut, Storrs, CT, 1958.

WALL, J: Play Experiences Handicapped Mothers may Share with Young Children. School of Home Economics, University of Connecticut, Storrs, CT, 1959.

WAGGONER, NR: Child Care Equipment for Physically Handicapped Mothers. School of Home Economics, University of Connecticut, Storrs, CT, 1961.

MAY, EE: Work Simplification in Child Care. Teaching Materials for the Rehabilitation of Handicapped Homemakers. School of Home Economics, University of Connecticut, Storrs, CT, 1962.

GARDNER, S: Having babies and other neat things. Paraplegia News, 31:359:33. August, 1978.

Equipment for the Disabled: Disabled Mother, 2 Foredown Drive, Portslade, Sussex, BN4 2BB England, 1978.

HEINTZMANN, L: Parenting from a wheelchair, Caliper, Winter 1979-80.

DUFFY, Y: All Things are Possible. AJ Garvin and Association, P.O. Box 7525, Ann Arbor, MI 48107. 1981.

Can a wheelchair bound woman have a baby? Accent on Living, 25:4. Spring, 1981.

HALE, G. (Ed): The Source Book for the Disabled. Bantam Books, Inc. 1981, pps 282–315.

ASRAEL, W: An approach to motherhood for disabled women. Rehabilitation Literature, July–August, 1982. Vol. 42. No. 7.8.

COLEMAN, B: Flyer, homemaker, engineer. Rehabilitation Literature, July-August. Vol. 43. N7-8. 1982.

MOYE, B & HUME, J: A second shot at life. Quad Wrangle, Aug-Sept. 1982.

11

Household Management

KITCHEN
   Kitchen Plans
   Kitchen Options

Kitchen Areas
Cooking Methods

Many quadriplegic homemakers with wrist extension will be able to do a major part of the cooking and cleaning if this is where they wish to use their energies. Those without wrist extension, but with elbow flexion may be able to do some cooking, but will require assistance with major cooking and cleaning.

KITCHEN

Some quadriplegic people may wish to cook complete meals or occasional snacks, and in this case the patient's existing kitchen plan should be drawn up to see what changes will be required. Planning may be facilitated by using scale cutouts to represent counter tops, appliances, and so forth, so that plans can be visualized and changed easily. Major alterations may be necessary if the patient is to be the homemaker, but if another person is to be the major homemaker these alterations may be modified for the convenience of both. Wheeling and turning must be cut to a minimum by thoughtful design of the kitchen, particularly for the patient who uses a flexor-hinge splint, since wheeling is usually difficult when wearing a handsplint.

Kitchen Plans

Five main layout designs of kitchens are possible, "U," "Corridor," "L," "Island" and Straight. The principles of any kitchen design apply to both disabled and nondisabled users, except that an "Island" design may be more of an obstacle to a wheelchair user. Generally a "U" design has the most efficient work triangle, but the corners are often wasted. A "Corridor" is the next most efficient unless the user must slide, rather than lift objects (Fig. 11-1). An L design may be excellent for a person who stays in one area and perhaps is not the main cook.

This efficiency rating must be modified by users' likes and dislikes, size of a family, cooking methods, and available space. There are many books on kitchen design and space saving storage available, which explain work triangles, and the principles of kitchen design. Some examples of kitchen designs for wheelchair accessibility can be found in the Appendix.

KITCHEN OPTIONS

Open-Under Type Counter with Upper Half of Kitchen Accessible

A kitchen may be built open-under, so that counter tops and overhead cupboards can be reached, and all cooking is done facing forward (Fig. 11-2). De-

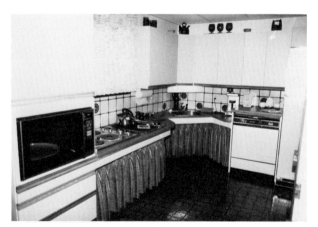

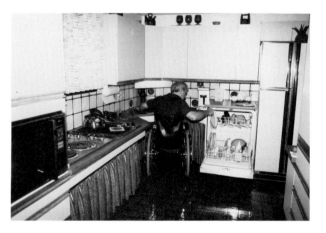

FIGURE 11-1 A

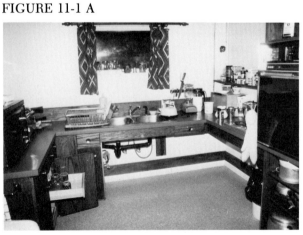

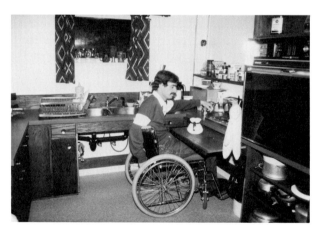

B

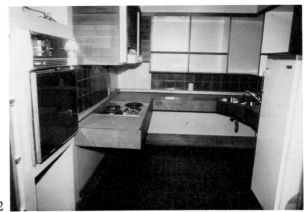

FIGURE 11-2

pending on the knee height of the user, shallow drawers may be built into the counters also. Extra depth counters may permit storage at the back; this is particularly useful if overhead cupboards are inaccessible. The open-under design allows easy maneuvering using the counters to push against, rather than the wheels, which may not be clean. This kitchen is designed with the wheelchair user as the main cook.

Pullout Kitchen: Lower Half of Kitchen Used

A kitchen can be adapted so that the counters and overhead cupboards are not in reach, but drawers, pullout shelves, pullout trolleys, and lap trays are used instead (Fig. 11-3). Small electrical appliances such as an electric frying pan or broiler are easily placed on these, at a convenient working height and may be used as substitute for range top or oven. If drawers are being built they should be built as far down as the user can reach. This design is particularly useful if there are several cooks requiring differing cooking height surfaces in the kitchen, but is usually less efficient if the wheelchair user is the prime cook.

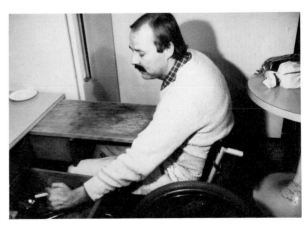

FIGURE 11-3

Adapted Areas

If the wheelchair user is adapting an existing kitchen, some undercounter cupboards can be removed, thus creating different work centers accessible to the wheelchair. The under-sink cupboard may be removed to make a clean-up center; the cupboard beside the cooking top may be removed for a cooking center (Fig. 11-4A).

An area may be built so that the cook can stay in one place, and use pull-out storage for most needs. This is especially useful if the disabled cook is not the prime cook, and does not have to use all appliances and storage. For a quadriplegic cook, the overhead cupboards illustrated would need to be lowered. (Fig. 11-4B).

Angled Approach to Counter Adaptation

Some kitchen designers for the disabled advocate large toe spaces under drawers for wheelchair footrests. This may be useful for some, but generally there is a danger of bumping shins, and the wheelchair user is always working twisted

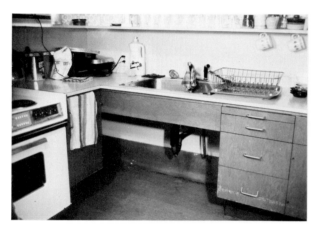

FIGURE 11-4 A

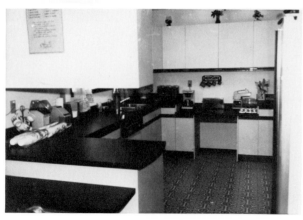

B

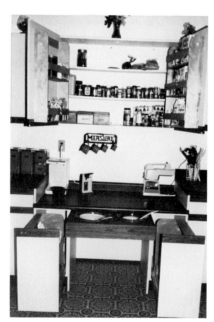

414

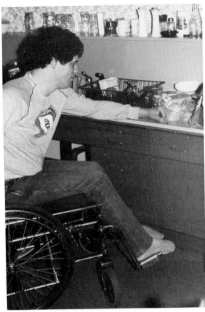

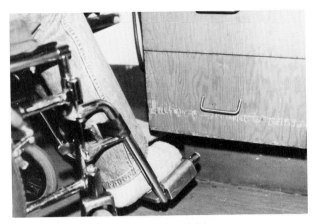

B. Extra Turning Room Available

FIGURE 11-5

A. Awkward Angle for Working

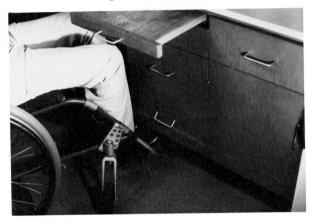

C. Improved with Pullout Board

towards the counter (Fig. 11-5A), a position which may be harmful if used over many years. It has the advantage over the open-under counter of adding storage space, particularly for a taller person who has lower footrests, and it may be useful if extra room is required for turning (Fig. 11-5B). If meal preparation is mainly done on a wheelchair tray or pullout board, this design may be useful (Fig. 11-5C).

KITCHEN AREAS

Sink and Clean Up Area

The sink and drain should be closed in or insulated to prevent burns (Fig. 11-6A); the taps should be within reach and easy to turn. Lever taps or a central control type may be easy to operate. A hose for filling pans with water to avoid lifting them will probably be useful also (Fig. 11-6B).

Shallow 6-inch (15.24 cm) sinks can be obtained to allow knees to go under. If a sink can be obtained with a drain at the back, this is ideal, provided the drain

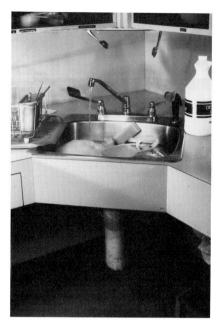

FIGURE 11-6 A

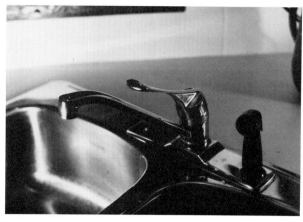

B

plug is accessible. The drain plug may require adaption with a rigid rod or a plastic loop handle riveted to it.

Dishwasher. The front-loading dishwasher with pullout shelves and front controls is very convenient for a wheelchair user (Fig. 11-7).

Cooking Areas

Range. Some quadriplegic people cook by approaching the range from the side, though this is difficult if two hands are required. In this case a reacher may be required for control knobs and a mirror may be required to look inside pans.

Cooktop. Ideally a cooking top should be set into a counter so that knees can go under for a close approach (Fig. 11-8A). The controls should be near the front, and may require adaptation; some newer controls must be pushed down and then turned, a difficult movement for many people. Universal switches may be purchased and substituted for the push and twist type. Lever-type switches are recommended (Fig. 11-8B).

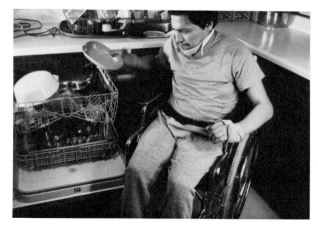

FIGURE 11-7

416

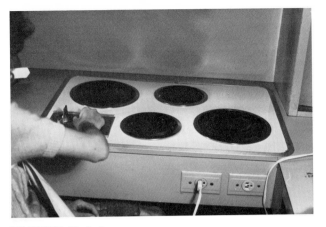

FIGURE 11-8 A

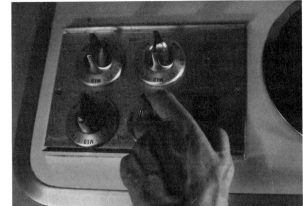

B

Portable Burner: Small Appliances. If a counter-top burner is not practical, a portable burner, broiler, or toaster oven may be used, set on a trolley or pullout board at a convenient height (Fig. 11-9). This method is excellent for many appliances, but care must be taken that the trolley is not moved while the cord is plugged in.

Ovens. Few quadriplegic people are strong enough to reach over an oven door to lift dishes out. More convenient and safer are wall ovens with a side hinged door (Fig. 11-10).

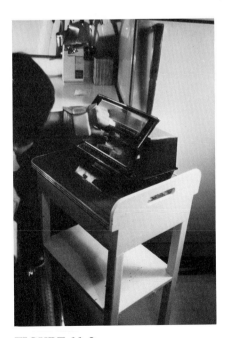

FIGURE 11-9

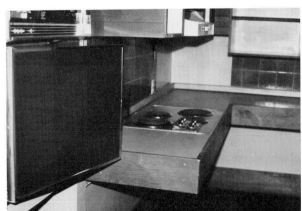

FIGURE 11-10

417

This enables the cook to get close enough to lift dishes onto an adjacent shelf, pullout board or trolley (Fig. 11-11). The oven base for the average patient in an active duty lightweight wheelchair should be 25 inches (63.5 cm) above the floor if the door is to clear knees. A pullout board beneath the oven will be useful for those who must rest elbows on a firm surface to enable them to lift.

An oven set 5 inches (12.7 cm) lower will bring the shelves level with the adjacent counter or pullout shelf, and will be more convenient for a person who can reach the oven from beside it.

Casseroles may be pulled out of the oven by pulling out the oven shelf with a hook or oven mitt (Fig. 11-12) and sliding the casserole straight onto a shelf, wagon, or wheelchair tray level with the oven shelf. A baker's peel, a wooden paddle with handles which can be slipped under the casserole, may be used to slide it onto the adjacent surface.

Ovens with a self-cleaning setting are very useful for the disabled home-maker.

Microwave Ovens. Microwave ovens are very useful for those with lack of heat and cold sensation, for those who are not strong enough to lift dishes, or for

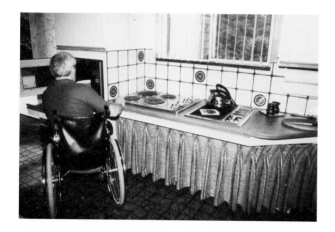

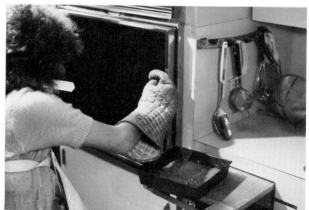

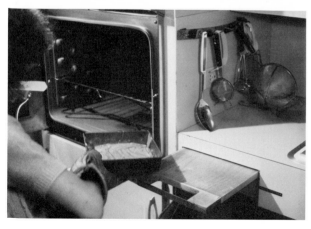

FIGURE 11-11

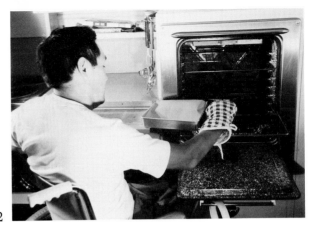

FIGURE 11-12

people who are in temporary accommodation with no heavy wiring. Side-hung oven doors, easy controls, and a flat oven floor are easiest to manage. Door handles and oven dials on older models may require adaptation with loop handles or levers. These ovens may also be used by people who do no other cooking, but who wish to heat prepared meals. A built up block may be slid into place after the door is opened to eliminate lifting, or bail-type handles may be added to a tray to make lifting easier (Fig. 11-13).

Electric Outlets. Electric outlets should be within reach (Fig. 11-14). An ideal position is on the counter front, but an overhang to prevent water running over and on to the plug is recommended. Plugs can be adapted, or the wire can be stiffened by taping on a stiff nonconducting material such as wood doweling. If the cook cannot push a plug in, a permanently plugged-in cord with a switch may be substituted.

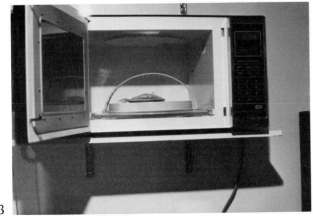

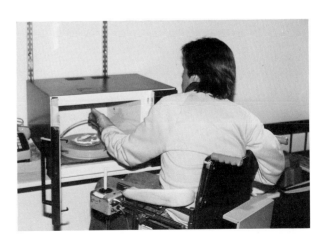

FIGURE 11-13

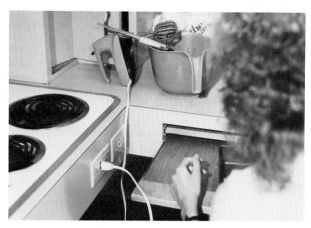

FIGURE 11-14

Storage Areas

Storage is a problem for most wheelchair users since so much of it is out of reach or must be eliminated to allow knee room (Fig. 11-15).

Overhead cupboards may be lowered to a more convenient 14 inches (35.56 cm) above the counter. These may be open shelving or closed cupboards with loop-handle doors. Space savers such as lazy susans, carousels, swing-out corner cupboards, pullout storage trolleys, and well organized pantries are helpful (Fig. 11-16). Even out-of-reach storage may be utilized for less used items, or for items used only when help is available.

A list of the most used utensils and ingredients for each area should indicate where storage would be most useful. These areas may be 'clean up', 'mixing', 'chopping', or 'heating', and each person's different styles of cooking will influence storage design, as well as the physical ability to reach and lift or slide equipment. People with small children will find low open storage an invitation to disaster, others will find it indispensable. Those who are unable to lift easily will require continuous counters, and storage on a deep counter. It is helpful for a patient to have the opportunity to work in a model wheelchair kitchen so that requirements can be assessed.

Refrigerator. Neither freezer nor refrigerator should be out of reach. A short refrigerator with a freezer area above, or a side-by-side type may be indicated. Slide-out refrigerator shelves or a combination sliding shelf and pullout shelf from the counter may be useful. In this case a side-by-side freezer-refrigerator would be inconvenient because the pullout shelf in the counter would be too far from the refrigerator shelf. The refrigerator door should open so that the opening is near the counter, and the door handle should be a metal loop-type pull. A leather or webbing loop may be fastened to the doorpull if the handle is solid, or awkward to hold (Fig. 11-17). An automatically defrosting refrigerator makes clean up easier.

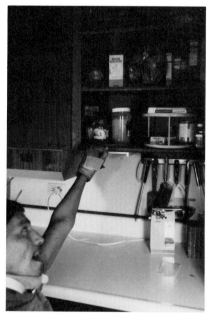

FIGURE 11-15

420

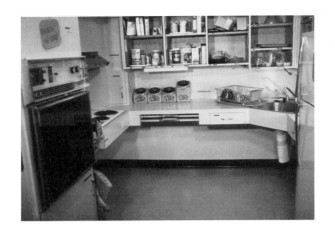

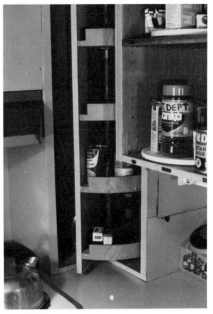

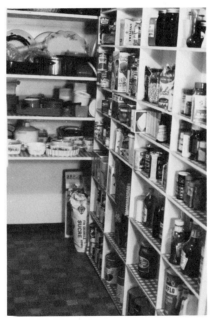

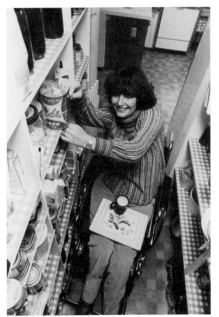

FIGURE 11-16

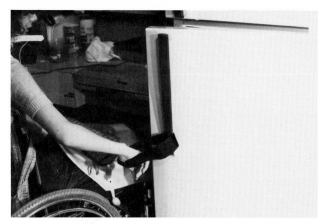

FIGURE 11-17

Countertop Height, Depth

If a kitchen is designed for an individual the counter height should be designed to suit. One person may prefer a low area for mixing and a higher one for cutting; others must have level counters so that dishes may be slid rather than lifted. A person in an active duty lightweight wheelchair usually finds 27 inches (68.58 cm) knee room below the counter and 33 inches (83.32 cm) countertop height sufficient. A person in a different wheelchair will require both measurements to be adjusted.

With the proliferation of wheelchairs of differing heights, it becomes very difficult to suggest countertop heights which would be suitable for group homes where different people use the kitchen, or for apartments designed 'in general', and not 'in particular' for a wheelchair user.

Systems are available that adjust the countertop height at the touch of a button, or at the turn of a crank. Cheaper systems require longer to adjust, but will be acceptable if the adjustment required is infrequent. Screw jack-type legs can be used on a straight counter, or U-shaped counter if the arms of the U are short. These jacks will require adjustment a few turns at a time in rotation. If a straight counter is used, adjustable table legs, or adjustments into solid ends can be used.

If a counter is adjustable, the plumbing from the sink must be flexible.

The depth of the countertop can be increased for those who must store items at the back of the counter, or for tall people who require foot room.

Lighting

Well placed and adequate lighting, including light from windows and skylights, can reduce fatigue and make a kitchen look cheerful. Switches must be within reach and operated by touch or lever.

Laundry

Washer and dryer should be accessible and have the controls within reach. A front-opening washer and dryer is ideal. Some makes of stacker washers and dryers used unstacked, side-by-side are very convenient for a wheelchair user.

422

Organization

The disabled homemaker cannot afford to be disorganized, because of the effort and time required for every task.

When planning, the tasks to be done should be divided into preparation, performance, and cleanup. Time is saved if all ingredients and utensils are brought to the cooking area in the fewest possible trips. Cleanup is easier if the minimum number of utensils is used, and if preparation is done close to the cleanup area. Performance is often easier if labor saving appliances can be used. All moves should be planned to save time and energy.

The kitchen areas should be organized so that minimal travel is required while doing any task. For instance, pots can be stored near the sink, or an urn of water may be stored near the burners. Extra utensils may be obtained so that duplicates may be used in more than one area, rather than carrying the one utensil to and fro.

The disabled cook may find it frustrating that tasks now take longer. Time must be taken to plan ahead so that some heavier jobs can be spread over several days, and others must be started earlier to avoid a disorganizing and frustrating rush.

Planning the daily routine needs will help in energy conservation; for instance, it is useful to plan for any assistant time, so that all the tasks required can be foreseen and completed while the assistant is available. Some jobs are best done by another member of the family or by paid help, and this is a good method of energy conservation. It can be very hard to ask for this help; but an effective way of asking for it is a valuable skill.

It is particularly important for those who have homemakers to learn to work with an employee (Fig. 11-18). Some people are diffident about asking for jobs to be done, or do not know what to do if they are unhappy with the standard of work. Many people have never been in a position of employing someone, and so have never acquired management skills. They may need assistance or training so that they can feel comfortable in this role.

Labor saving by eliminating tasks may call for adaptability and some thinking on the part of the disabled homemaker and the family. For instance, the home-

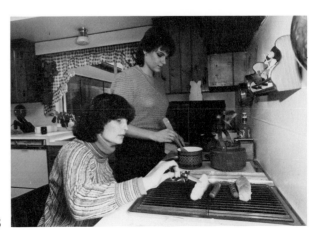

FIGURE 11-18

maker may wish to eliminate the chore of peeling potatoes, but if there is a family to cook for, they must cooperate with the decision. Sometimes if the family is asked to help solve the problem, members will have excellent ideas, and will be more willing to cooperate.

Cutting down the number of times a task is done is another excellent labor and energy saver. An example is the use of a continental quilt to save daily bed-making, or perhaps the meticulous housecleaner may reduce the frequency of cleaning slightly.

Many shortcuts or energy savers do not involve anything more than good planning. Many meals can be made in bulk and frozen for future use, or mixing bowls or cooking utensils can be used for several similar dishes without being washed between times.

Prepared packaged meals are usually more expensive than home-cooked meals, but can save a great deal of time and energy. They are sometimes not as tasty as home-cooked dish, but cooks must decide which is more important, their time and energy, or their pocketbooks and their families' tastes.

Safety

The cook who cannot distinguish hot or cold must take great care when handling hot utensils. Some quadriplegic patients seem more sensitive to heat than is normal, and blister after touching almost tepid objects. Oven mitts should be worn when handling hot objects, and should be checked often for worn spots and wet areas. They may be adapted to be worn over a flexor-hinge splint. This is done by splitting them longitudinally over the leverage mechanism and rebinding the edges.

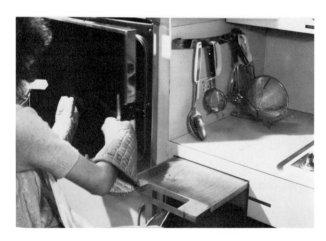

FIGURE 11-19

Extra-long oven mitts can be obtained, and provide good protection for the arms (Fig. 11-19).

A waterproof apron should be worn when handling hot items. Safety aprons are available which are large enough to cover a person seated in a wheelchair, so that there is protection if hot liquids are spilt.

Hot items must never be carried directly on or between the knees. A lap tray or trolley cart should be used.

Fire. A suitable fire extinguisher adapted for easy use should be kept in the kitchen. A handily-placed opened box of bicarbonate of soda is also useful for damping small fires, such as a fire in a frypan.

COOKING METHODS

Cutting

Knives with sawing blades or sharp slicing blades may be used. They will usually need handle adaptations for holding or for modifying the angle of cutting.

Use of food processors will save time and energy. The ability to operate the machine and wash it must be checked out. Features are changed from time to time, and such changes do not always make the machine easier for a disabled person to use.

Used utensils or sharp knives may be placed in the pocket of a splint safely by folding a paper towel over the working end of the utensil (Fig. 11-20).

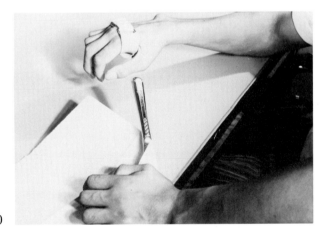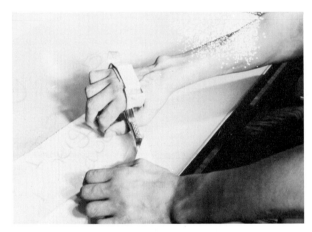

FIGURE 11-20

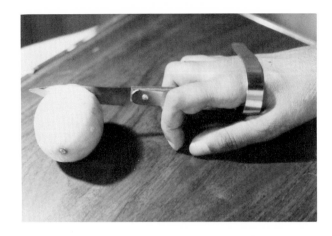

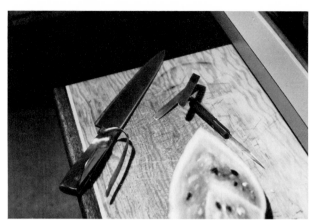

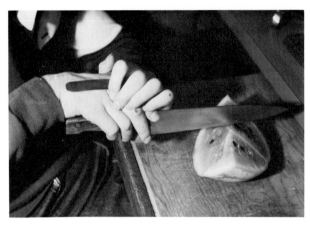

FIGURE 11-21

The angle of this paring knife has been found to be very useful by many people (Fig. 11-21). Since the weight of the hand is the main power, the knife must be kept very sharp.

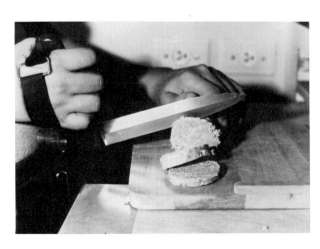

FIGURE 11-22

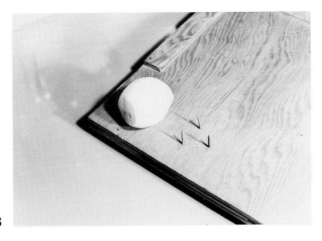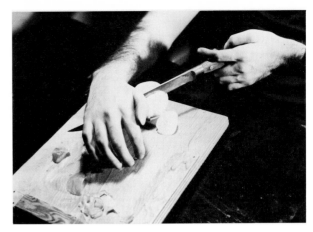

FIGURE 11-23

The upright knife handle allows a very natural and comfortable hand position (Fig. 11-22).

A cutting board with galvanized or stainless steel nails protruding up through it may be used to impale vegetables and similar items, freeing both hands (Fig. 11-23). The board is held in place with suction cups or a nonslip pad. A small rim on two sides of the board may be useful for wedging food, for instance, as when buttering bread.

Another type of functional cutting board may be made by drilling the tip of a sharp knife and bolting it to the cutting board between two corner brackets. This forms a fulcrum so that very little pressure is required to slice food (Fig. 11-24).

A swivel in conjunction with stainless steel nails on a cutting board gives good leverage and control (Fig. 11-25). A person who has no wrist extension as well as those who have this advantage can slice effectively if the knife is sharp.

An appliance to slice or shred can be most useful (Fig. 11-26). Such appliances should be tested to make sure that the cutters can be removed, that bowls are not too heavy for lifting and that the appliance can be assembled and taken apart for easy cleaning.

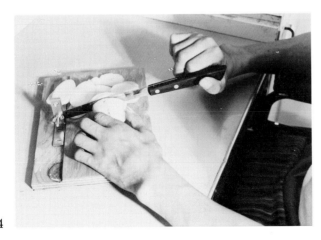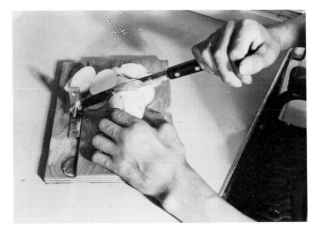

FIGURE 11-24

427

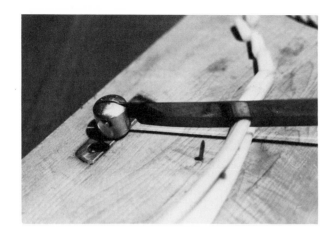

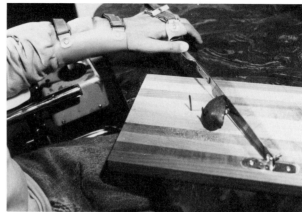

FIGURE 11-25

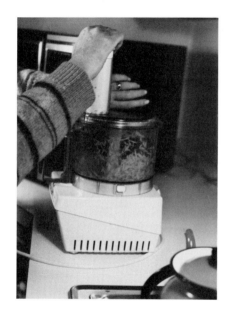

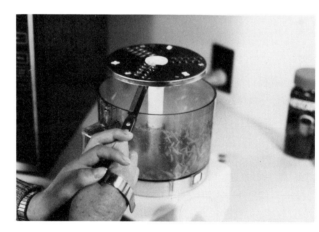

FIGURE 11-26

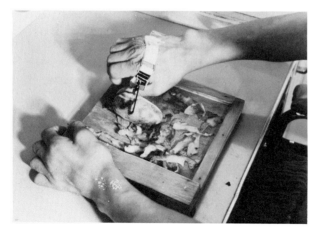

FIGURE 11-27

428

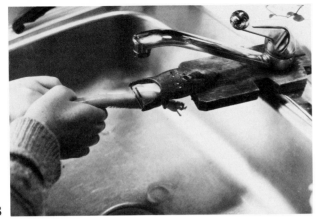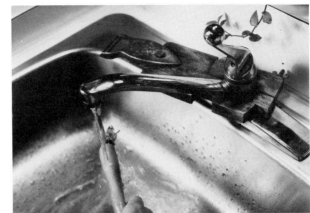

FIGURE 11-28

Peeling

Vegetables can often be scrubbed and left unpeeled. A scrub brush on suction cups may be useful for this. If vegetables must be peeled a choice may be made to fix the vegetable down, or to fix the peeler.

In Figure 11-27 the potato is impaled on stainless steel nails on a cutting board, and the peeler is held in a suitably adapted holder. The board may be placed on a nonstick mat, or suction cups or a clamp may be used. An advantage of this method is that vegetables may also be held easily for slicing.

In Figure 11-28 a swing-away peeler is used and the vegetable is drawn under it. This peeler is more suitable for longer, easily held vegetables such as carrots or parsnips, and the former (see Fig. 11-27) may be more easily used for large, awkward vegetables such as large turnips, swedes, or rutabagas.

Pouring and Draining

A kettle or teapot tipper may be used with oven mitts or a cloth (Fig. 11-29). The cook shown in Figure 11-30 pours by resting the plastic base of an elec-

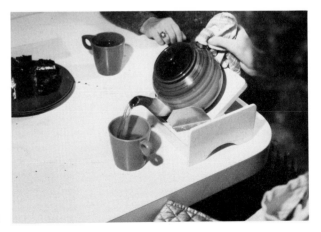

FIGURE 11-29

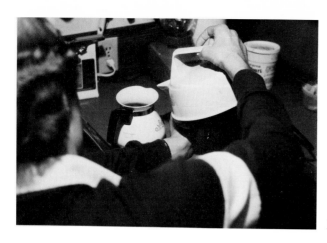

FIGURE 11-30

tric kettle on his bare hand, and has done this for several years with no ill effect. It is recommended that a person with good sensation test the kettle for heat before this method is used by a person with anaesthesia. This method must never be tried with metal kettles or with a kettle that drips.

A person who uses a great deal of hot water may find an urn safe and convenient (Fig. 11-31A). The smaller, press-down top dispenser can also be convenient, but requires a higher reach (Fig. 11-31B).

Pots and pans should have large handles, double handles, bail handles (see Fig. 11-13) or loop handles (Fig. 11-32). A small bailer or ladle can be used to substitute for pouring when the pot cannot be lifted.

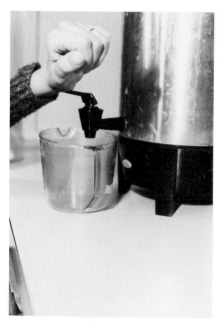

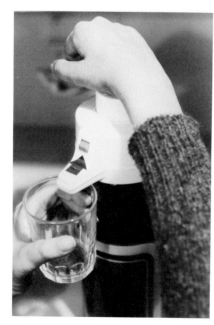

FIGURE 11-31 A   B

430

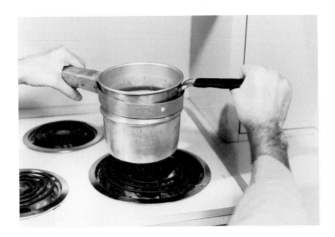

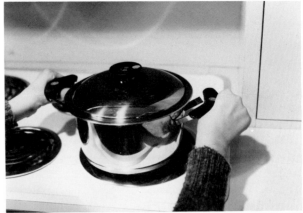

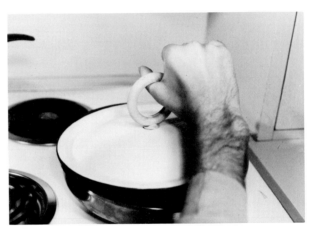

FIGURE 11-32

Vegetables that must be drained can be cooked in a sieve or steamer ready to be lifted out of the pot (Fig. 11-33).

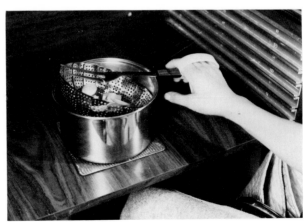

FIGURE 11-33

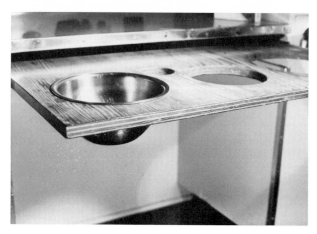

FIGURE 11-34

Mixing

A lower counter is frequently easier to mix on, for both disabled and able-bodied cooks. Since disabled cooks usually need to stabilize bowls also, a good solution is to use the cut out area in a pullout board, which both lowers and stabilizes a bowl (Fig. 11-34). Some carpenters cut the hole with a sloped edge so that a fitted lid can be placed over the hole when it is not needed. The lid can be pushed out from below. This creates more working area, but can harbor food scraps if not well cleaned.

Mixing bowls can be obtained with handles and with nonskid bases. Metal or plastic bowls that can be drilled and riveted may be adapted with a handle. Non-slip mats are also useful.

Tools for mixing may require adapted handles, and electric beaters, hand held or in a stand may be useful (Fig. 11-35). The cook should test that the beaters can be inserted and ejected before deciding to purchase a particular model.

When emptying a mixing bowl it is sometimes impossible to hold it and

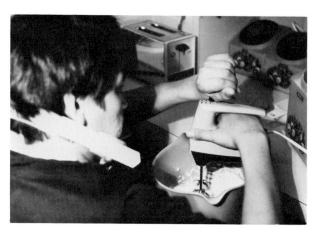

FIGURE 11-35

scrape at the same time. A hole may be drilled near the edge of the bowl and the full bowl hung from a heavy cup hook (Fig. 11-36). If more stabilization is required, two holes and two cup hooks may be used.

When hot items are mixed, nonstick type pans may be useful because many quadriplegics are unable to stir fast enough to prevent sticking.

Opening Containers

Opening packages, cans, jars, and frozen food cardboard cans can be an exercise in coping with frustration, particularly if they contain the prepared, low-effort food recommended to save energy.

Many of the methods worked out by or for one-handed people can be used by the quadriplegic cook. Once a utensil or package is stabilized, two hands are free to work.

Jars. Lids can sometimes be made easier to open by standing the jar in cold water while hot water is run onto the lid to expand it. A sharp tap on the lid in the opening direction may also help to loosen it.

The jar may be placed on a nonslip pad to leave two hands free to turn the lid (Fig. 11-37).

A second nonslip pad may be used to hold the lid (Fig. 11-38).

A wedge box lined with nonslip padding at the sides and base gives good purchase (Fig. 11-39). Emptying packages into jars with easy opening lids, or having a helper loosen all jars in advance may be the solution; particularly if child proof lids are used, as these often prove to be adult proof also.

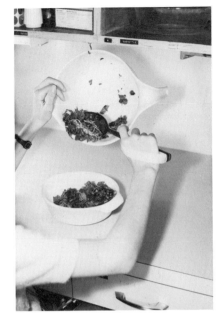

FIGURE 11-36

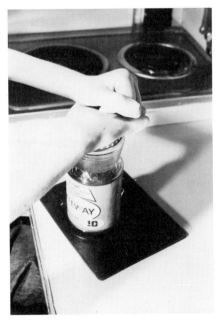

FIGURE 11-37

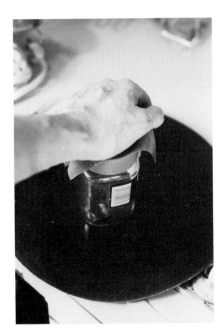

FIGURE 11-38

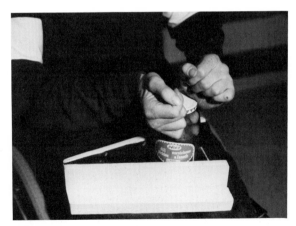

FIGURE 11-39

433

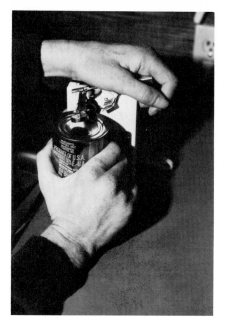

FIGURE 11-40

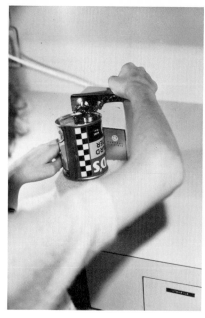

FIGURE 11-41

Cans. Cans may be held using tenodesis (Fig. 11-40), or they may be rested on sponges to bring the can to the right height. The springiness of the sponges helps to keep the can in place (Fig. 11-41).

Boxes and Packages. Cardboard boxes can often be opened using a sharp knife. A series of careful stabs with the point will make a perforation that can be cut or torn more easily.

Some larger boxes can be stabilized for opening by placing them in a drawer that is held closed against the box by wheeling against it.

Using leverage rather than a direct cut can make it easier to slice cardboard

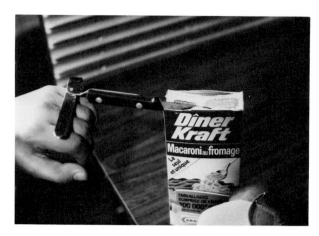

FIGURE 11-42

434

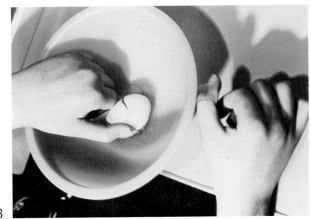

FIGURE 11-43

(Fig. 11-42). A saw type knife edge requires less pressure than a sharp knife, and works well on some types of cardboard.

Bottles. Bottle openers may be stabilized so that both hands can be used to hold the article. For instance, pop bottle openers can be fastened to the wall. Bottle openers or can openers with handles can also be lengthened for greater leverage.

Breaking Eggs

Eggs may be broken open by dropping them from about 12 inches (30 cm) above the pan (Fig. 11-43) and picking out the eggshell.

A sharp tap with a knife on the side of the egg will cut the shell sufficiently to allow the knife tip to be inserted (Fig. 11-44). The shell may be levered open slowly so that, if desired, the yolk may be separated.

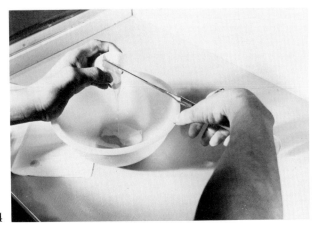 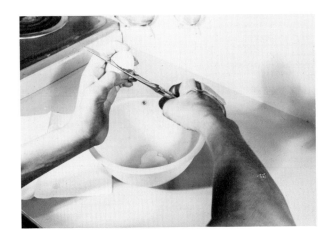

FIGURE 11-44

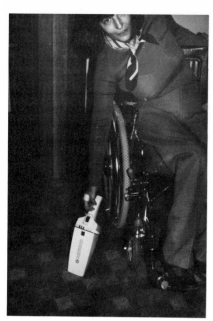

FIGURE 11-45

Cleaning Up

Much cleaning can be avoided or minimized by careful selection of appliances and surfaces. If finances permit, easily cleaned nonwax flooring, a self-cleaning oven, frostless refrigerator, nonstick pans, and wipe-down counters will save a great deal of time and effort, and will eliminate the need to employ someone to do this cleaning.

Vacuuming and Sweeping. A quadriplegic homemaker who does some cleaning usually finds that a central vacuum system with a wall socket is convenient, and saves dragging a vacuum cleaner around.

A small, hand-held vacuum is adaptable for the homemaker with some wrist extension who cannot manage a bigger vacuum. This type of vacuum is also useful for the lower-lesion homemaker, for small clean up jobs (Fig. 11-45). Cleaning under furniture may be eased if a flexibly handled mop is used, but moving furniture and doing thorough cleaning is beyond the physical capabilities of the complete lesion quadriplegic person.

Picking Things Up from the Floor. Scissor-type pickup sticks are useful for those who have balance and control adequate to use two hands. A magnet may be stapled to one blade to pick up small metal objects. Barbeque tools, both spatula and fork, are useful depending on what is to be picked up.

Mops with flexible handles can be useful to recover objects that have rolled under furniture.

Shopping

Phone-in shopping with delivery service is effortless, and is available in some areas. In many cases a store will make a special effort to accommodate a disabled customer, to pick up and deliver goods, or to assist the customer in the store.

The main shopping problems are transport and access to the store, reaching items required, transport of groceries, access to the cashier, and handling money.

Some of these problems may be solved by asking for help, by using stores that are accessible, or that will adapt their layout for disabled customers. Wheelchair bags are generally not large enough for groceries, but a basket may be held on the lap. A purse or wallet on a chain may be pulled out of a pocket easily for the cashier to sort.

USEFUL REFERENCES AND AIDS

American Heart Association; The Heart of the Home, 44 East 23rd Street, New York 10, New York. (Has useful ideas for energy saving and organization. General, not specifically for people in wheelchairs.)

BLAKESLEE, ME: The Wheelchair Gourmet, General Publishing Co. Limited, Don Mills, Ontario, 1981. (Many excellent tips for cooking from a wheelchair.)

Kinger, J: Mealtime Manual for People with Disabilities and the Aging, Institute of Rehabilitation Medicine, New York University Medical Center, and Campbell

Soup Company, 1978. (An invaluable book with many ideas and excellent illustrations. Highly recommended for excellent ideas, recipes and easy reading.)

McCullock, HE and Farnham, MB: Kitchens for Women in Wheelchairs, University of Illinois, College of Agriculture, Extension Service in Agriculture and Home Economics, Circular 841, 1961. (Much useful information and ideas for storage.)

Wheeler, HW: Planning Kitchens for Handicapped Homemakers. Rehabilitation Monograph XXVII. The Institute of Physical Medicine and Rehabilitation, New York University Medical Center, New York, 1965.

Small Kitchen Appliances and the Disabled, Manitoba Hydro Customer Service, 1983. (Useful information—plans are made to keep the information up to date.)

Homemaker with Weak Upper Extremities. (M-2241-X) 28 min. color film. Media Resources Branch, National Medical Audiovisual Center. Station K, Atlanta, Georgia, 30324, 1971. (Demonstrates meal preparation activities, kitchen planning and selection of equipment for use by quadriplegic people. Focuses on a college-age quadriplegic who lives independently in his own apartment. Also demonstrates car transfer and driving skills.)

12

Car Transfers and Driving

CAR TRANSFERS

EQUIPMENT

A bridgeboard is usually needed in car transfers. Such boards may be of different types.

A rectangular bridgeboard, 10 inches by 30 inches (25.40 cm by 76.20 cm), may be made of ¼-inch (.635 cm) tempered hardboard, beveled at the ends and with all edges rounded (Fig. 12-1). The only finish required is polish, which may be either a good car polish or talcum powder, or both.

A tempered hardboard bridgeboard is rounded at the ends to make it easy to slide under the buttocks and is shaped for the individual's car (Fig. 12-2).

These boards are light and easy to handle, and can accommodate differences in height between wheelchair and car seat. Note that untempered hardboard is not strong enough for any but the lightest individuals. If tempered hardboard cannot be obtained, a stainless-steel board may be substituted, but care must be taken that the edges have a slight downward curve to protect the skin from dam-

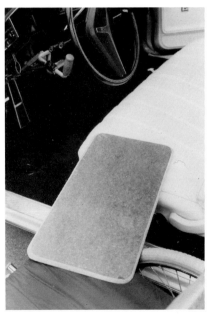

FIGURE 12-1

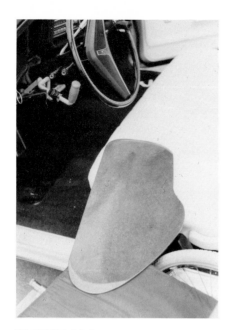

FIGURE 12-2

age. If the person is prone to pressure areas on the buttocks, padded transfer boards should be used.

A rectangular bridgeboard may be made of 3/8-inch (.95 cm) plywood cut to 10 inches (25.40 cm) by 30 inches (76.20 cm) with the edges beveled and sanded. The top surface and the edges are padded with 1/4-inch (.64 cm) foam rubber and covered with nylon material (Fig. 12-3A). Nonslip matting may be applied to the undersurface at either end (Fig. 12-3B).

A bridgeboard with a post and flange to fit into the front wheelchair arm socket and a cutout to accommodate the wheel of the wheelchair, overlaps both wheelchair cushion and car seat. It may be made of unpadded, tempered hardboard or it may be 3/8-inch (.95 cm) plywood with the edges chamfered; the board is padded with 1/4-inch (.64 cm) foam and nylon covered. This board should be only lightly padded or it will create a high ridge to slide over, since it does not abut to the seats. The floor flange is fastened to the board with countersunk flathead bolts (Fig. 12-4A). The part of the pipe that has not been machined down acts as a stop, which regulates the height of the bridgeboard. The machined part should be short enough so that it does not extend below the wheelchair arm socket. The board, when in position, extends about 2 inches (5.08 cm) over the wheelchair cushion, and about 4 inches (10.16 cm) on to the car seat, depressing both slightly (Fig. 12-4B).

A very stable bridgeboard, similar to the previous board, including the projection fitting into the wheelchair arm socket, has a leg by the front corner of the car seat, which extends from the bridgebord to the car floor, and another leg projecting down from the back corner of the bridgeboard, resting on the doorsill.

The palette-shaped bridgeboard is made of 1/2-inch (1.27 cm) plywood, the

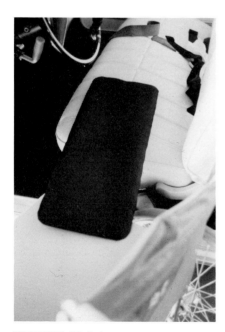

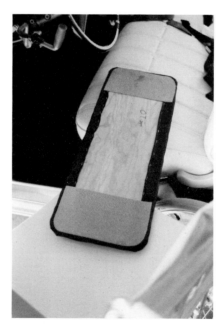

FIGURE 12-3 A   B

440

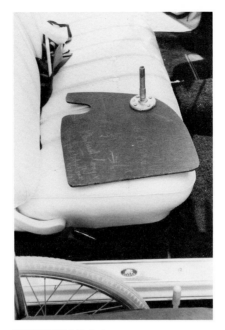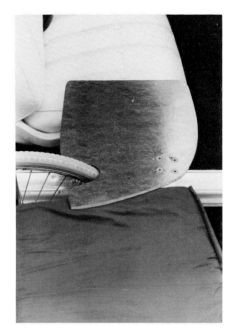

FIGURE 12-4 A   B

edges of which are chamfered and smoothed. A length of ³/₄-inch (1.91 cm) pipe is machined to fit into the front wheelchair arm socket and is threaded into a floor flange (Fig. 12-5). The position of the floor flange on the underside of the board is determined by placing the board between wheelchair and car and placing the

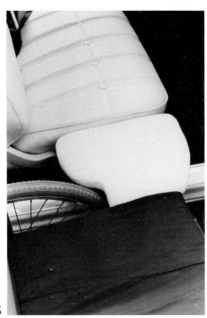

FIGURE 12-5

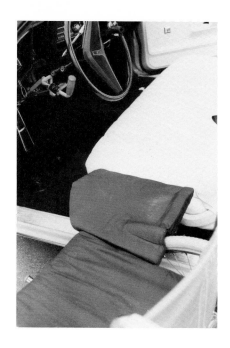

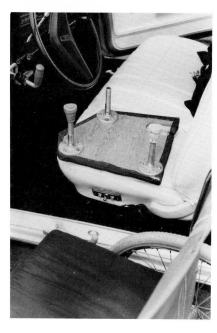

FIGURE 12-6

pipe in the wheelchair arm socket. Another floor flange and pipe are placed as a leg to the floor of the car to provide stability. This board may be padded and covered.

The board can be padded and nylon covered, with an extra roll of padding at the rear to prevent the patient from sliding off the back of the board. This board

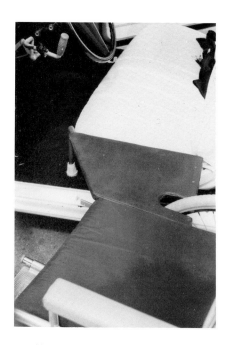

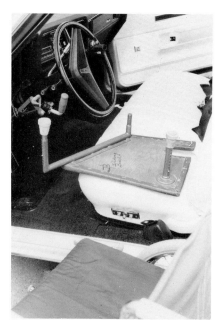

FIGURE 12-7

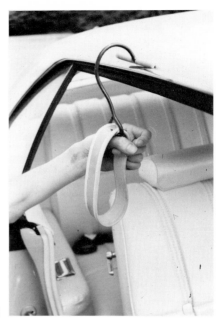

FIGURE 12-8

does not project over either car seat or wheelchair cushion; it abuts on both. The board should extend from the front edge of the wheelchair seat to the front edge of the car seat (Fig. 12-6).

Different makes of cars may necessitate some modification of design (Fig. 12-7).

An overhead strap may be required. It may be permanently fixed to the ceiling of the car or detachable, with a hook which will fit into the guttering over the car door (Fig. 12-8).

Bridgeboards and car seats may be sprayed with silicone or dusted with talc to facilitate sliding. The type of clothing worn and the type of seat covering must be taken into consideration. While the patient is first learning transfers, a synthetic and cotton-mix material for pants, or a nylon material which will move with the patient, can be effective to reduce friction. A hard nylon fabric is preferable for car seats, since vinyl tends to become sticky and plush-type material tends to cling.

CHAIR TO CAR

It is often easier to transfer on the driver's side so that the steering wheel may be utilized as an aid for pulling.

Quadriplegic individuals use parking lots whenever feasible to eliminate variations in levels. However, if street parking must be used, it is safer to use the curbside door.

In all transfers the patient opens the car door and wheels his chair as close to the seat as possible, turning the front of his chair towards the car at about 30°. He applies the brakes and removes the wheelchair arm nearest the car.

443

Method 1. (Fig. 12-9)   The patient who is able to do a pushup will probably use no sliding board. He places his feet in the car before transferring because he gains a mechanical advantage as he flexes his trunk forward, placing a significant amount of weight on his feet. To transfer, he places his hands well back, one on the chair and one on the car seat. Flexing his trunk forwards, he depresses and flexes his shoulders and twists his upper trunk away from the car to pivot onto the seat.

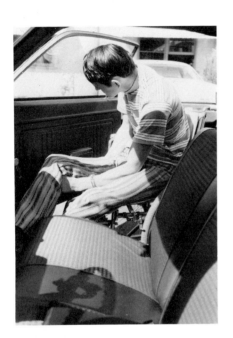
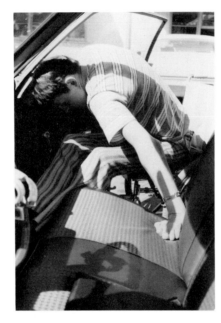
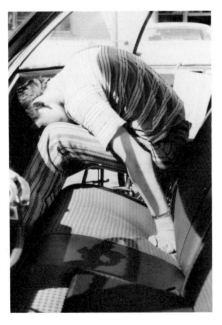
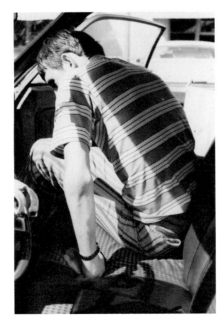

FIGURE 12-9

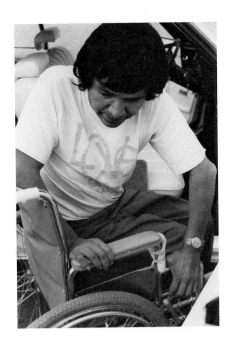 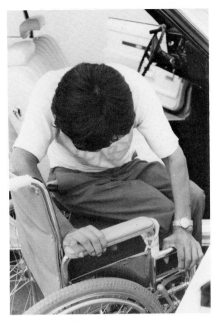 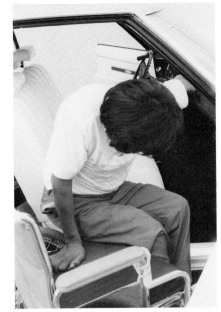

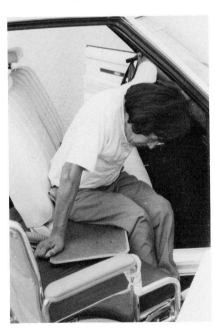 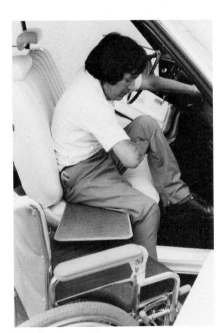

FIGURE 12-10

Method 2. (Fig. 12-10)   The bridgeboard is placed in position first; then the patient turns away from the car and places both hands against the chair arm rest or on the cushion against the chair arm. He leans away from the car, pushing himself backwards towards the car, using his shoulder and elbow flexors. He repositions his hands, one on the dashboard or on the door, and the other hand close to his buttock. He leans towards the chair and pushes his buttocks onto the car seat. He now lifts his legs into the car.

445

Method 3. (Fig. 12-11) The patient leans away from the car to insert the sliding board well underneath his buttocks, with the other end resting on the car seat. He shifts forward in the chair and lifts both feet into the car. He must place his feet so that his knees will flex when he transfers, or he may find that he is blocked by a knee locked in extension. He leans on one elbow on the car seat and hooks the other wrist through the steering wheel. He pulls with both arms to slide

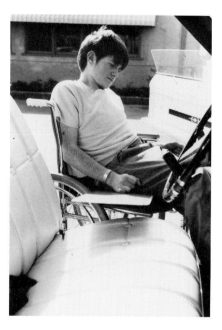
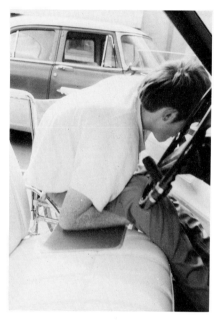
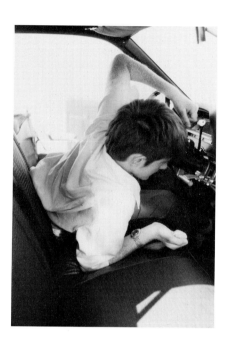
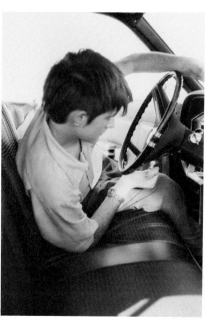
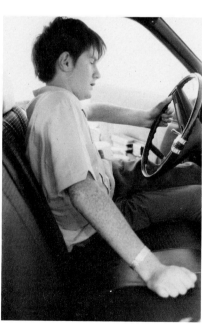

FIGURE 12-11

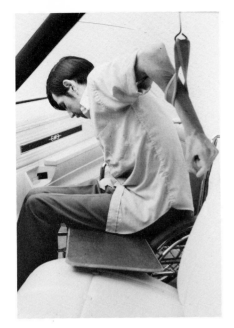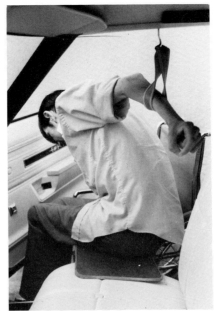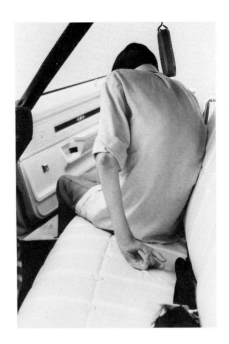

FIGURE 12-12

onto the car seat. He pulls himself partially upright with the arm near the chair, using the steering wheel or the doorframe; this enables him to lock his other elbow and stabilize his position.

Method 4. (Fig. 12-12)   The patient leans away from the car to place the bridgeboard in position. He hooks his sling into the car roof gutter and places his forearm in it to maintain balance while he leans away from the car again. He places his thumb web against the front upright of the chair arm, pushing strongly with this arm while the arm in the sling is internally rotated to pull and swivel him into the car. He then lifts his legs into the car.

CAR TO WHEELCHAIR

Some patients will not be able to turn the castors of the wheelchair forward, and must transfer being careful not to put too much weight onto the footrests. The door of the car will block the front of the chair and increase stability.

Foot Position

The feet may be lifted onto the footrests at the beginning or the end of the transfer, or one foot only may be lifted out before transfer. The latter is the most common method because it can help to lever the patient towards the chair by blocking the calf against the doorsill when the trunk is rotated. Balance may be easier in this position because of the wide base and the elimination of a position which could trigger spasm.

The patient who places both feet on the footrests before transfer may do so because he has long legs that can be difficult to move under the controls when

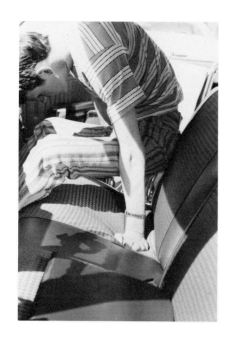
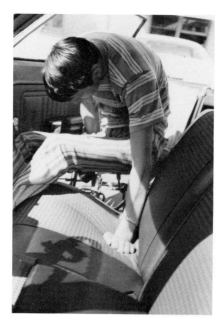

FIGURE 12-13

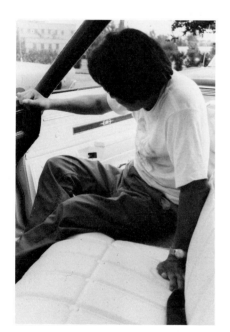
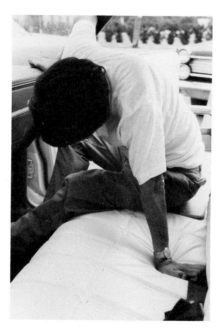
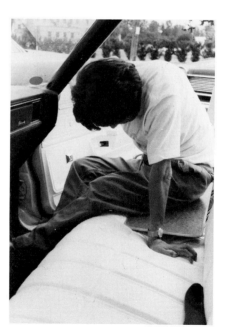

FIGURE 12-14

448

transferring. He may be a patient who has tight hamstrings or one with flexor spasms that could pull him forward off the seat of the chair if he leaves his feet inside the car.

Method 1. (Fig. 12-13) The patient who is able to do a pushup will probably use no sliding board after he has mastered this technique. His feet remain in the car while he places his hands, one on the car seat close to his buttocks, and one on the chair seat as far away as possible. He flexes his trunk forward and pushes up with his arms while he turns his upper trunk toward the car to pivot onto the chair seat.

Method 2. (Fig. 12-14) The patient places his bridgeboard in position. He places one hand on the dashboard and one hand on the car seat and flexes his trunk forward. This movement helps to pivot him as he pushes himself backward out of the car.

Method 3. (Fig. 12-15) The patient leans away from the chair to place one end of the bridgeboard underneath him with the other end resting on the wheelchair. He places the hand furthest from the chair by his buttock and locks the elbow. The other hand is placed on the dashboard or the wheel to maintain balance and to assist him to twist his trunk away from the chair. He throws his weight over the locked arm and flexes the shoulder of that arm strongly. Simultaneously, the shoulder of the arm nearest the chair is internally rotated, bringing the elbow up, permitting strong elbow flexion and shoulder adduction to push the patient towards the chair. At the halfway point the hand near the chair may be moved to the door windowsill to gain new purchase.

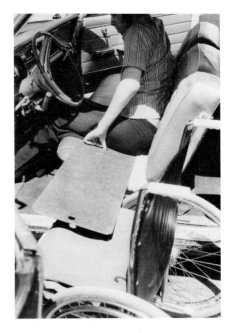

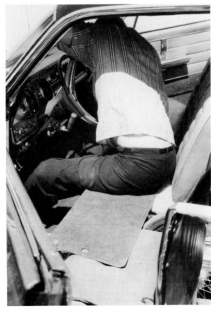
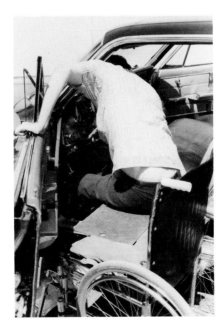
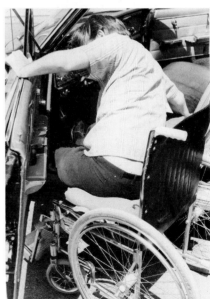

FIGURE 12-15

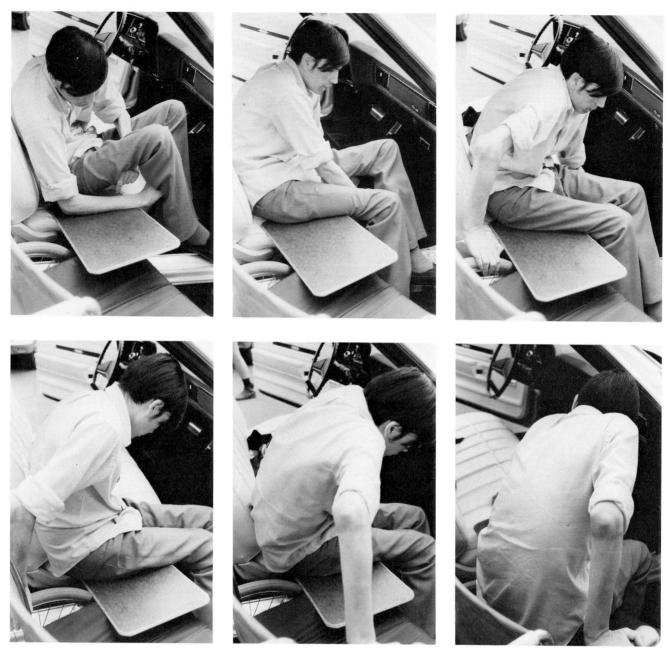

FIGURE 12-16

Method 4. (Fig. 12-16)   The patient places his bridgeboard in position and lifts his feet onto the footrests of the chair. Since his legs are blocked by the doorsill of the car, they act as a fulcrum to assist him to pivot out of the car. He flexes his trunk forward and places one hand on the chair wheel or back and the other on the car seat close to his buttock. He externally rotates the shoulder nearest the car and flexes and abducts it to push. His arm on the chair is internally rotated and adducts to pull him towards the chair.

450

Method 5. (Fig. 12-17)   The patient lifts both feet out of the car and places the forearm nearest the chair in the overhead strap. He leans away from the wheelchair and places his elbow on the car seat, relieving some of the weight from his buttocks. A combination of a pull with the arm in the strap and a push with the arm on the car seat will twist and lever him towards the chair. He sits himself

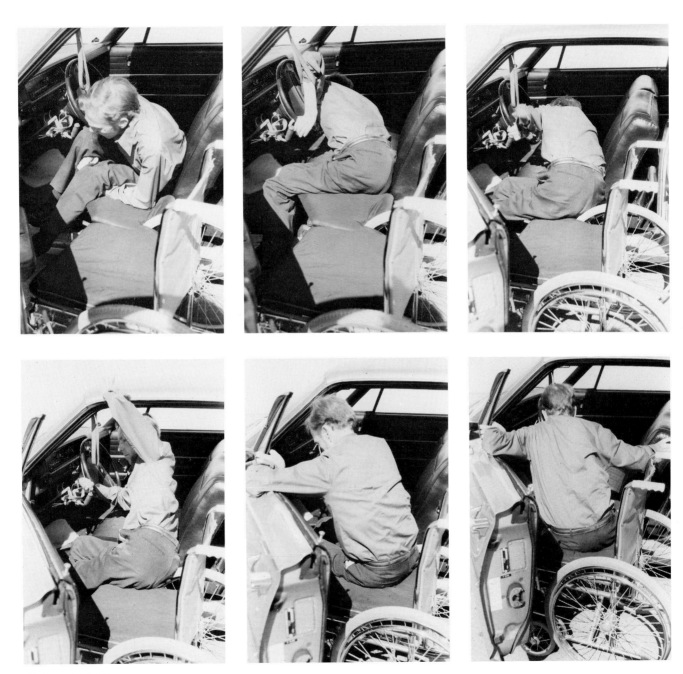

FIGURE 12-17

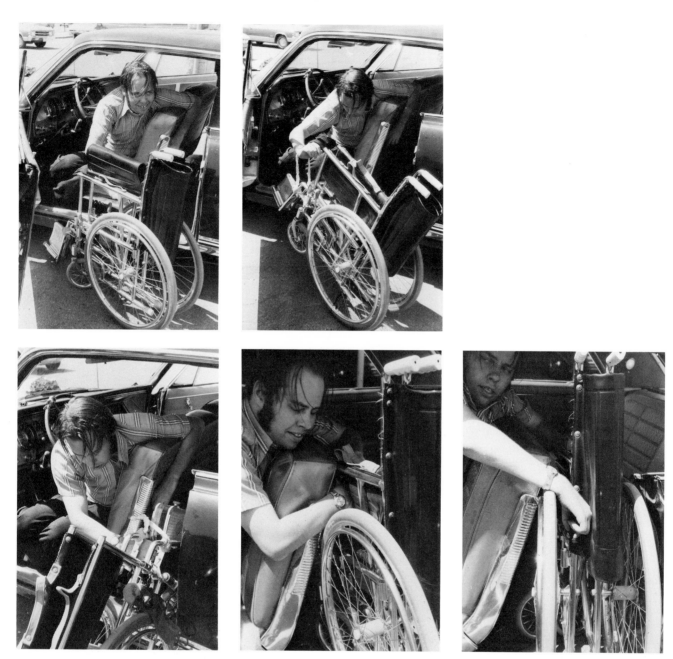

FIGURE 12-18

up by either pulling on the strap, or hooking a wrist around the wing window frame, the front door post, or the roof of the car. He completes his transfer by placing a hand against the wing window frame and the other against the side of the car seat. When he flexes his trunk and pushes with both arms, his buttocks are moved back onto the chair.

LOADING THE WHEELCHAIR INTO THE CAR

It is almost impossible for a quadriplegic person to load a wheelchair into the back of a four-door car because of the interference of the center post. Therefore, directions are given for loading the wheelchair behind the driver in a two-door car or beside the driver in a two- or four-door car.

Loading the Wheelchair Behind the Driver in a Two-Door Car

To facilitate loading and unloading the wheelchair, the well between the doorsill and the drive shaft housing can be filled in with plywood to within ¾-inch (1.9 cm) of the top of the doorsill. The slight drop at the doorsill prevents the chair from rolling away when loading and unloading the chair.

The quadriplegic driver first removes the bridgeboard and places it and the cushion beside him. He then leans over and releases the wheelchair brake on the side nearest him, enabling him to swing the chair around so that it faces him. He unlocks the other brake, swings his footrests up and places his wrist under the chair seat and lifts it to fold the chair (Fig. 12-18). He now lines the chair up with the gap between the car seat back and the doorjamb. He leans over and hooks his wrist under the leg strap of the chair to lift the front wheels of the chair over the sill. In a car with a split seatback, he may move over toward the other side and tip the seatback forward to allow more room for the wheelchair. In a car with electrically controlled seats he need only move them into the forward position. He leans toward the chair over the seatback and catches the leg strap again. By pulling and leaning back, he rolls the chair into the car. He then moves back into the driver's seat and shuts the door.

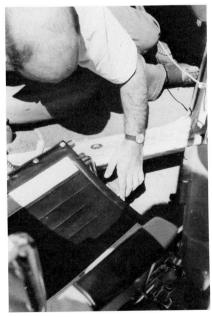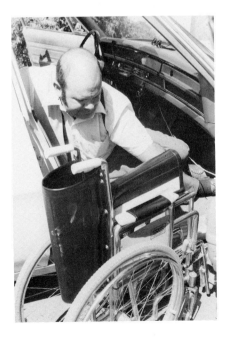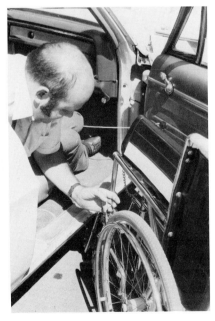

FIGURE 12-19

453

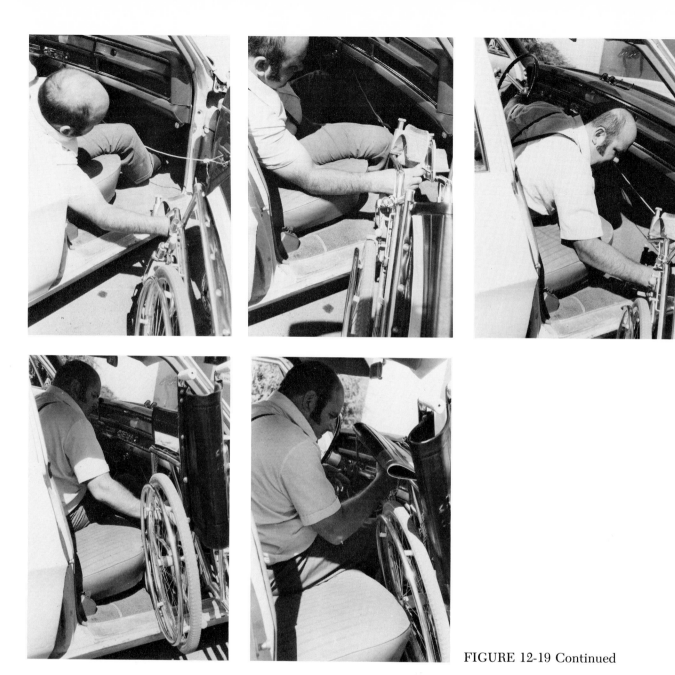

FIGURE 12-19 Continued

Loading the Wheelchair Beside the Driver in a Two- or Four-Door Car

The person who enters the car from the curb side may place his chair behind the front seat as described, or he may place it on the floor beside him.

Having transferred into the car, the quadriplegic driver maintains balance with his right arm over the seatback while he hooks his left wrist under the

454

wheelchair seat and raises it to fold the chair. He maneuvers the chair so that it faces him (Fig. 12-19). He now releases the chair seat and disengages the brakes. He moves himself further into the car and reaches down with his right arm to the leg strap or chair-front upright to lift the front wheels of the chair onto the doorsill. He moves toward the driver's side and maintains balance with his left arm on the steering wheel, or over the seat back. He then leans down to hook his forearm behind the front chair upright, so that when he pulls himself erect with his left arm and pulls on the chair with his right arm, the chair rolls into the car. A long cord, permanently fastened to the door and conveniently placed on the dashboard, will enable him to close the door.

Unloading the Wheelchair from the Two-Door Car

The driver opens the car door and slides onto the other seat in order to pull the seat back forwards or he moves an electrically operated seat forwards (Fig. 12-20). He leans over the seatback and pushes the chair out carefully until the back wheels are on the ground and the front castors are hooked over the doorsill. The chair remains in this position while he moves across toward the door. He reaches around the seatback and places his wrist under the closest seat rail. As he lifts the chair so that the castors clear the doorsill, the chair will start to open as it is rolled back. This lessens the danger of the chair tipping over. As he lowers the chair he swings the front towards himself. He pushes down on the seat rail nearest him, partly opening the chair, and then puts on the far brake while it is still within reach. This will not prevent his maneuvering the chair, which he does by pushing

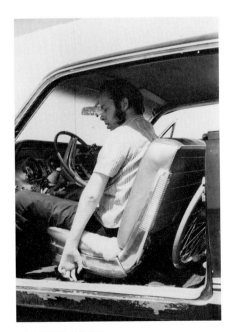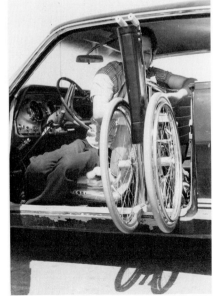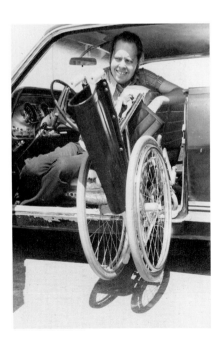

FIGURE 12-20

455

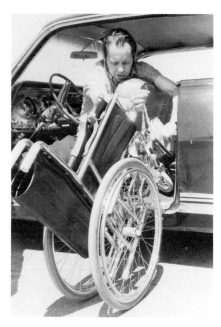 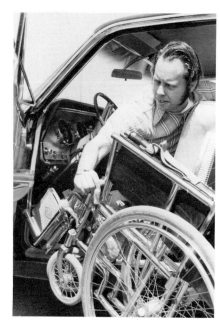 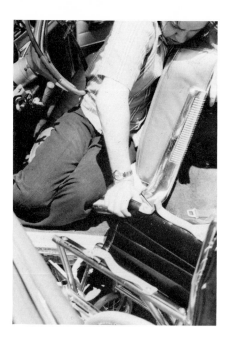

FIGURE 12-20 Continued

again on the rail nearest him and jiggling the chair into position. He then applies the near brake and puts the cushion and bridgeboard in place.

Unloading the Wheelchair From Beside the Driver

The person leans across and opens the door. He maintains balance with the arm near the chair over the back of the car seat, a position which allows him to push against the chair front with the other arm (Fig. 12-21). When the chair is balanced on the doorsill, he moves over towards the door. He now stabilizes himself by placing the arm near the driver's side on the dashboard or by hooking it through the steering wheel. The other arm controls the chair while the back wheels are lowered to the ground. He changes arms once again and places the arm near the chair over the car seatback while the other arm lowers the front castors. The chair is opened by pushing down and jiggling a seat rail; it is worked into position for transfer. The changes of arm position are necessary to secure a strong and stable hugging action throughout the maneuver.

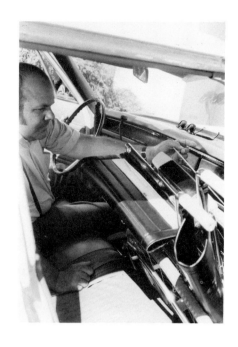 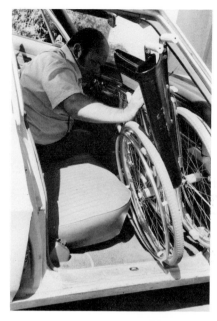 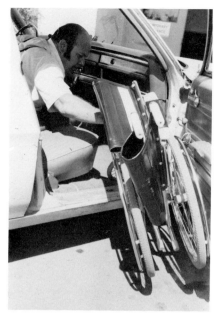

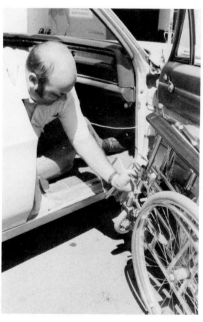 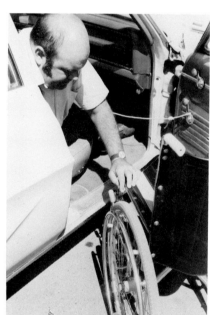

FIGURE 12-21

457

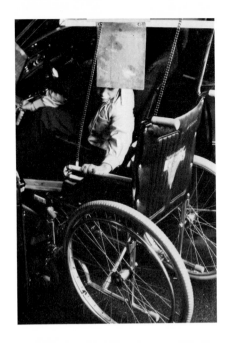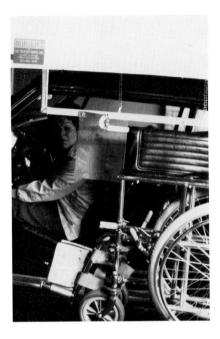

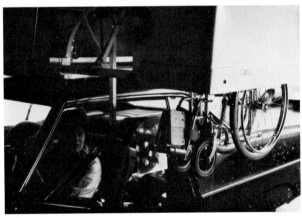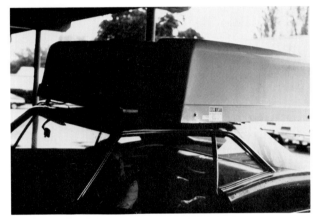

FIGURE 12-22

Loading a Wheelchair Using Apparatus

A patient may use a mechanical hoist to load the wheelchair into a car top luggage holder (Fig. 12-22). She removes the cushion and activates the mechanism to lower the hook and chains. She swings the hook so that it catches under the fabric of the wheelchair seat. She activates the "up" switch, and the wheelchair is automatically folded and hoisted up into the box. When closed, the box is weatherproof.

When unloading the wheelchair, the only difficulty may be in unfolding the wheelchair.

The Patient Who Cannot Load His Wheelchair

Using two wheelchairs is a satisfactory solution for the patient who drives himself to work. One chair is used at home and one at the office. If there is a carport, he can leave his chair in position and back up to it with the car door open when he returns. If there is no carport, there should be no problem in having the chair delivered to him on arrival. If the patient can afford only one chair, someone else must load and unload it for him.

DRIVING

The person who must rely on public transport will find that its accessibility for a person in a wheelchair varies greatly depending on geographical location. In one area, transportation may be unobtainable, in another, transportation must be booked days or weeks ahead, and in some of the more progressive centers, buses or taxis may have been converted for easy wheelchair access. This allows the disabled person to make spontaneous arrangements, as most people do. Many disabled people feel trapped if they are unable to accept last-minute invitations because of a lack of transport. Converted taxis or personal transport are best suited to the needs of most disabled persons.

The ability to drive a car or van is a great asset to many, giving them independence, vocational opportunities, and social outlets.

While driving the physical ability of the driver is not readily apparent and this can provide a great psychologic lift for the disabled driver.

POSITIONING

Adjustment of the seat position is important. Generally, a quadriplegic driver handles the controls best when the seat is in the forward position. However, care must be taken that the steering attachment is not so close that it will catch on clothing. The tilt of the seat is usually fairly upright, as in the wheelchair. The seat may require raising so that greater mechanical advantage is obtained when turning the steering wheel. This will aid in turning the steering wheel through the dead spot that sometimes occurs near eleven o'clock. All the positioning may be tried out using cushions initially if the car has no electrical adjustment for the seats. Once the optimum position is determined, the seat should be permanently adjusted by a mechanic.

The armrest on the door frequently is used by the driver as a fulcrum to gain leverage when managing the controls. It is possible that the armrest may require repositioning.

It is essential that the quadriplegic driver be stabilized in his driving position, or he will lose leverage on both controls and steering wheel. The combination seat and over the shoulder safety belt will often suffice (Fig. 12-23A), but if the patient still loses balance, a shoulder and lap combination may be used with one additional belt. This belt runs from the doorpost, around the driver below his arm pits, and back to the doorpost (Fig. 12-23B and C). This belt prevents a fall to the right when the car is turned to the left, and also stabilizes the upper trunk, allowing more power to be applied to the steering wheel. Even greater stability can be

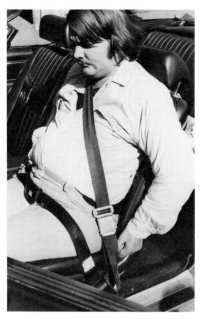 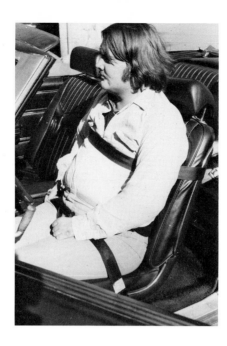 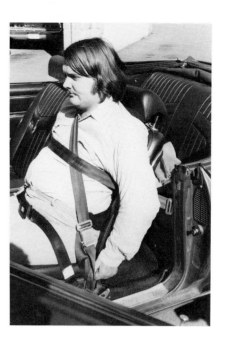

FIGURE 12-23

obtained by securing a padded upholstered block on the seatback to hold the driver's rib cage from armpit to waist. This block must be thin enough not to interfere with the driver's arm.

Sometimes a thumb loop must be fastened to the belt near the buckles to permit the driver's fastening his belt. A push-button type buckle is easily released. If the button is too deep to be pushed easily, a plastic knob may be glued on to raise it.

STEERING

Power steering is required. If the resistance is too great to overcome, the steering can be modified. A qualified mechanic may machine down the spool valve in the steering box, which will reduce the effort considerably. A minimal effort steering option is available; a backup power unit must be installed to work steering and brakes in case of a power failure. Since the backup system must also be manageable by the quadriplegic driver, the expense is high.

A joystick control is in development.

The position of the steering wheel may be modified. Some steering wheels have an adjustable tilt, which may also be useful in transfers. The steering wheel may have to be adjusted forward or back by lengthening or shortening the steering column. This may be required when driving from the wheelchair in a van.

The wheel size may be changed: larger for greater leverage, and smaller for those with less range.

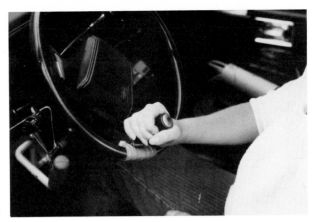

FIGURE 12-24

Hand Attachments

Position. The steering attachment can be moved to various places on the wheel to increase the comfort of the driver and to facilitate the turning of the steering wheel.

Swivel Post Attachment. A swivel steering post may be made for the person with tight finger flexors or spasticity, or for one who has some active grip (Fig. 12-24).

"U" Attachment. (Fig. 12-25) 'U' shaped open-top steering attachments, or an oval-shaped attachment, are commercially available and are easily fastened to a steering wheel. The U shape is suitable for a person with triceps and wrist extension so that his hand will remain in the U during turns. The flattened oval is suitable for a person with wrist extension who has a tendency to pull his hand away from the wheel.

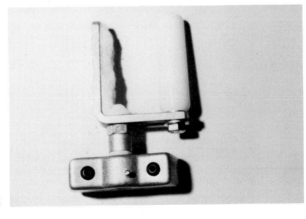
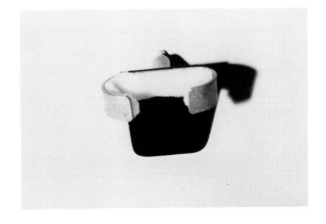

FIGURE 12-25

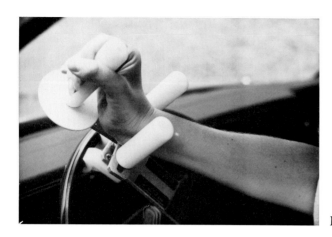

FIGURE 12-26

Three-Post Attachment. A three-post grip (Fig. 12-26), adjustable to the individual's hand, is commercially available. The grip swivels on a bar which has an adjustable spring clip for attachment to different sizes of steering wheel. This

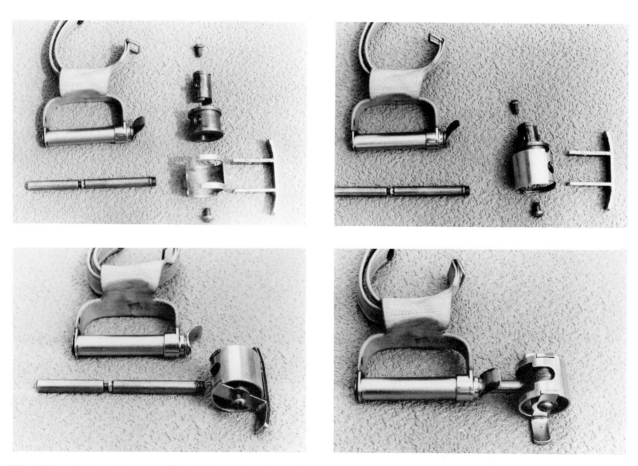

FIGURE 12-27.   Steering Wheel Swivel and Hand Attachment

462

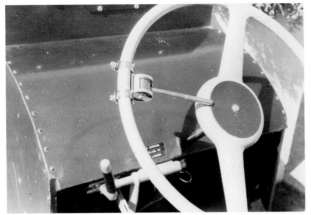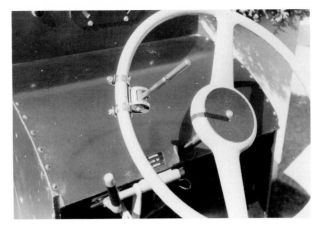

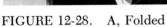

FIGURE 12-28.   A, Folded   B, Unfolded

steering attachment is intended for the person with triceps, so that the steering hand will not pull out during a turn.

The three posts act as a hand splint to keep the wrist in extension and the fingers locked onto the post, thus allowing the arm to relax while driving.

Locking Attachment. This attachment is in two parts—a steering-wheel swivel and a hand attachment (Fig. 12-27). When the two are mated, the hand is locked to the wheel.

The swivel is clamped to the inner border of the wheel. It is usually placed at one o'clock and then adjusted to the individual's needs (Fig. 12-28). The hand attachment (Fig. 12-29) consists of a tube fastened to a dorsal splint, usually extending no further than the wrist. The splint is the only part of the attachment that must be individually fitted.

The wheel attachment is normally in the folded position so that it does not interfere with the transfers (see Fig. 12-28). To lock the two parts together the stem is partially raised and the tube slipped over it until the flange on the tube

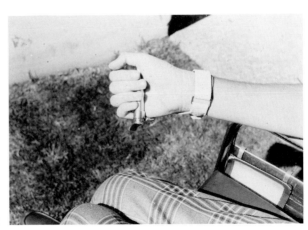

FIGURE 12-29.   Hand Attachment

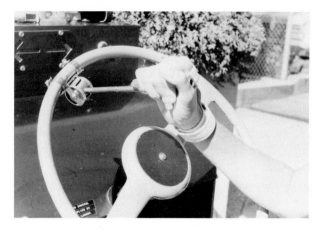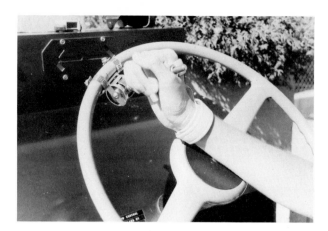

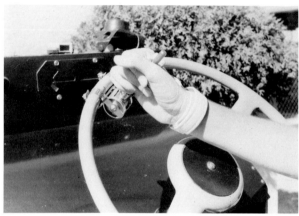

FIGURE 12-30.   Engaging the Swivel and Attachment

matches the slot in the wheel attachment (Fig. 12-30). The stem is then swung up to a right angle to the wheel. It is now locked. To release the lock, the plunger on top of the stem must be pushed down with the other hand, the forehead, or the chin (Fig. 12-31).

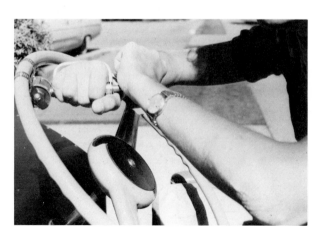

FIGURE 12-31.   Disengaging the Swivel and Attachment

Two-Plane Hand Control. There are many different hand controls available. A commonly used mechanical type requires a forward thrust for the brake and a downward motion for the throttle (Fig. 12-32). This may be satisfactory for the driver who has triceps.

Rocker Hand Control. Another type of hand control has a rocking action on a vertical plane—the driver pulling back and down for throttle and pushing forward and upward for brake; a push is the natural stopping reaction. The rocker action makes an ideal device for the quadriplegic driver because he can use biceps and shoulder flexion to apply his brakes. The hand does not slip off the lever because the angle never reaches vertical when the brakes are fully on. The throttle is applied by shoulder extension aided by the weight of the hand and arm. If the patient has wrist flexion this is also used. Endurance on long drives is much enhanced by the relaxed position of the arm that maintains throttle by the use of gravity (Fig. 12-33). The simplicity of design involving few moving parts makes this a particularly safe and troublefree device.

Reducing Effort Required. If a person cannot supply enough power to apply the brakes adequately, a qualified mechanic may reduce the power required for braking by machining down the booster cylinder of the car.

Electronic Control. If this power reduction is insufficient, electrically powered controls may be required.

Handle Adaptation. If the driver cannot easily maintain his hold on the brake, the hand piece can be adapted with a loop or 'U' handle (Fig. 12-34).

Parking Brake. Some people may be able to handle a parking brake using a

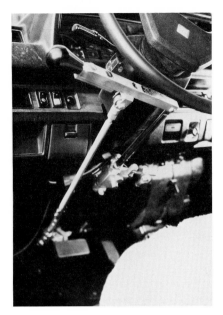

FIGURE 12-32

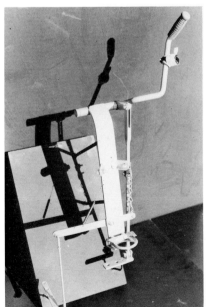

FIGURE 12-33.

A, Control Mounted in Car

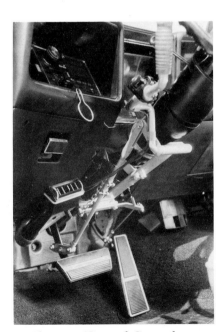

B, Close-up View of Control

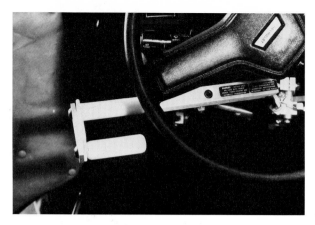

FIGURE 12-34

hand extension, others will require an electrically operated brake. In the illustration the control switch for this can be seen on the door (Fig. 12-35A). The cable and motor to apply the brake can be seen in Figure 12-35B.

SWITCHES — KEYS — DOORHANDLES

Switches, keys and doorhandles may be modified by adding loops, knobs, levers, extensions, and chains. Some switches may be modified to be voice activated.

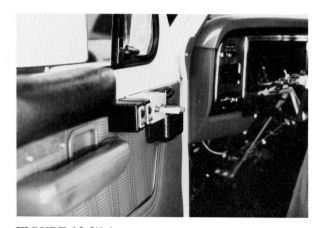

FIGURE 12-35 A

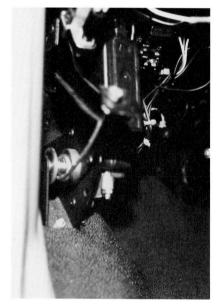

B

466

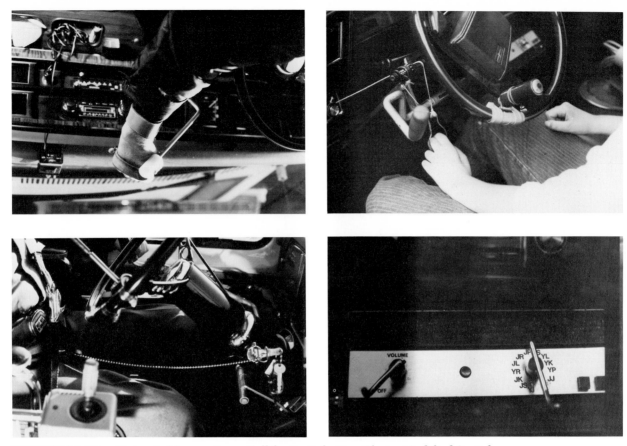

FIGURE 12-36.   Extended Lever Loop Pull for Switch Key Chain Modified Switches

Note the key attached to a chain (Fig. 12-36) which is attached to a spring return carried on the waist belt. This allows easy retrieval, with tension off the chain while driving.

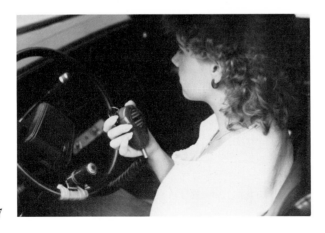
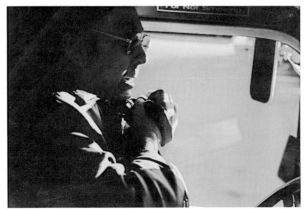

FIGURE 12-37

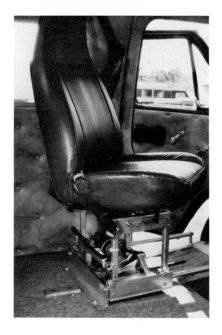
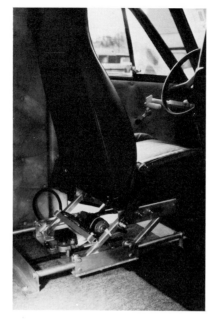

FIGURE 12-38

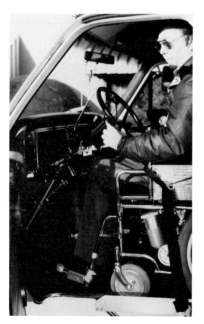

FIGURE 12-39

OTHER EQUIPMENT

Side mirrors and electrically operated windows are most useful.

A radio telephone is a convenience for many quadriplegic drivers and can be invaluable in an emergency (Fig. 12-37).

VANS

Powered lifts are required for all quadriplegics to get into the van.

Powered Seat. The patient may drive from the van seat provided that the seat is powered, so that it can roll back on a track to allow transfer from the wheelchair (Fig. 12-38). The seat must also adjust up and down to accommodate both transfers and driving positions.

Driving from the Wheelchair. If the driver is unable to transfer, the van must be adapted so that he can drive from his wheelchair (Fig. 12-39). In order to accommodate the extra height of the wheelchair, channels may be installed in the floor of the van provided that there is sufficient room between the floor and the chassis. A dealer accustomed to modifying vans for the disabled will be able to advise on available suitable models. Channels may be electrically powered to raise and lower the wheelchair so that the floor will be level for wheeling.

Adaptation for Tall Person. A tall person may also require a raised roof and windscreen so that vision is not obscured (Fig. 12-40).

Steering Column. Figure 12-41 shows the lengthened steering column, often required for the person driving from a wheelchair.

Tie-Downs. Tie-downs are mandatory for the wheelchair driver; these may be electrically operated at the push of a button (Fig. 12-42).

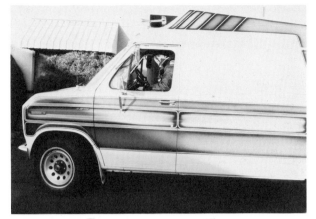

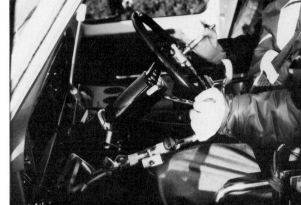

FIGURE 12-40

FIGURE 12-41

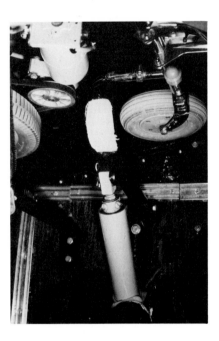

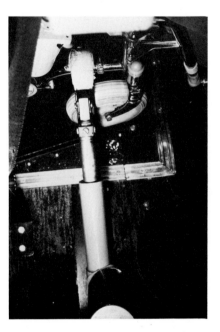

FIGURE 12-42

Seating. Driving for long distances from a wheelchair is not comfortable, as it is not sprung. Pneumatic tires on the wheelchair provide some resilience. To increase comfort and balance the wheelchair may be inclined back by modifying the floor of the van.

USEFUL REFERENCES AND AIDS

BUTLER, C AND KENEL, F: The Handicapped Drivers Mobility Guide. Falls Church, Virginia, Traffic Safety Department, American Automobile Association,

1981. (A complete list of where driver training equipment, advice and general information can be obtained by correlating a code with a comprehensive list of facilities.)

CRUGOLD, GD, HARDEN, DH: Assessing the driving potential of the handicapped. The American Journal of Occupational Therapy, Vol. 32, No. 1, January 1978.

GAREE, B: Going places in your own vehicle. Bloomington, Illinois: Accent Special Publications, Cheever Publishing Inc., 1982. (Good practical update on what is available on the market plus other helpful information.)

KRAEMER, DG: Driver Education for the Handicapped Manual. Menomonie, Wisconsin, Center for Safety Studies, Stout Vocational Rehabilitation Institute, University of Wisconsin, Stout, 1980. (Some excellent guidelines for conducting driver training.)

MENAHEM, L, et al: Teaching Driver Education to the Physically Disabled. Albertson, New York, Human Resources Center, 1978. (Very good basic information, done in an easy to understand way.)

OLSON, DA, HENIG, E, AND REISS, RG: Proceedings of a National Symposium on Driving for the Physically Handicapped at the Rehabilitation Institute of Chicago. Chicago: Education and Training Center, Rehabilitation Institute of Chicago, 1981. (Comprehensive information.)

REGER, SI, ET AL: Aid for Training and Evaluation of Handicapped Drivers. Bulletin of Prosthetic Research, 35–39, Fall 1981. (Excellent and a very thorough study of the abilities of quadriplegic driver candidates. The study utilized an elaborate assessment tool.)

SCOTT, M, AND PRIOR, RE: Mobility Aids for the Severely Handicapped: A Status Report. Bulletin of Prosthetics Research, 192–213, Fall, 1976. (A research report on the marrying of wheelchair and van. A very interesting discussion of problems encountered and their solutions.)

Quadriplegic Functional Skills: Driving. Color film, 17 mins. Producer: McLean, Elmer, Nugent. National Medical Audio Visual Center, Washington, DC 20409, or Atlanta, Georgia, 30333. 1974.

13

Housing

OPTIONS TO CONSIDER
  Types of Housing
  Types of Construction
  Outside the House
  Ramps

Escalators and Elevators
House or Apartment Entry
Inside the House or Apartment
Kitchens
Home Adaptation Measurements

Houses are seldom built with a wheelchair in mind; therefore modifications are usually required. This chapter gives some guidelines on alternatives for these modifications.

A patient may return to his home, his parents' home, a group home, or a specially designed home for the disabled. The permanence and quality of adaptions will depend on the particular needs of the patient and family, the projected length of stay, and on the available finances.

OPTIONS TO CONSIDER

1. Alterations to the main floor of the house may be indicated.

2. Basement conversion is particularly useful for a young person who would normally have preferred to live away from family, or who would have moved out of the family home shortly.

When a basement conversion is done, placement of plumbing to ensure drainage governs the placement of the bathroom and the kitchen.

A kitchen may be roughed in during a major conversion for a single person in case he wishes to share or become more independent at a later date. A basement may be gloomy unless the windows can be made low enough for a person to see out from a wheelchair. An excavated area outside glass doors leading to it may be possible in some cases. This may make the apartment feel less like a basement.

3. An extension may be built, perhaps containing a bathroom and bedsitting room. A possible need for a work area and for an extra storage area should be considered, and also the possibility that the patient may wish to share the apartment later.

4. Consider advising the family to buy or build a more suitable house for wheelchair living.

TYPES OF HOUSING

Cross Section	Type	Advantages	Disadvantages
	Flat on concrete pad	Level or near level entry.	Plumbing hard to move
	Concrete footings, full basement	Apartment possible in basement	Elevator or ramp required for main floor.
	Concrete footings, crawl space.	Plumbing, wiring possible to move	Some steps to main floor.
	Split Level		1. Often difficult for elevator to reach all floors. 2. There may be a lack of head room for an escalator. 3. Any one accessible floor may be too small for conversion.
	Apartment	Usually has accessible entry and elevators.	May be difficult to remodel.
	Mobile Home	May be purchased to suit. May be double wide.	Hard to fasten bars, etc., to walls. May require ramp or elevator.

472

Types of Construction

Wood Frame:  Uprights are usually (but not always) 16 inches (40.64 cm) from center to center. They may be covered on the inside with gyproc or with lath and plaster in an older home. Nothing weight bearing can be fastened directly to either of these finishes; the uprights (studs) or the rafters must be used. Many houses and some apartments are of wood frame construction.

Concrete: Often built using weight bearing pillars and solid floors. The ceilings are often false. It can be difficult to fasten grab bars to walls, move plumbing, and place poles. Studs may be metal and easy to find with a magnet, but require drilling and tapping to accept bolts.

Outside The House

Pathways should be smooth, level, and at least 36 inches (91.44 cm) wide and should run from the car to the house entry. It is desirable to have a hard-surfaced area outside for recreation. Sheltered access to the house directly from the garage or carport adjoining the house is most suitable for a quadriplegic person's use.

There must be sufficient room to provide wheelchair space alongside the car for transfer and for putting the wheelchair into the car.

If a van is used, a garage or carport may require a higher roof.

The type of garage door that opens and closes by radio beam is ideal, but an overhead door that is operated by electric motor and push button may be adapted. If there is a garden, a pathway may be constructed to reach it.

Ramps

Ramps must be at least 36 inches (91.44 cm) wide and may be built of wood, concrete or expanded aluminum (Fig. 13-1). They should be made slip resistant,

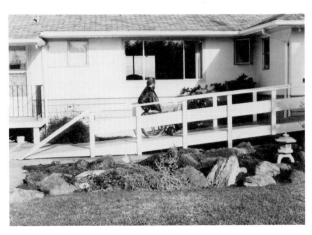

FIGURE 13-1

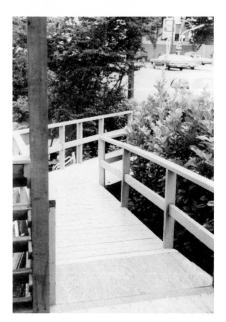

FIGURE 13-2

by applying indoor-outdoor carpeting or nonslip strips. Slats may be used in the center of the ramp for a pusher to gain good purchase. The edges of the ramp must have guard rails to prevent the wheelchair from rolling off. There must be a flat area at the top of the ramp so that the wheelchair does not roll back while the door is opened. If the ramp must be doubled back on itself to gain length, the turn area should be level.

A grade slope which can be managed by the individual must be worked out carefully. Quadriplegic patients generally are not able to handle more than a minimal grade even when commercial hill holders are used.

Sometimes it is necessary to bridge the gap between the porch and the sidewalk or pathway where there is a sunken area (Fig. 13-2). This bridge should have guard rails.

Where icy conditions or other weather considerations warrant, a covered ramp may be indicated. Building regulations may not allow this to extend to the street without a special permit.

Ramp Grades

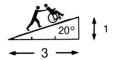

Can be managed over a short distance by a strong paraplegic person if he uses momentum. This is very steep even for a person pushing a wheelchair (see Fig. 13-1).

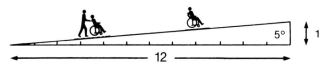

This grade can be managed by most paraplegic people, and by most pushers (see Fig. 13-2).

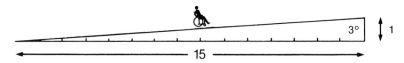

A one in fifteen grade can be managed by a low lesion quadriplegic person; he may require grade aids. This is an easy grade for a pusher.

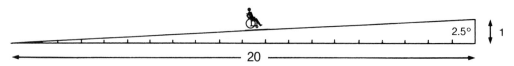

This grade can be handled by a quadriplegic person with a low lesion easily. Grade aids will be an assist to many people. This grade is easy for almost any pusher.

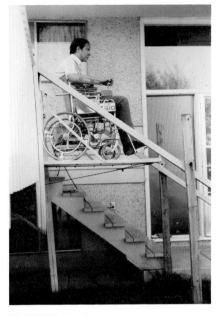
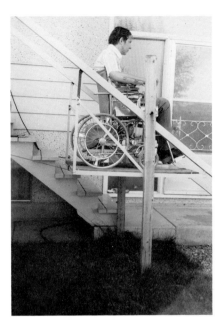
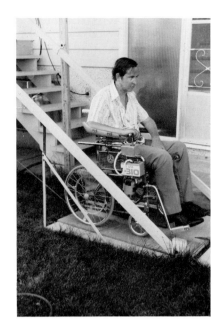

FIGURE 13-3

Note that these numbers may be used with any unit of measurement. For example, twenty feet to one foot, or twenty metres to one metre.

ESCALATORS AND ELEVATORS

There are several types of escalators and elevators that may be used inside or outside the house.

An electrically-powered wheelchair escalator may be built over stairs, while still allowing the stairs to be used. (Fig. 13-3). This escalator runs on two rails so that the stairs can only be used when the platform is at the bottom.

Some escalators run on rails on one side of the stairs and are capable of going around curves. These leave the stairs free when the platform is folded up (Fig. 13-4).

The appearance of the house and how alterations may affect its resale value should be considered, as well as convenience when placing an elevator.

An elevator may be installed indoors, or it may be installed in a covered area, perhaps up through a deck or from a carport or garage (Fig. 13-5).

The concrete pad underneath the elevator should have a recessed well so that the entrance is level.

If possible, the elevator should have the entrance and exit in line. If the wheelchair has to turn to exit, a turning radius must be allowed. See "Home Measurements", page 482. The controls should be at one side inside the elevator and within easy reach. Built up control buttons or a lever may be required.

Ideally the elevator should be enclosed, lighted, and have safety features to prevent it descending onto someone below. It should also have safety gates for the

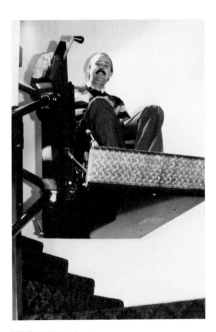

FIGURE 13-4

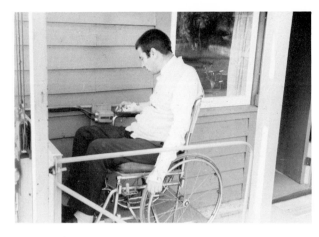

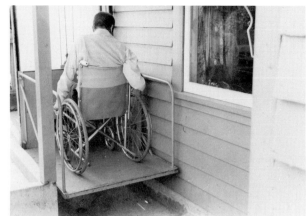

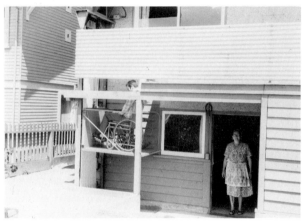

FIGURE 13-5

open elevator shaft. If the elevator is not to be permanently installed, see-through flooring such as expanded aluminum, and safety gates will prevent accidents (Fig. 13-6). It is mandatory for all elevators to have a safety stop so that in the event of mechanical failure the platform will not drop.

HOUSE OR APARTMENT ENTRY

Many quadriplegic patients cannot wheel over small obstacles such as door-sills. These can be eliminated where there is a covered porch. There should be room for turning outside the door to permit the door to be closed.

INSIDE THE HOUSE OR APARTMENT

Doors

Doors should be a minimum of 30 inches (76.20 cm) wide for a direct approach. Angled approaches may require a wider doorway. Door knobs may be

476

exchanged for lever handles, which are easier to operate. A handle 12 inches (30.48 cm) from the hinge side of the door, wide enough to insert a wrist, will aid in closing the door. Alternatively, a looped rope can be used to pull the door shut. Folding or sliding doors with large handles are easy to open and close.

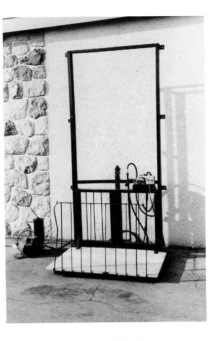 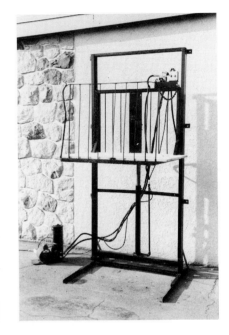

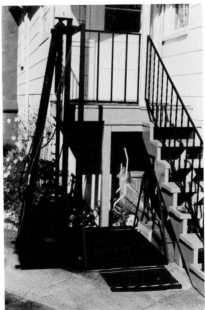 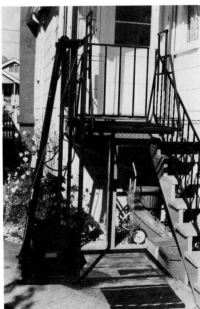

FIGURE 13-6.   Transportable Electric/Hydraulic Elevator

A telephone control for unlocking doors may be installed in a house, or environmental controls can be used for this purpose. The doors may also be opened by electric motor using a control near the door. This is particularly useful for the person in a powered wheelchair who cannot open the door manually.

Floor Surfaces

Slip mats and deep pile rugs are obstacles and should be removed. Wood or linoleum floor surfaces are the easiest to wheel on, followed by indoor-outdoor carpeting, since this has a very short pile. The deeper the pile of a carpet the harder it is to push the wheelchair over it.

Hallways and Corridors

Corridors should be wide enough to allow the wheelchair to turn and approach doors directly. Areas of the walls and door jambs that may be scraped by the wheelchair may be covered with a protective material.

Furniture

An adequate passageway should be left between pieces of furniture so that the wheelchair can be easily maneuvered. One chair may be removed from dining and family areas to provide wheelchair space and avoid conspicuous furniture moving each time the room is used. Dining tables should be high enough to clear the patient's knees.

Windows

Because temperature changes plague the quadriplegic patient so much, he should be able to control the windows or temperature control independently, particularly in his bedroom. The swing-out window with a lever or crank control is the easiest type to handle.

Bedroom

There must be room for the patient to maneuver easily into position for bed transfers and to gain easy access to the clothes cupboard and chest of drawers. The clothes rail must be lowered to within reach. Drawer pulls may be adapted by adding a loop of strong material such as webbing, leather, or tape. A large drawer may have a strap fastened between the two pulls; this strap should not be so loose that it can be caught in the drawer below. Ideally the drawer pulls may be changed to metal loop handles.

Bathroom

Bathroom fixtures must often be moved to accommodate a wheelchair. This may involve a minor change such as pivoting the toilet a quarter turn on its mount, or it may involve relocating fixtures or replanning the bathroom.

Often it is preferable and cheaper to build an additional bathroom. Since a quadriplegic patient will spend some time in the bathroom, a second bathroom may be a great asset in a family home. The placement of plumbing will depend upon the method of transfer used by the patient. Due consideration is given to the layout of the individual's bathroom when the method of transfer is worked out; for instance, if before his return home the patient can transfer equally well from the left or right side of the toilet, the transfer appropriate to his own bathroom is perfected. If a wheelchair shower is used it should be incorporated into the bathroom if possible.

Planning. It is often useful to map the outline of the bathroom and the fixtures on the floor with tape, so that the patient can wheel from fixture to fixture. Changes are easily made at this stage, and the whole layout is easier for the patient to visualize when it is full scale.

Doors. Bathroom doors are sometimes narrower than other doors in the house, a particular problem if the corridor is also narrow.

Doors can be widened slightly by having a second set of hinges brazed to the first set so that the whole door moves back (Fig. 13-7). Alternatively, strong offset hinges designed for cupboards may suffice. If this does not allow adequate room, the whole doorway may need enlarging. Swing doors, sliding doors, or bifold

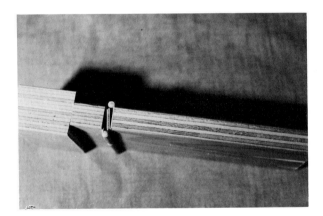
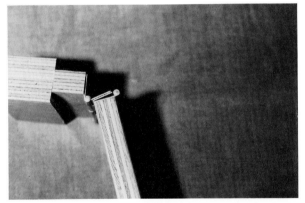
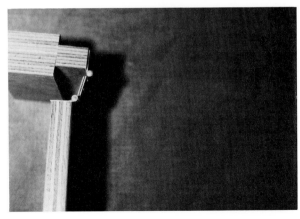

FIGURE 13-7

doors will be chosen depending on cost and space requirements. The bathroom door should swing outward if there is a possibility of a person's falling and blocking the door.

Toilet. Access to the toilet should be checked. Thirty-two (81.28 cm) to 35 inches (88.9 cm) will accommodate an 18-inch (45.72 cm) standard wheelchair angled less or more beside the toilet. The patient may need room beside the toilet for toileting and cleaning equipment. Sometimes a cupboard can be placed by the toilet which will accommodate both balance requirements and storage. Generally, toilets in a home, purposely designed housing, or institution should not be raised for the disabled person. A correct height, removable toilet seat can be provided for the individual. The gap under this raised seat allows independent or dependent bowel management, and perineal care. In addition, a raised toilet seat can be removed for traveling, thus allowing versatility.

If the toilet is to be installed in a basement, a contractor or plumber should be consulted regarding placement and the height of the toilet which will allow sufficient drainage.

Commodes. Some specially designed housing may have raised toilets which may need lowering to normal height. A toilet must be low enough to allow a commode chair to wheel over it. If the commode is propelled by the patient, the water tank should be checked to ensure that it is not too wide for the wheels to straddle it. The approach should, if possible, be straight. Room should be allowed at the side for those who require help, or for those who must lean sideways when toileting.

Grab Bars. Bars may be fixed, swing away, or swing up. Overhead bars that project forward should either swing away or have a padded end. If overhead bars have a long span, they may require an extra hanger. Bars must be fastened into studs.

If the studs are not in the most convenient place, the bars may be firmly bolted to a length of wood, which is then fastened into the studs. Lag bolts, strong expansion bolts, or heavy screws may be used as fasteners. The bar should be tested to ensure that it cannot be torn away from the wall. Bars should be thick enough to provide a comfortable hold, at least 1¼ inches (3.175 cm) diameter, and the gripping surface may be cross-hatched or rubber covered.

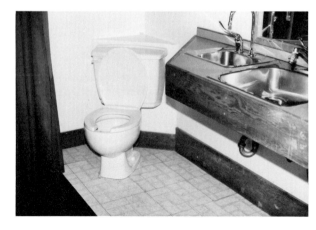

FIGURE 13-8

480

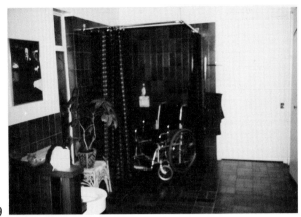

FIGURE 13-9

Bathtubs. Room should be made for a straight-on approach, which is easier if a person transfers from wheelchair to tub bottom; angled approaches may be possible for some if there is no room for a straight approach. The bathtub may be raised to wheelchair height to make the transfer easier. If a bathseat is used, room for an angled approach may be required.

A hand-held shower with a diverter valve and a thermostat is convenient for use with a bathseat, in which case shower curtains should also be installed.

The taps and the drain plug should be within reach and easy to operate.

Wall grab bars, overhead bars, or a trapeze may be required. If an overhead trapeze is used it must be bolted through a beam in the ceiling.

Wash Basin. The basin should be open underneath with knee clearance, and the pipes insulated (Fig. 13-8). The mirror, razor outlets, taps and storage should be within reach. Lever taps with a heavy duty stem may be required, or taps may be custom adapted. An extra basin may be useful for soaking and washing urinary apparatus, and a bar over the basin for drying this equipment is also useful. If there is adequate room left in the bathroom for a turning space, drawers may be installed at the side under the counter. If necessary, a foot clearance may be left underneath, if the extra few inches are required for turning. The corner of the cabinet in this case should be rounded, and if possible a rubber protector applied.

Wheel-in Shower. The best design is one that allows the patient to wheel in and out without turning. Lips, ledges or rims should not be installed. A shower may have minimum 30-inch (76.20 cm) walls on the narrow sides, but is better with more room, especially if the patient is dependent and may require room for a helper (Fig. 13-9).

The whole bathroom floor, or just the shower area, may be tiled and slightly sloped to drain in a corner. The patient may wish to have a divider between toilet and shower, but it is more versatile without. The larger the area, the less slope required. A 2-inch (5.08 cm) drop to the drain is usually required. Where the toilet is included as part of the shower area, the shower hose may be placed within reach, so that the patient can shower on the toilet.

Cedar or plastic duck boarding with narrow spaces 1/4 inch (.64 cm) between slats may be used to provide a completely level surface. This must have a recessed area beneath for drainage. This type may be preferred by the patient who has a

481

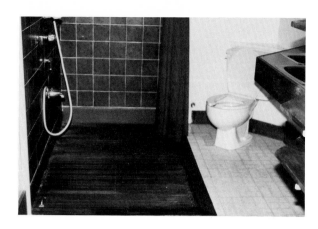

FIGURE 13-10

rigid commode chair that does not wheel easily on an uneven floor, or if the slope of the floor makes a toilet transfer difficult (Fig. 13-10).

Mixer valves shoud have a reliable temperature control; this may be a simple cutoff switch for the hot water if too high a temperature is reached. A flexible shower hose with a telephone shower head is convenient for many patients.

Curtains. The curtain rod may require custom building. In a small bathroom, curtains may not be required at all, and the shower area may include the toilet.

Examples of bathroom plans may be found in the Appendix.

KITCHENS

Kitchen modifications may be required, depending upon the present kitchen layout, and on the amount that the wheelchair user plans to use the kitchen. These modifications are discussed in Chapter 11. Examples of plans may also be found in the Appendix.

HOME ADAPTATION MEASUREMENTS

Measurements are based on 18-inch (45.72 cm) E & J active duty lightweight wheelchair with standard desk arms.

Note: Some types of electric wheelchairs and E & J Sports models are 1 inch (2.54 cm) higher. Measurements must be adjusted according to the wheelchair used.

Average counter top height	33″	(83.82 cm)
Average under counter height - knee height	27″	(68.58 cm)
Depth of counter required for a desk arm chair (a patient with a deeper chair seat or long feet will require more depth)	24″	(60.96 cm)

Recommended turning area	5′	(152.4 cm) diameter circle
Minimum turning area	4′8″	(142.24 cm) diameter with maneuvering
Minimum with jumping (for temporary accommodation)	4′	(121.92 cm) with much maneuvering
Corridor to door turn	5′8″	(172.72 cm) minimum total of door and corridor
Recommended door width	30″	(76.2 cm)
Room required beside toilet to permit angled approach	32″-35″	(81.28-88.9 cm)
Room required beside toilet on nontransfer side	7″	(17.78 cm) if no help required (minimum)
	21″	(53.34 cm) if help from side required
Room required for a commode wheelchair on either side of the toilet	6″	(15.24 cm)
Wheel height	25″	(63.5 cm)
18″ (45.72 cm) wheelchair width (deduct 1″ (2.45 cm) for wheelchairs with wrap around arms	26″	(66.04 cm)
18″ (45.72 cm) back width	19″	(48.26 cm)
Seat rail height	19½″	(49.53 cm)
Seat height with compressed 4″ (10.16 cm) foam cushion	20½″	(52.07 cm)
Outside paths	36″	(91.44 cm)

USEFUL REFERENCES AND AIDS

Building Standards Branch, Ministry of Municipal Affairs, Parliament Buildings, Victoria, British Columbia, V8V IX4: The Section 3.7 Handbook: Building Requirements for Persons with Disabilities Including Illustrations and Commentary

1984. (Excellent illustrations and clear explanations. Useful handbook even where the regulations are not applicable.)

Canada Mortgage & Housing Corporation: Housing the Handicapped, 1974, 75, 77, 84. Ottawa, Ontario, K1A OT7.

FOOTT, SYDNEY: Handicapped At Home, Design Council, 28 Haymarket, London, England. SWIY 450. 1977. (Good ideas and illustrations—many ideas suitable for North America—some available or applicable only for Europe.)

KUSHNER, C, FALTA, PL, AITKENS, A: Making Your Home Accessible: A Disabled Consumer's Guide. Canadian Housing Design Council and Policy Research, Analysis and Liaison Directorate, Policy Coordination Bureau, Consumer and Corporate Affairs Canada, Minister of Supply and Services Canada, Ottawa (Ontario) K1A OC9. 1983.

SMALL, R AND ALLAN, B: An Illustrated Handbook for Barrier Free Design; Copies available from: The Easter Seal Society for Crippled Children, 521 Second Avenue West, Seattle, Washington, USA, 98119, 1978. (Public areas mainly—excellent illustrations.)

WALLER, FELIX: An Introduction to Domestic Design for the Disabled, Disabled Living Activities Group, Central Council for the Disabled, England, 1968.

14

Recreation

SPORTS
- Archery
- Billiards, Snooker, Pool
- Excercising
- Field Events
- Fishing
- Flying
- Kayaking or Canoeing
- Motor Ball
- Quad Rugby (Murder Ball)
- Sailing
- Sledge Hockey
- Sit-Skiing
- Sporting Rifle
- Swimming
- Table Tennis
- Tennis
- Volleyball

HOBBIES
- Board Games
- Card Playing
- Carpentry
- Ceramics
- Computers
- Gardening
- Leatherwork
- Playing Musical Instruments
- Painting
- Photography
- Reading
- Radio, Tape Deck, Television
- Social Times

Recreation should be introduced early because recreation, socialization, and fun are vital for a balanced life, and because recreation can be an excellent gateway for disabled persons to integrate into society and to help them adjust to a new life style.

Often the most difficult step for a disabled person is that of entering the community, learning how to cope with physical obstacles, and learning how to adjust to other people in a new role. Old friends may drift away because of interests and sports in which the disabled person can no longer participate. Although a person does not necessarily start a job or sport in order to meet people, this is probably how most people meet new friends. A disabled person may be limited in opportunities to work and play, and may have to make a conscious effort to learn how to participate in the community. Many newly disabled people do not realize how many barriers there are and how to overcome them until they have completed a graduated "community living" course. People who are learning these skills must put them into practice to consolidate their knowledge, and this can often be best done through learning recreation skills and options.

As skills are learned they must be applied in real situations (Fig. 14-1). For instance, a person who has increased wheeling endurance could use this to go to the local store, and combine the endurance test with meeting the store clerk, and handling payment, and perhaps learning to ask for help in the store. A person wishing to go to a football game or theater will learn to phone for a ticket, make sure that the stadium or theater is accessible, and perhaps that toilets are also accessible. The person may also need to arrange transport, or make sure that a parking space is available close to the destination. When in public, the person in a wheelchair may need to ask for help, or perhaps decline the offer of help, and may have to explain to the curious child why he is in a wheelchair, at the same time perhaps attempting to relieve the embarrassment of the parent. The skills required for arranging an outing, whether the arrangement is done independently, or by asking for physical assistance, are best learned before discharge from any rehabilitation center, and frequently prove to be a most valuable bridge to living in the community.

It is useful at first for the disabled person to go on an outing with a group of other disabled people as an introduction to the "outside world", but when he returns home, he may be the only disabled person around and will not be able to

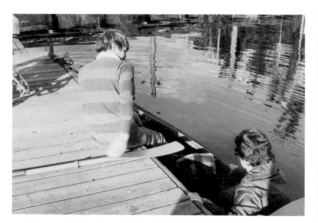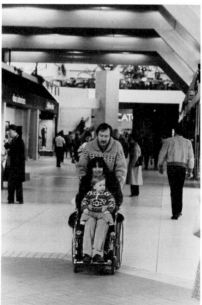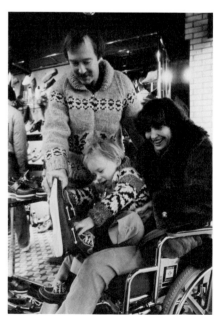

FIGURE 14-1

486

take refuge in a group. Therefore, an organized program to encourage the newly disabled person to take steps into the community will be invaluable. When he returns home "discharge shock" will be reduced, and he will be better prepared for his return. Some of the possible activities and some adaptations are shown in this chapter to indicate some of the activities that are participated in by quadriplegic people. It is hoped that these examples will help others to find interests and "gateways".

SOME RECREATIONAL ACTIVITIES PARTICIPATED IN BY QUADRIPLEGICS

Sports Involvement	Personal Hobbies	Social Activities
Archery	Adult education	Camping
Billiards	Animal breeding	Church groups
Boating (towing waterskiers, etc.)	Astronomy	Discussion groups
Driving (car rallies)	Beadwork (Indian)	Drama (directing, etc.)
Exercising	Bird watching	Education programmes
Fishing	Board games	Hobby clubs:
Flying	Card playing	Gardening
Kayaking and canoeing	Carpentry	Photography
Sailing	Carving—wood, clay or soapstone	Stamp collecting
Sledge hockey	Ceramics	Archery, etc.
Shuffleboard (table)	Collecting (stamps, etc.)	Organizing
Sit-skiing	Computers	Pen pals
Sporting rifle	Cooking	Service clubs
Swimming	Driving—rally, cross country, etc.	Singing and music
Weight lifting	Flying model airplanes	Social functions and parties
Wheelchair table tennis	Gardening	Spectator sports
Wheelchair rugby	Ham radio	Theatre
Wheelchair track and field	Lapidary work	Visiting and entertaining
Wheelchair volleyball	Leather work	Volunteer work: (Cubs, Scouts, Y.M.C.A.,
Sports:	Model building	Boys Club, Red
Organizing	Model road racing	Cross, etc.)
Refereeing	Mosaic tile work	
Coaching	Music	
Judging	Painting	
Time keeping	Photography	
Score keeping	Reading	
Starting	Traveling	
Tournament official	TV viewing	
Managing	Weaving	
Public relations	Writing	
Fund raising		

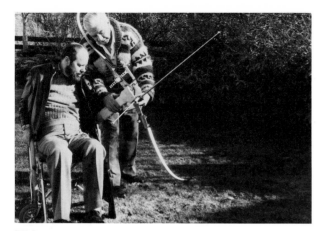

FIGURE 14-2

SPORTS

Archery

Archery can be enjoyed in competition with others or as an individual sport (Fig. 14-2). A simple bow may be used for beginners; "equipment hounds" can use counter balance arms, telescope sights, or fold away bows.

A commercially available trigger, the "Fletch-o-matic", can be released easily by gentle pressure on the archer's cheek (Fig. 14-3).

A piece of aluminum is bent at a right angle and a "V" cut into the aluminum

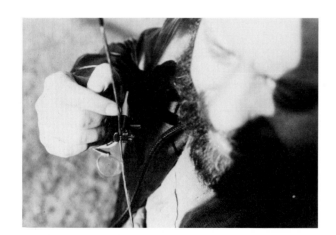

FIGURE 14-3

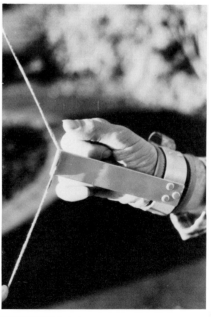

FIGURE 14-4

488

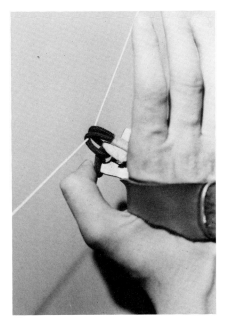 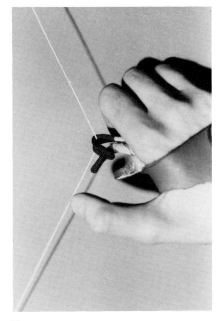 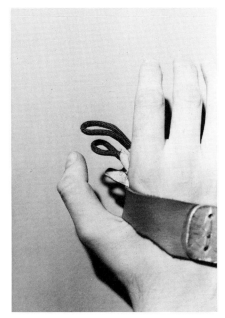

FIGURE 14-5 A   B   C

with the corner of a file on the inside of the right angle from top to bottom, to accommodate the bow string. The edge of the aluminum is then cut at a slight angle, cutting through the bottom of the V. As the archer raises his elbow the bow string slides by the end of the aluminum to release (Fig. 14-4).

This splint for holding and releasing a bow string is simple and has a smooth release action. Two loops of fine shock cord are attached to a metal hand splint with a trigger-shaped projection. The larger loop is placed over the bow string and the smaller loop is pushed through the large loop and over the trigger (Fig. 14-5A). A small movement of the hand (Fig. 14-5B) will release the bow string (Fig. 14-5C).

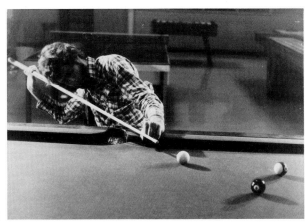

FIGURE 14-6

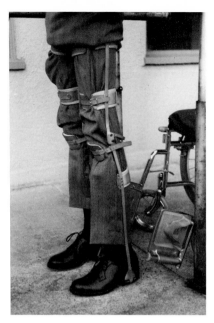 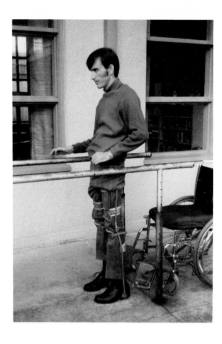 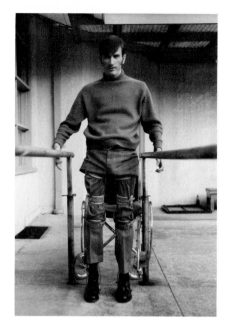

FIGURE 14-7

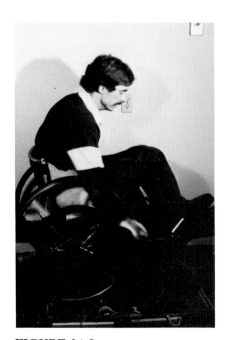

FIGURE 14-8

Billiards, Snooker, Pool

Some quadriplegic players will require splints for stabilizing the cue, or will require cue rests for reach. Pool is included in the disabled games (Fig. 14-6).

Exercising

Standing in braces can be regarded as a recreational exercise for some low-lesion quadriplegic patients (Fig. 14-7). Mental and physical benefits are derived from the change of posture. The braces, with sole plates and anterior and posterior stops, are the type used by paraplegics. A standing table may be used instead of parallel bars so that study, reading, or other hobbies may be carried out at the same time.

Exercising (Wheelchair)

Training for racing can be done indoors, perhaps during poor weather, on a commercially available exerciser (Fig. 14-8). These exercisers have different features: resistance, locking rollers, odometers, and so forth.

Those who do not race may also enjoy this activity for the exercise value, comparable to the person who enjoys a workout on a stationary bicycle.

Field Events

Sports events draw people together, and can foster competition, friendship, fitness and pleasure. This friendly group of Manitobans came to compete in British Columbia, and left with most of the prizes in field events.

490

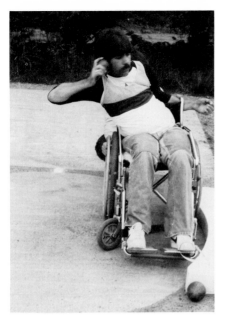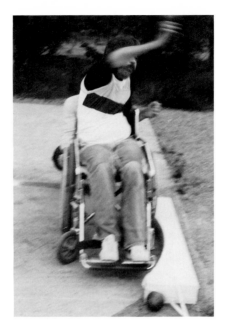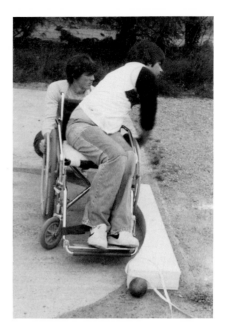

FIGURE 14-9

Shot Put

The shot is pushed off the shoulder very much in the normal manner (Fig. 14-9). The angle of the wheelchair can be varied.

Javelin

The javelin is not adapted, though the cord wrap is useful to stop its slipping through the hand with a tenodesis or weak grasp (Fig. 14-10). The javelin used in competition is the Women's Olympic Javelin.

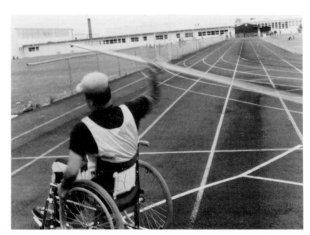

FIGURE 14-10

491

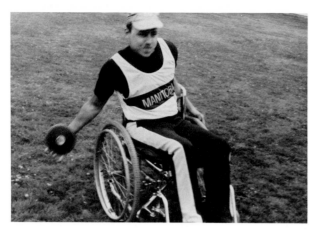

FIGURE 14-11

Discus

The women's weight discus is used in competition. No hand splints are allowed. The discus must be thrown across the body, so the angle of the chair is important (Fig. 14-11).

FISHING

Some quadriplegic people own and operate their own boats and can adapt the boat for their own needs. Some people have a derrick rigged to hoist themselves into position. Others enjoy lake or river fishing from the shore (Fig. 14-12). Rod holders for rods will be useful for many. A star drag reel is often easily converted, or electronic reels may be used.

FLYING

At least one make of small plane, the Aercoupe, has been flown by quadriplegic pilots. Quadriplegic pilots have been licensed by the Canadian Department of Transport.

Ultra lights have been flown by muscular dystrophy quadriplegic people, and as illustrated, by paraplegics (Fig. 14-13). There is no reason why low lesion quadriplegic people could not fly them also.

KAYAKING OR CANOEING

A sport that is very relaxing and enjoyable is kayaking. This sport can be enjoyed by the quadriplegic person with very little modification to equipment (Fig. 14-14A).

This quadriplegic man is able to get into a stabilized kayak unassisted, but most will require help (Fig. 14-14B). The seat and backrest have been padded with closed cell waterproof foam to prevent pressure areas. Adaptations for gripping the paddle may be required.

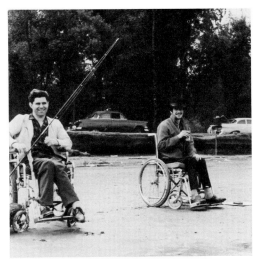

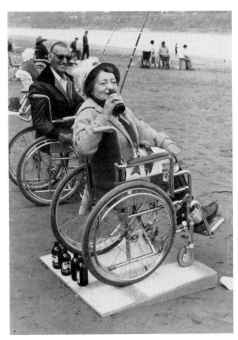

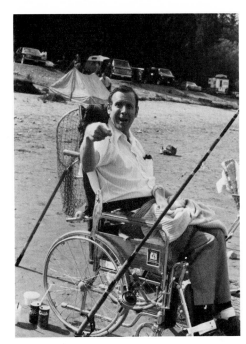

FIGURE 14-12

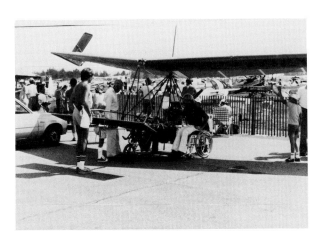

FIGURE 14-13

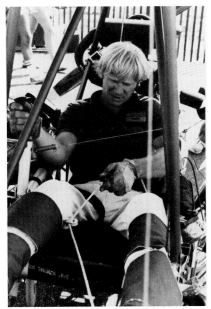

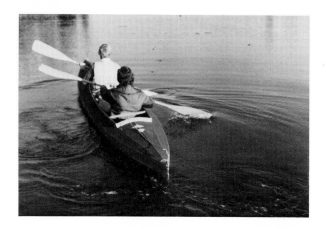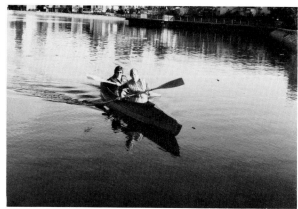

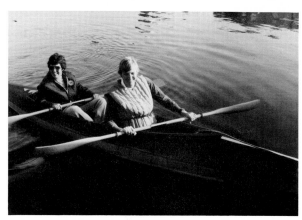

FIGURE 14-14 A

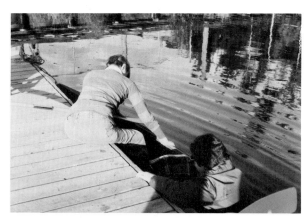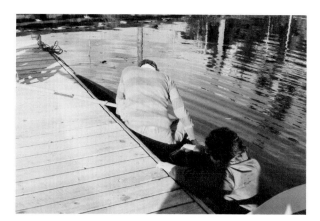

B

Getting out is harder than getting in, and assistance may be required (Fig. 14-14C). The method of getting out should be worked out before the start of the expedition, preferably on land.

494

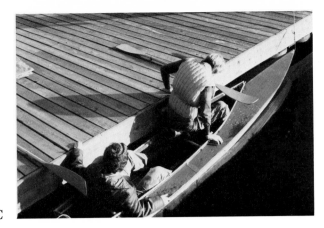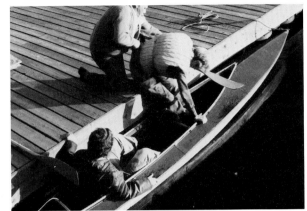

FIGURE 14-14 C

MOTOR BALL

This game allows the person in a powered wheelchair to take part in an active team game, where a large ball is "bunted" with a hoop attached to the wheelchair leg rests (Fig. 14-15). This loop also protects the players feet. Some of the players even use head control units and can become skillful tacticians and control the ball well.

QUAD RUGBY (MURDER BALL)

This game is somewhat similar to wheelchair basketball (a game which can also be played by the low lesion quadriplegic person). The game is played using a volley ball in a basketball court, with twenty foot (6.10 m) wide goals at each end. The ball may be carried but must be bounced or thrown every ten seconds. Goals are scored by carrying the ball through the goal (Fig. 14-16).

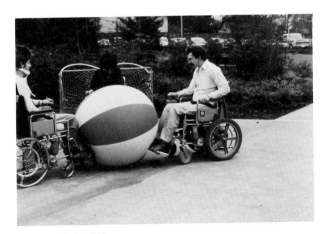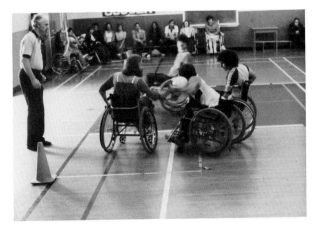

FIGURE 14-15   FIGURE 14-16

495

This sailor climbs aboard his catamaran when it is still on the dolly on the dock (Fig. 14-17). The majority of quadriplegic sailors will require help to get

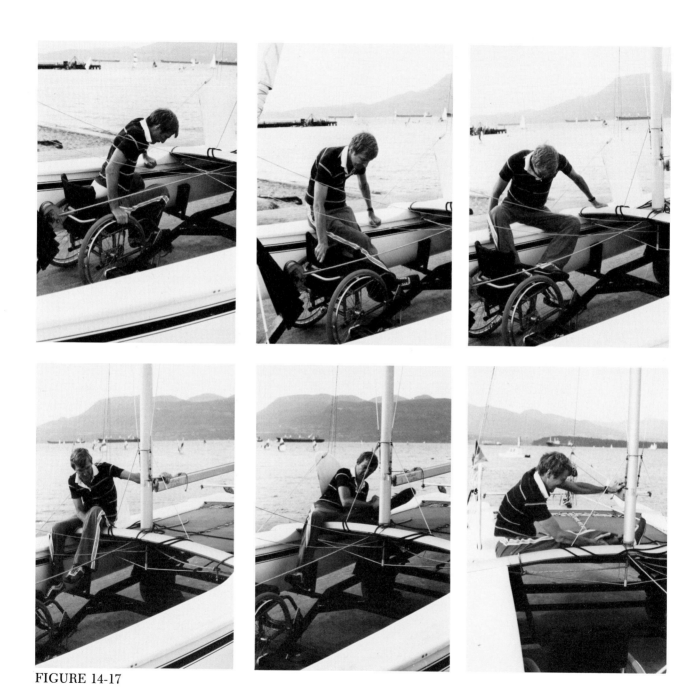

FIGURE 14-17

496

aboard, and all will require help with rigging the boat and putting it in the water. Most helmsmen will not be able to manage both tiller and sheet because of insufficient balance. It is safer and more fun to have two or more people in the boat.

SLEDGE HOCKEY

This is a fast moving team game similar to ice hockey. The sled has skate blades under the seat and skids at the front. The sledge is propelled by means of hockey stick handles with sharp picks at the end. The regulation hockey puck is hit using the same ice picks. The quadriplegic player requires a higher back on the sled, and also safety straps. The ice pick has been adapted with a rubber ball as a hand stop and the player has a golf glove with tapes from fingers to wrist (Fig. 14-18) which has also been taped with adhesive tape for extra stability. The quadriplegic player must hold the pick low to maintain control, but has a much shorter stroke than the paraplegic in the background. Steering and stopping are done by leaning. This game is very fast and exciting for both player and spectator. It is fascinating to watch the puck being flicked under the sled to another player, making it very hard to follow.

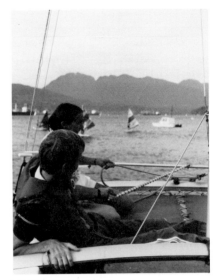

FIGURE 14-17 Continued

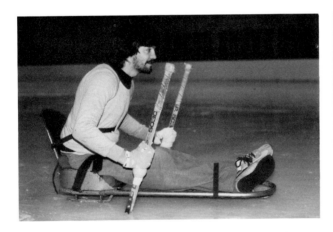

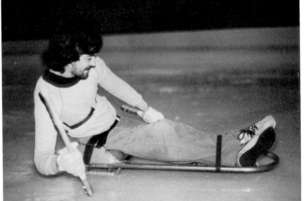

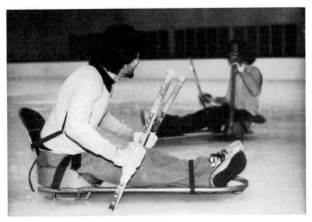

FIGURE 14-18

497

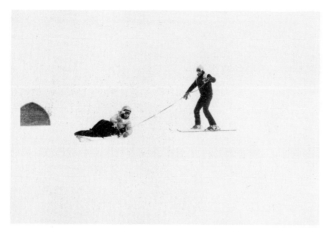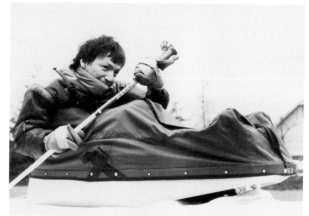

FIGURE 14-19 (Photo by G. Anderson)

SIT-SKIING

Sit-skiing can be great fun for the spinal cord injured, including the low-lesion level quadriplegic person (Fig. 14-19). There are many different makes of sit-ski, all of which have some features in common. The inside of the sit-ski should be well padded to protect pressure areas, and the cover should fit well to protect insensitive parts of the body from cold and wet. In addition, very warm clothing should be worn, and legs should be checked to ensure that they are not cold or in danger of frost bite. A higher back and fastening straps are required for the quadriplegic skier.

The quadriplegic sit-skier usually skis with an able-bodied skier behind holding onto a tether rope, and he steers using kayak-type poles, thrusting one end of the pole into the snow and leaning into the turn. Most people will require adapted or taped ski mitts for control of the pole. Loading and unloading the sit-ski at the chair lift requires two people, usually the chair lift attendant and the tetherer, who with practice will be able to load and unload the sit ski without stopping the lift. A safety strap is required for the chair once on the lift, and equipment must also be on the sit ski for use in a possible chair lift evacuation.

SPORTING RIFLE

The quadriplegic marksman may be at no disadvantage competing against able-bodied marksmen in sporting rifle shooting, but is at some disadvantage in skeet shooting because he cannot turn far enough to follow the complete arc of the target. (A gold shield has been won in open competition by the marksman who supplied this information.)

The quadriplegic rifleman will require some modifications for steadying the rifle. A firmly fixed, carpeted lap board and a padded armrest is used by this gold medalist. He has also put his spotting telescope on a flexible stand attached to the lap board (Fig. 14-20).

498

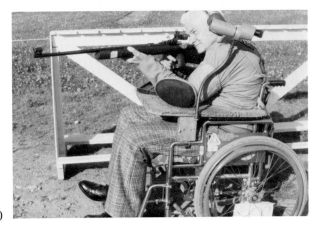

FIGURE 14-20

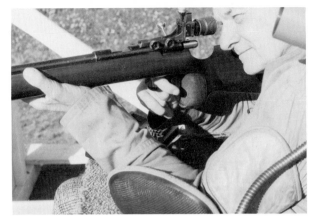

The higher lesion quadriplegic rifleman may require an adjustable stand on his lap board. This must be able to take fine adjustments and yet remain stable (Fig. 14-21).

Regulations in sports meets will specify how much, and what type of apparatus may be used, but any apparatus that will enable a person to enjoy a sport may be used noncompetitively.

SWIMMING

The quadriplegic swimmer, even though skilled before his accident, must be supervised when he is introduced to swimming again. An instructor will progress him by starting him floating on his back, and then to sculling on his back, up to the old English back stroke (Fig. 14-22). This stroke is introduced because the bilateral movement allows him to control the roll of his body. Later, alternating strokes, such as back crawl, can be introduced when the swimmer has learned to compensate for the lack of leg and trunk movement.

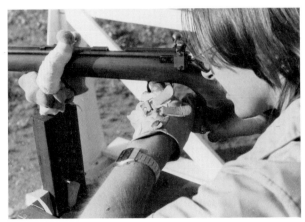

FIGURE 14-21

499

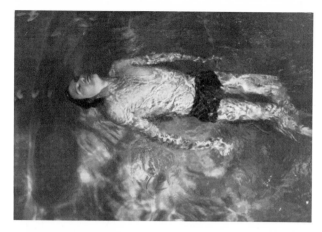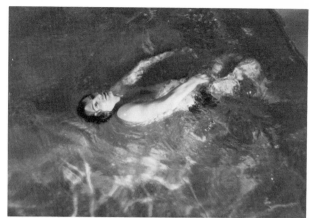

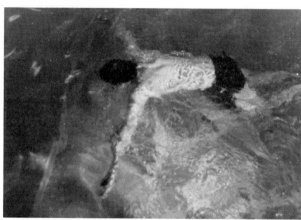

FIGURE 14-22

When the swimmer is relaxed and at ease in the water, swimming face down can be started. Once controlled breathing has been mastered, breast stroke and butterfly stroke are possible, followed by the free style crawl if the swimmer has a low lesion.

Under a good swimming coach, style and speed can be improved so that competition or recreation can be more enjoyable.

TABLE TENNIS

A table tennis paddle may be held by bandaging the hand around the handle with an elastic bandage, or it may be held as in Figure 14-23 with masking tape. Both methods allow the paddle to be adjusted while being held firmly.

TENNIS

The rules for tennis for the disabled are the same as regulation tennis except that the ball is allowed to bounce twice for the wheelchair player. The lower lesion quadriplegic with control of pronation and supination will be able to hit the

500

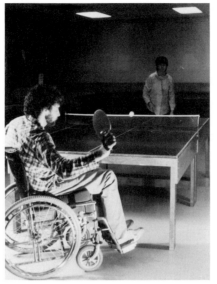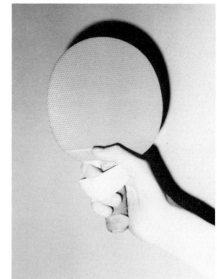

FIGURE 14-23

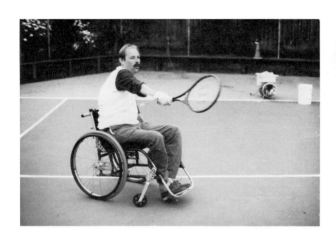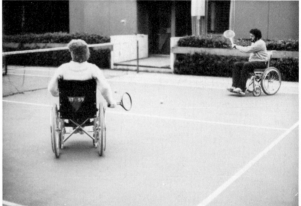

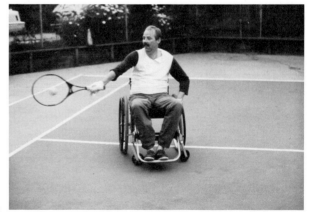

FIGURE 14-24

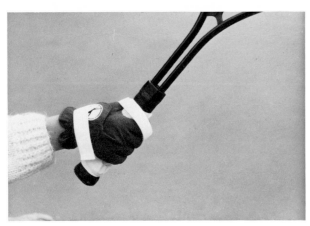

FIGURE 14-25

ball with a fair degree of accuracy (Fig. 14-24). Able-bodied ball boys will be an asset to keep the game moving if there is a wheelchair foursome.

The hand must be firmly fastened to the racket using an adapted glove and tape or elastic. Resin also helps to keep the gloved hand in position (Fig. 4-25).

VOLLEYBALL

This is an excellent team game which can be played with large numbers of people if the players are stationary (Fig. 14-26). The players can have varied disabilities, or no disability, and the rules can be varied to suit each person's disability. In this game an able-bodied person stands behind each team to catch overthrown balls, and to ensure that all players are included in the game.

When the game is played as a competitive sport there are five players on each side, with two forward players and three people at the back, all of whom are allowed to move all over the court. The rules are similar to regulation volleyball rules.

HOBBIES

BOARD GAMES

A large size crib board with ¼-inch (0.64 cm) diameter pegs is easier to manage than standard boards (Fig. 14-27). Large chessmen, adapted checkers, etc., may enable the player to make moves more easily.

This man relaxes by pitting his wits against a computer in a computerized chess game, practicing so that he can beat his live opponents later (Fig. 14-28).

CARD PLAYING

Card holders may be purchased or made. Figure 14-29A shows a card holder that may be used to turn cards face up with the use of hand or mouthstick. Figure 14-29B shows a small box turned upside down with the cards held between cover and box. Figure 14-29C shows a board with diagonal saw cuts and a commercially

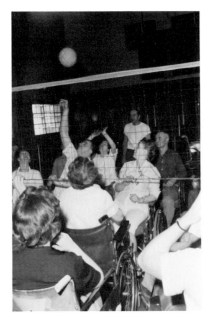

FIGURE 14-26

502

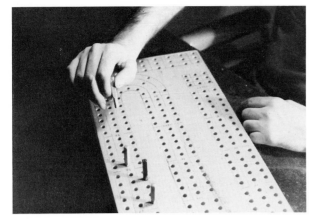

FIGURE 14-27

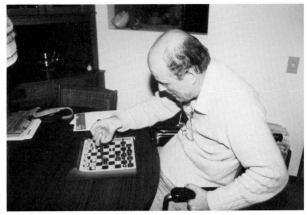

FIGURE 14-28

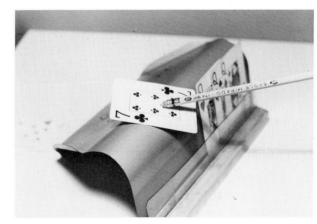

FIGURE 14-29 A

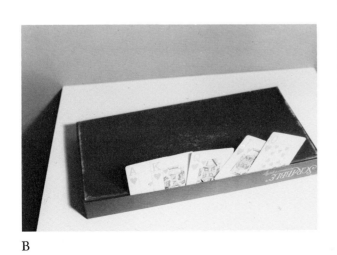

B

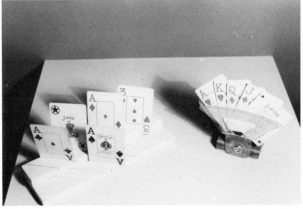

C

available plastic card holder fastened to a homemade base. Card shufflers may also be purchased.

CARPENTRY

Equipment such as band saws, and drills mounted in stands, enable a quadriplegic person to do some carpentry with little effort (Fig. 14-30). He will be lim-

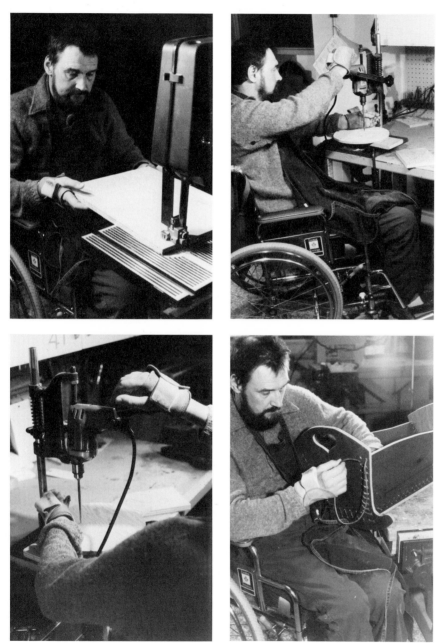

FIGURE 14-30

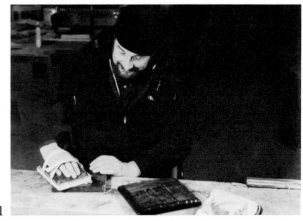

FIGURE 14-31

ited by the inability to use hand-held power tools such as circular saws and routers.

Hand sanding, sawing, and finishing can be done with some adaptations for holding (Fig. 14-31). Attention must be given to work bench heights and to the types of clamps and vises used.

CERAMICS

Ceramic painting and glazing can be done with good control, even using a brush held in the teeth (Fig. 14-32). This girl also does some clay carving using a mouth stick. Some excellent work has been done by quadriplegic people using the technique of carving rather than modeling in soft clay.

COMPUTERS

Computers used for games or for more serious pursuits can be all-absorbing, and can be used by very high lesion quadriplegic people, provided that the interface is suitable.

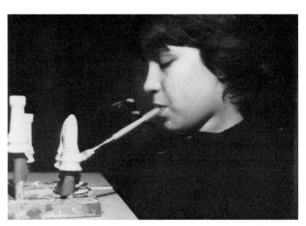

FIGURE 14-32

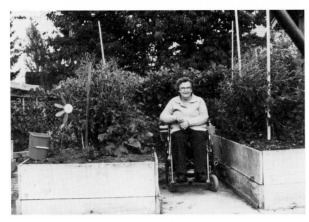

FIGURE 14-33

GARDENING

This gardener has grown large quantities of vegetables in plots raised to wheelchair height (Fig. 14-33). She had the plots built up so that she could reach the center from either side, and has a sprinkling system which can be controlled from the house.

Many lightweight or easy to hold tools are suitable for disabled gardeners; specially designed tools are also available (Fig. 14-34).

Some gardeners may need to approach work closely, and will find it easier to have a table garden, so that their knees can go under (Fig. 14-35). Pots and hanging baskets can also be planted on a tabletop, and can provide an artistic outlet and great pleasure.

LEATHERWORK

Thonging, carving, or stamping and tooling have all been hobbies done by quadriplegic people, and some have turned their hobby into a paying job. Leather

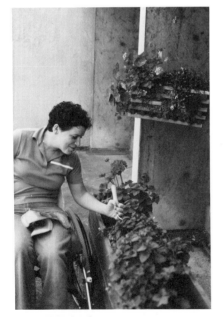

FIGURE 14-34

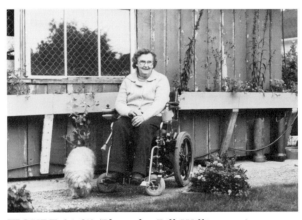

FIGURE 14-35 (Photo by Bill Williamson)

506

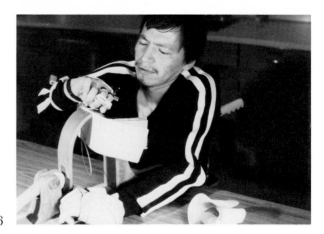

FIGURE 14-36

clamps and adapted tools may be required (Fig. 14-36). For instance, one arm of a leather punch may be clamped down, and the other arm elongated by slipping a pipe over it to improve the leverage.

PLAYING MUSICAL INSTRUMENTS

Instruments which do not require finger dexterity can be played satisfactorily; the trombone and harmonica, or mouth organ, are examples. In some cases the instrument must be adapted for holding. Some wind instruments may not be suitable, depending on the person's breathing capacity.

Even with two fingers, or two typing sticks, electric organs can also be very satisfying to play. Excellent music can be produced using various automatic accompaniments initiated by the mere push of a button. The organist shown spends hours playing and singing, often entertaining family and friends, leading them in sing-a-longs (Fig. 14-37).

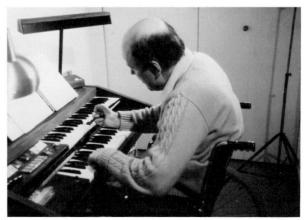

FIGURE 14-37

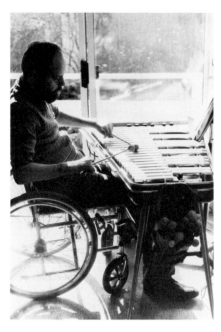

FIGURE 14-38

Many electronic instruments take little physical effort and can often be adapted. This vibraphone has had the resonator bar moved so that it can be held down with an elbow (Fig. 14-38).

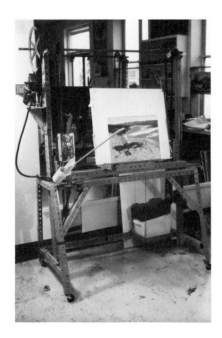
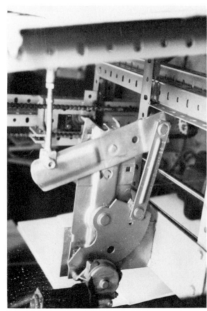

FIGURE 14-39

508

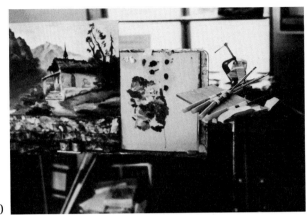

FIGURE 14-40

PAINTING

A painter who is very disabled, and is using a mouthstick will find an electrically driven easel a great advantage, particularly for larger canvases. This easel was built by the artist's father. It can be adjusted up or down, and the tilt can be varied by using an electric wheelchair toggle switch (Fig. 14-39).

This artist has had a stand placed at mouth height on the right of the easel with a variety of brushes positioned so that a minimum of cleaning is required when changing colors. His palette is set up for him and positioned by his painting so that he can concentrate on his art with minimal movement and maximal independence (Fig. 14-40).

This young man enjoys doing caricatures, using artist's felt pens. Two electric cable clips are fastened to a wrist splint that fits these pens and enables him to change colors independently (Fig. 14-41).

Painting or sketching can be developed as an extremely satisfying hobby that may be a mere pastime, or a full-time, all-absorbing occupation.

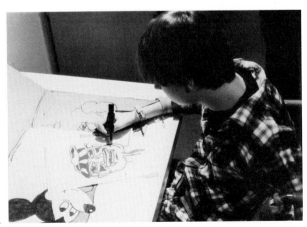

FIGURE 14-41

509

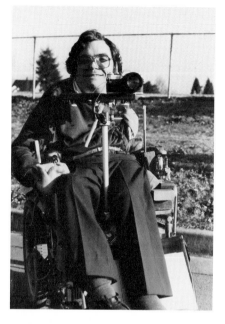

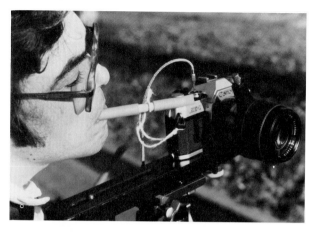

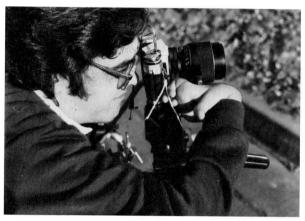

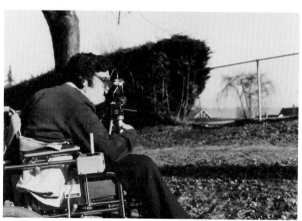

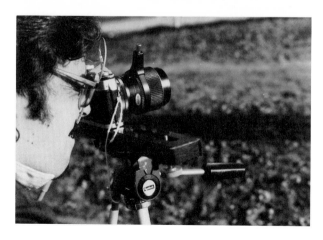

FIGURE 14-42

510

A commercially available head from a tripod may be fitted into a specially made sleeve adaptation on the wheelchair. Some people will fit the tripod onto the arm or side frame of the wheelchair (Fig. 14-42).

The tension on the tripod head is adjustable, and can therefore be set so that the camera can be swiveled and tilted.

A zoom lens is very necessary for a person who cannot change lenses, and who cannot physically approach many of his subjects easily. The lens pictured (a Tamron lens) has an adjustment similar to an F-stop ring, and can be zoomed by turning the ring with a large lever.

A mouth stick may be required to adjust the F-stop, shutter speed, and flash adjustment.

A cable release is usually required and may be operated by two hands, one hand and a chin, or, as in the photograph above, by teeth and tongue.

READING

A reading stand may be bought or made. If a mouthstick or headstick is used to turn the pages, it is often necessary to stretch an elastic over the pages which have not been read. If the stand is nearly vertical, other elastic strips are used to retain the book cover in position (Fig. 14-43). The type of swingaway clip used on a music stand may be attached to a reading stand to keep the pages down.

If a stand is used in bed, the book will be facing downward (Fig. 14-44). In this case both the elastic and the music clips will be required. If the patient uses an overhead bar, a book holder may be suspended from it, and two legs may be added to rest on the bed to adjust the angle and stabilize the stand. If a page turner is required, the eraser end of a pencil may be used, or a wad of electrical and moisture insulator gum which remains slightly sticky may be pushed onto a suitable length of doweling.

There are several makes of electric page turners that can be used by severely

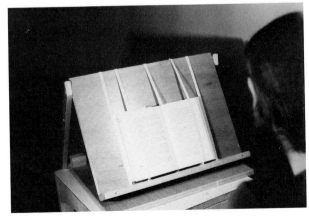

FIGURE 14-43

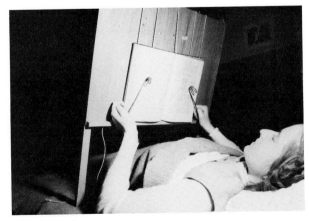

FIGURE 14-44

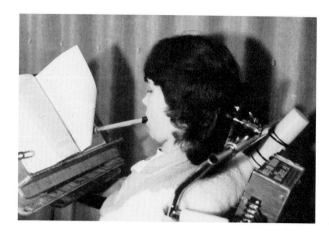

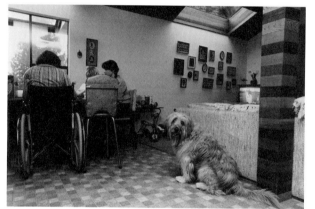

FIGURE 14-45

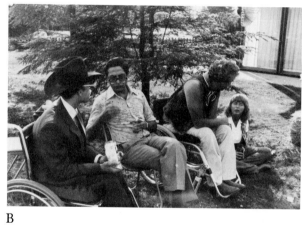

FIGURE 14-46 A

B

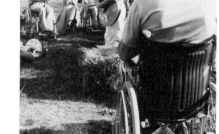

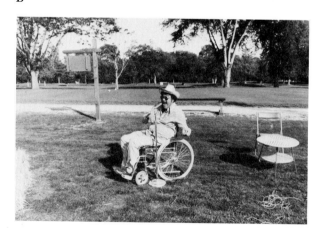

C

D

(A, photo by P. Battistone; B, C, and D courtesy of Canadian Paraplegic Association, B.C. Division)

512

disabled patients, with a suitable interface, but great care must be taken in selection of a suitable model. The turner should be able to take various sizes and thicknesses of books and magazines and should turn a single page reliably at any part of the book. It should not take a great deal of time or skill to set up or adjust. If a person using the page turner is studying, it is an advantage if the machine can turn the pages backwards as well as forwards. A stand for hand turning or mouthstick turning is usually more reliable than a mechanical page turner, and should be the first choice (Fig. 14-45).

RADIO, TAPE DECK, TELEVISION

Knobs or switches of radios, record players, or televisions, may require adaptation. Some plastic knobs can be drilled to take a short length of metal rod to add leverage.

SOCIAL TIMES

Social times may range from having a neighbor over for a cup of coffee (Fig. 14-46A), to a quiet chat with a few friends (Fig. 14-46B), or to a large party (Fig. 14-46C) complete with a master of ceremony (Fig. 14-46D).

USEFUL REFERENCES AND AIDS

ADAMS, RC ET AL: Games, Sports and Exercises for the Physically Handicapped, Lea and Febiger, Philadelphia, 1982. (Some useful adaptions and ideas.)

ARMSTRONG, M: A Community Integration Program for the Spinal Cord Injured, S.C.I. Digest, Summer, 1981.

Athletic Training Manual, Canadian Wheelchair Sports Association, B.C. Divison (Undated).

AXELSON, P: Sit-Skiing, Sports 'n Spokes, January-February, 1984.

Barrier Free Leisure Facilities, Recreation Council for the Disabled in Nova Scotia, 1977.

CECCOTTI, F: Electronic fishing reels, Sports 'n Spokes, July-August, 1982.

COLE, JA ET AL: New Options. The Texas Institute of Rehabilitation and Research, Houston, Texas, 1978. (Community skills program, discussion and modules.)

CRASE, N: Miya epoch fishing reels suitable for electronic usage. Sports 'n Spokes, July-August, 1982.

CROUCHER, N: Outdoor Pursuits for Disabled People. Woodhead-Faulkner Ltd., 1981.

DRAAYER, E (Ed): Sport and Recreation for the Disabled, An Index of Resource Materials, Sport Information Resource Centre, Ottawa, 1979.

Getting it Built—Accessible—A Guide to the Planning and Design of Recreation Facilities, Canadian Parks/Recreation Association, 333 Riger Road, Vanier, Canada, 1983.

GORDON, S ET AL: Adaptive device for the quadriplegic golfer, Archives of Physical Medicine and Rehabilitation, Vol. 66, July 1985.

GUTTMAN, L: Textbook of Sport for the Disabled, H.M.&M. Publishers Ltd., Milton Rd., Aylesbury, Bucks, England, 1976. (Many options shown, including rules for disabled sports.)

Introduction to Archery, Canadian Wheelchair Sports Association, B.C. Division. (undated)

Introduction to Riflery, Canadian Wheelchair Sports Association, B.C. Division. (undated)

Introduction to Swimming, Canadian Wheelchair Sports Association, B.C. Divison. (undated)

Introduction to Table Tennis, Canadian Wheelchair Sports Association, B.C. Division. (undated)

Introduction to Track and Field, Canadian Wheelchair Sports Association, B.C. Division. (undated)

Introduction to Weightlifting, Canadian Wheelchair Sports Association, B.C. Division. (undated)

KELLY, SL: Adaptations for independent use of cassette tape recorder/radio by high-level quadriplegic patients. The American Journal of Occupational Therapy. Vol. 37, No. 11. Nov. 1983.

PANDAVELA, J ET AL.: Martial arts for the quadriplegic. American Journal of Physical Medicine. Vol. 65, No. 1. Feb. 1986.

ROGERS, JC, FIGONE, JJ: The avocational pursuits of rehabilitants with traumatic quadriplegia. The American Journal of Occupational Therapy, Vol. 32, no. 9, October 1978. (An informative survey.)

SATALOFF, RT, ET AL: Rehabilitation of a quadriplegic professional singer. Arch Otolaryngol Vol. 110, Oct. 1984. (Useful information for those who wish to sing or play wind instruments.)

SLATTER, ER, GIBB, MM: A table tennis glove for tetraplegics. Paraplegia, Vol. 17, no. 2, July 1979. (A good pattern for holding and well described.)

Sports 'n Spokes, 5201 North 19 Avenue, Phoenix, Arizona 85015. (Excellent—many ideas for sports and equipment.)

SZATO, A: Hunting rifle for quadriplegic patients, Archives of Physical Medicine and Rehabilitation, Vol. 60, September 1979. (Detailed instruction of how to modify and adapt the rifle for the quadriplegic person.)

Transportation in Canada, A guide for Travellers with Special Needs, Transportation Development Centre, 1000 Sherbrooke St., W., P.O. Box 549, Place de l'Aviation, Montreal, Quebec.

WHITE, AS ET AL: Easy Path to Gardening, Readers Digest, 1972. (Informative book for disabled gardeners printed in England.)

15

The Dependent Patient

Methods used for transferring a dependent patient should be selected using mechanics best suited to the build of the patient and his helper. For example, the patient with a long trunk may have his trunk bent forward onto his thighs. His head and shoulders will then counterbalance his bottom, making his buttocks easy to move (see Figure 15-41). A patient who has a short trunk, or who cannot bend forward, may be better managed with a "thigh pivot slide transfer" (see Figure 15-42).

The patient should learn to apply mechanical principles to his own transfers, so that he understands how to teach people who are unfamiliar with transfer techniques. This also involves him in the selection of his particular transfer techniques, and will allow him to adjust the type of transfer to the build and ability of his helper and to various situations.

Patients should learn how best to teach helpers. For instance, one helper may find a set of photos of transfers helpful, another may find a verbal explanation sufficient. The patient will also find it essential to learn how best to ask for assistance, or decline offers of help, how to ask for changes in methods, and when to give appropriate thanks.

While it is hoped that transfers will require minimum effort because of the use of good mechanics, the assistant must still use good lifting techniques. Feet should be slightly apart for comfort and balance, and comfortable nonslip shoes should be worn. The assistant must keep her back straight and her pelvis tucked under, and should avoid twisting her back. The main effort should be made by the legs rather than the back or arms.

ADJUSTING POSITIONS IN THE WHEELCHAIR

The patient must be positioned in the wheelchair in a posture which will allow him to maintain balance, with maximum mobility and comfort (see Chap-

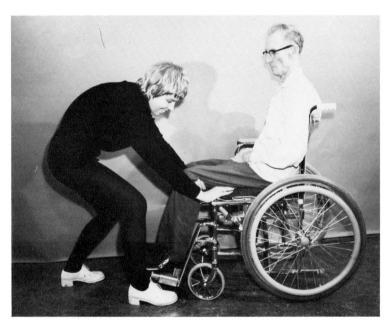

FIGURE 15-1

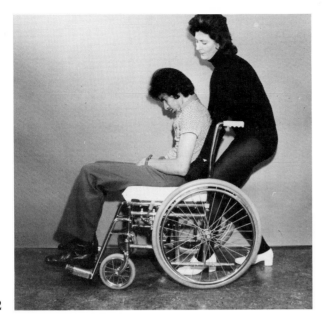 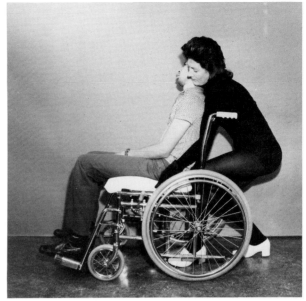

FIGURE 15-2

ter 2). The front castors of the wheelchair should be turned forward while positioning the patient. This lengthens the wheelbase and prevents the wheelchair from tipping forward. The brakes must be applied to prevent the wheelchair from moving, and during transfers the castor locks should also be engaged.

MOVING THE PATIENT FORWARD

Method 1: Pull from Front. Small adjustments forward and adjustments to square the patient in the chair may be made by pulling the patient from behind his knee with one hand and pushing against the chair seat beside the knee with the other hand (Fig. 15-1). There is little strain on the back because mainly the arms are used.

Method 2: Push from Rear (Arms). Sometimes it is desirable to move the patient forward while standing behind the wheelchair. The helper places her hands, palm up, under the buttocks. This places her elbows against the back of the wheelchair for leverage. Flexion of the elbows will now move the patient forward (Fig. 15-2). The helper's arms may be placed over the upper arms of the patient first if the patient requires stabilization.

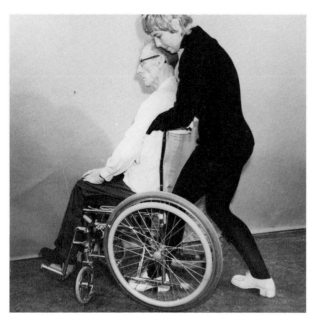

FIGURE 15-3

Method 3: Push from Rear (Legs). A patient may be moved forward slightly if the helper places a foot well under the wheelchair so that her thigh can be used to push against the bottom of the wheelchair back. The helper holds the patient under the arms to pull back slightly and to maintain the patient's balance (Fig. 15-3).

Straightening the Slacks While Avoiding Moving the Patient Forward. The slacks are grasped on the inside of the knee, avoiding any urine collecting apparatus, and the other hand is used to stabilize the cushion and to avoid any back strain while pulling the slacks (Fig. 15-4). This method has the advantage that wrinkles are pulled away from the groin area.

To straighten the wrinkles without moving the patient forward, the stabilizing hand may be placed against the knee, lifting it slightly. It may also be necessary to reverse hands to pull on the outer side of the slacks.

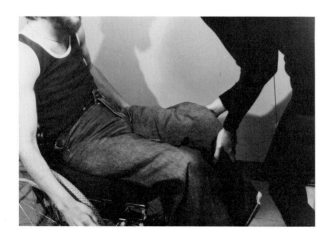
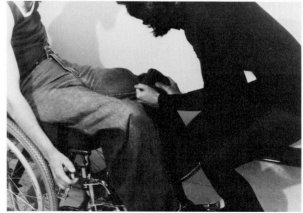

FIGURE 15-4

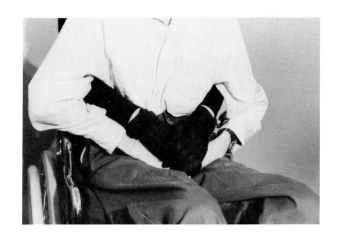

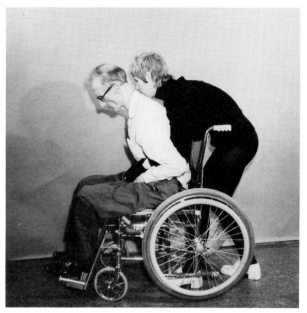

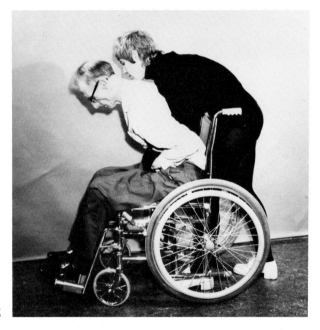

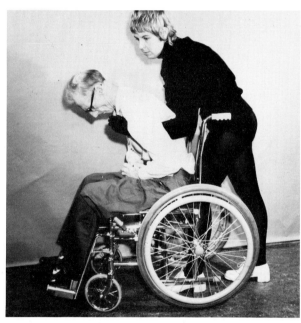

FIGURE 15-5

Moving The Patient Backward

Method 1: Lever I (Fig. 15-5).   Minimum effort for the maximum movement is expended in this method. The helper stands behind the chair with her
arms underneath the patient's upper arms while the patient remains leaning back
in the chair; the patient's hands are placed one on top of the other over the lower
abdomen. The helper's hands are placed over the patient's hands and the patient's

521

trunk is flexed forward. The forward flexion is controlled by the adduction of the helper's arms. The forearms are now placed below the patient's rib cage. By adducting the arms and straightening the elbows the patient is levered back into the chair. The rib cage provides a fulcrum and the pubis symphysis provides the point of leverage. When a large patient is moved, one hand may be positioned on the patient's hands and his trunk flexed forward before positioning the second hand.

Method 2: Lever II (Fig. 15-6).   If a patient cannot tolerate being bent forward, an alternative hand placement is possible which permits the helper to use her arms to keep the patient more upright. The helper stands behind the wheelchair and places her arms under the patient's arms, and sits him upright. She supports his trunk with her arms while she reverses her hands to slip them under his thighs. By leaning forward and shrugging, the helper levers the patient back using his ribcage as a fulcrum point.

Method 3: Knee Shoulder Rock I.   The assistant stands in front of the patient and stabilizes his knees between her own. She places her palms against both sides of the patient's upper rib cage. The assistant abducts her shoulders so that her elbows protrude, enabling the patient to place his arms over the assistant's elbows. The patient flexes his elbows as strongly as possible and hugs with his shoulders,

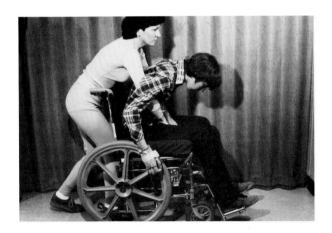

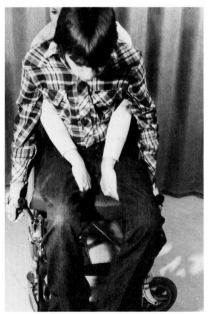

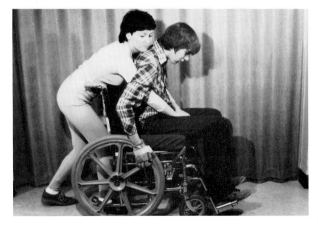

FIGURE 15-6

522

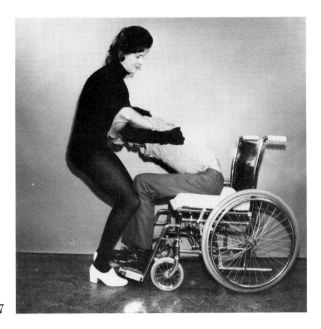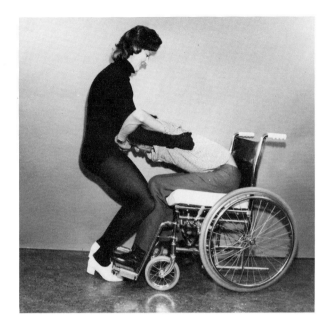

FIGURE 15-7

thus helping the assistant. The patient's trunk is pulled forward and simultaneously the assistant flexes her knees, thus using body weight to move the patient back into the chair (Fig. 15-7).

Method 4: Knee Shoulder Rock II. The assistant stands in front of the chair and stabilizes the patient's knees with her own. She slips her hands over the patient's shoulders and grasps the patient's upper arms close to the axillae. The assistant must straighten her arms at this point or she will lose most of her leverage.

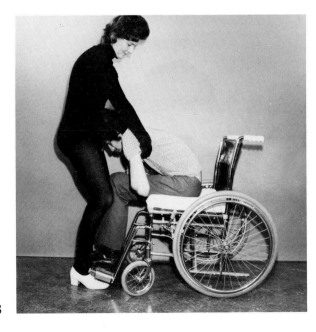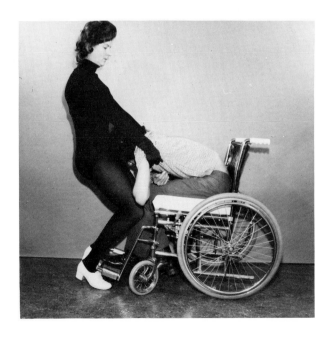

FIGURE 15-8

The assistant rocks her weight back and flexes her knees simultaneously, moving the patient back into the chair (Fig. 15-8). This method is most suitable when managing a heavy patient or a patient with very weak upper extremities. A shorter assistant may use the same method, but slip her hands under the patient's axillae from the front.

A patient may be positioned and centered by movement of the helper's knees in this or the previous method.

Method 5: Two Person Knee Shoulder Rock. The very heavy patient may require two people to move him (Fig. 15-9). One person stands behind the chair and the other in front. The person in front prevents the patient from sliding further forward by squeezing the patient's knees between her own. The front assistant now pulls the patient's trunk forward into flexion and holds him in this position. The assistant behind the chair grasps the slacks at the outside seam anterior to the hip joints and, with a combined pull and lift, moves the patient back in the chair.

Method 6: Two Person Slide. Two assistants may be necessary when a patient has been placed in an easy chair or in a high-backed or old-fashioned wheelchair (Fig. 15-10). They stand one on each side and in front of the patient, the outside foot forward and the knees flexed. The inside hand is placed under the patient's axilla, grasping the upper arm; the outside hand is placed under the patient's midthigh and the assistant's elbow rests on her own knee. The patient is pulled forward with the inside hands at the same time that he is pushed back with the outside hands. This must be done by both assistants simultaneously, using a preplanned signal.

Method 7: Quad Lift (Fig. 15-11). Another method that may be used by two assistants is especially useful if a cushion is inclined to shift, or needs to be replaced by a third person. The assistants stand in front of the patient and place

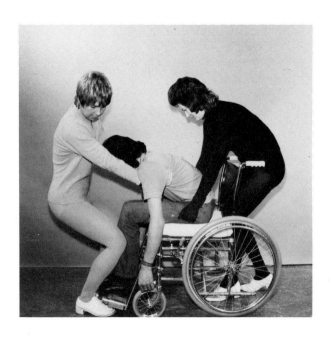
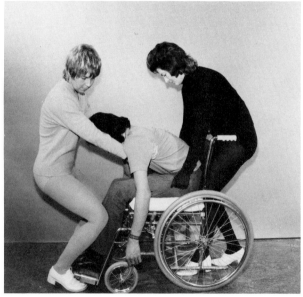

FIGURE 15-9

524

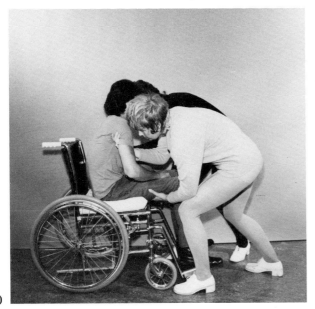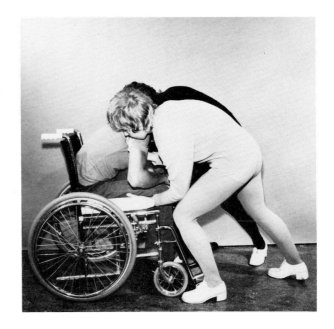

FIGURE 15-10

their inside hands under his midthighs from the inside. The patient is leaned forward so that his shoulders rest against the assistants' arms. Both assistants grasp the back of the patient's slacks. When the patient is lifted, he may be positioned very accurately. Where slacks are not worn, a towel placed under the buttocks may be used instead. This is a useful lift, comfortable for both assistants and patients. It has the advantage of avoiding any stress on the patient's shoulders.

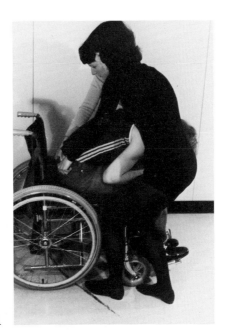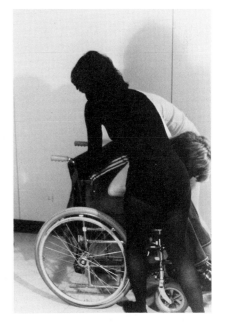

FIGURE 15-11

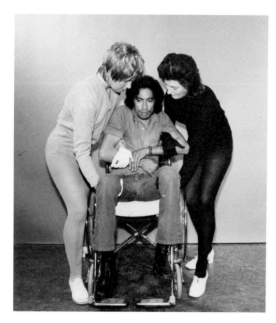 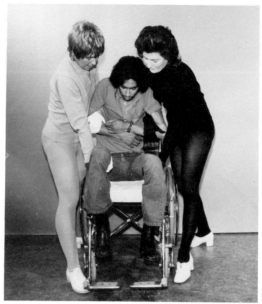

FIGURE 15-12

Method 8: Forearm Lift.   Two assistants may stand one on either side of the patient facing in the same direction as the patient. The hand closest to the patient is placed underneath the patient's axilla from behind and over the patient's forearm near the elbow. This is a flat handhold with the thumb aligned with the fingers. The other hand is placed under the thigh near the knee. The patient is levered back into the chair as both assistants lift, straightening their arms (Fig. 15-12).

Method 9: Tip Back.   There is an easy way to retrieve a patient who has slid forward so far that he cannot be sat upright on the seat of the chair. The assistant tilts the chair far back by stepping on the tipping lever and pulling back on the pushing handle (Fig. 15-13). The patient will slide back into the chair far enough to make one of the previous methods possible.

Method 10: Emergency Retrieval.   If the chair is in such a location that it cannot be tipped back, or, if the patient must be retrieved immediately, he must be pulled up from behind (Fig. 15-14). The belt may be grasped, or, if there is no belt, the wrists may be grasped by reaching under the axillae. Because a pull in this position is not easy, the patient should be pulled back just far enough for one of the other methods to be used to position him.

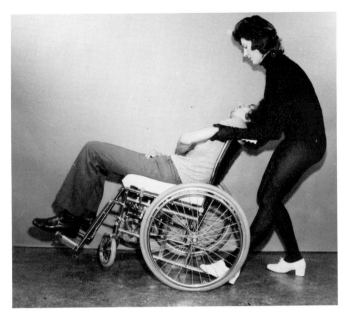

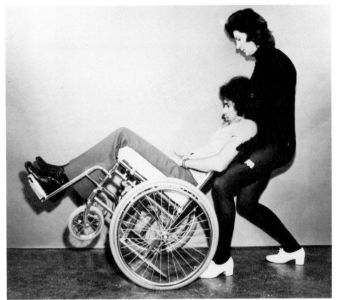

FIGURE 15-13

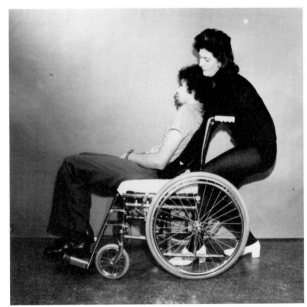

FIGURE 15-14

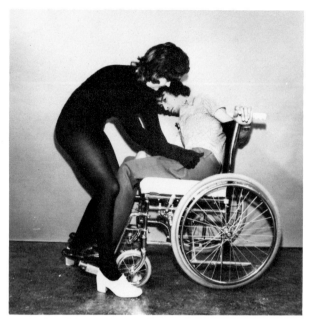

FIGURE 15-15

MOVING THE PATIENT SIDEWAYS

Method 1: Lean and Slide I.   The patient should be leaned sideways away from the proposed direction of travel before his slacks are grasped at the hip (Fig. 15-15). The patient may help to maintain his balance by flexing his elbow around the pushing handle on the side he is moving towards.

Method 2: Lean and Slide II.   The helper may stand behind the chair and grasp the slacks just forward of the hip. The other hand is placed on the opposite side of the patient, on the cushion by the trochanter. By the helper's pulling up on the slacks and pushing down on the cushion, not only will the patient slide over, but his slacks will be unwrinkled beneath him (Fig. 15-16). If the assistant's grip is not adequate, an object such as a cigarette lighter may be placed in the patient's pocket and the slacks may be grasped around it.

MOVING THE PATIENT IN THE BED

TURNING THE PATIENT

Supine to Prone

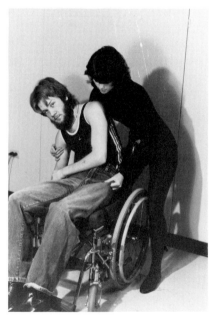

FIGURE 15-16

Method 1: Hand and Hip Pull (Fig. 15-17).   The helper places the patient's near arm under his buttock with the hand palm up and crosses his far leg over the near one. She grasps the patient's far arm with one hand and his thigh with the other. A pull will roll the patient over.

Method 2: Lever Over.   A patient may be turned with greater control and increased mechanical advantage using this method (Fig. 15-18). The patient's far

528

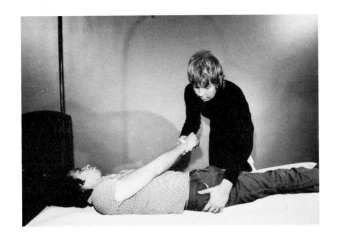

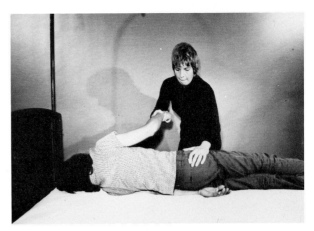

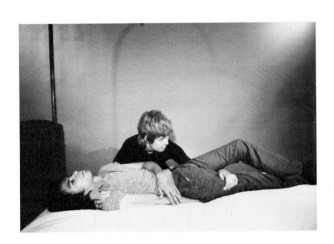

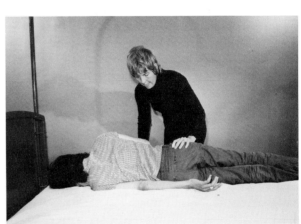

FIGURE 15-17

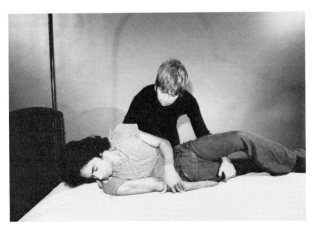

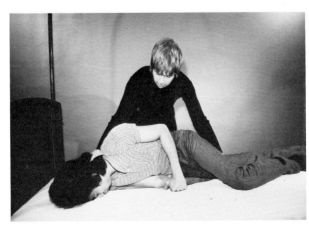

FIGURE 15-18

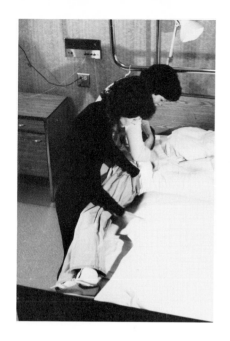
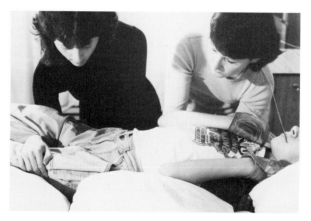
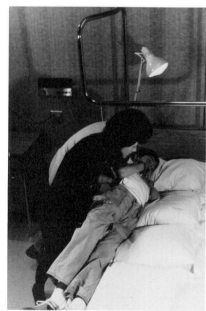
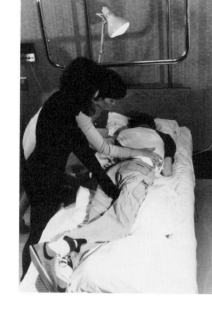
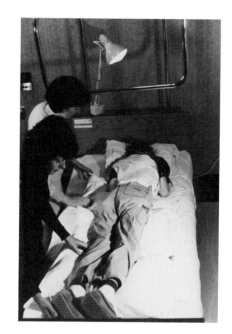

FIGURE 15-19

530

hand is placed palm up under his buttock, and his near leg is crossed over the far one. The helper places one hand under the patient's near leg and over the far leg, placing the crook of her elbow under his near buttock. The helper's other arm is placed under the near shoulder and her hand is placed on his far shoulder. When the helper's arms are straightened the patient is levered over.

Method 3: Two Person Lever Over.   Some patients must lie prone on pillows to relieve pressure areas or for urine drainage.

The patient is moved close to the side of the bed and the pillows are placed in their approximate positions. The patient is then rolled toward the helpers and is kept on the bed by the helpers' thighs while they reach over to tuck the top pillows under the patient. When the patient is allowed to roll back, the pillows will be partly beneath him. The patient's far hand is placed palm up under his buttocks and the helper near his knees places one hand under the patient's near leg and over the far leg, placing the crook of an elbow under his ischium. The helper's other hand is placed under the small of the patient's back as an extra lever. The other helper slides her arm nearest the patient's head, right under the patient's shoulders to grasp his far shoulder, while the other hand is placed under the patient's back to assist. On the count of three, both helpers stand to lever the patient up and over onto the pillows. This turn is easier if the patient is flaccid. One person may turn a lighter patient, using Method 2 (Fig. 15-19).

Method 4: Sheet Roll.   A heavy patient may be turned using a sheet which remains on the bed. The sheet edge is pulled out from under the mattress and folded over the patient. The helper blocks her knees against the side of the bed and uses her body weight rather than her arms to pull the patient onto his side. If a separate sheet is required, a nylon material is easiest to slip under the patient (Fig. 15-20).

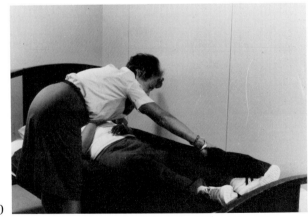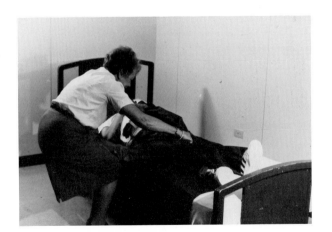

FIGURE 15-20

Prone to Supine

Method 1: Hand Hip Pull (Fig. 15-21).   The patient's head is turned towards the helper, and his far hand, palm up, is placed under his thigh as far under as possible. The near leg is crossed over the far leg. The helper reaches under the near thigh and grasps the patient's hand. Pulling on the hand and pushing on the pelvis will roll the patient over.

Method 2: Lever Over (Fig. 15-22).   The patient's head is turned towards the helper, and his far hand, palm up, is placed beneath his thigh as far under as possible. The near leg may be crossed over the far leg. The helper places an arm under the near thigh with the hand over the far thigh. The other arm is placed under the patient's axilla from the direction of the foot of the bed. The helper's arm continues through, placing her arm behind the patient's neck and onto his far shoulder. When the helper's arms are straightened, the patient is levered over. If, at the same time, the helper pulls, the patient may be positioned in the center of the bed.

Method 3: Two Person Lever Over (Fig. 15-23).   Two people may turn a very heavy patient. His head is turned towards the helpers and his far hand is

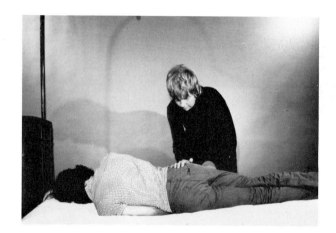
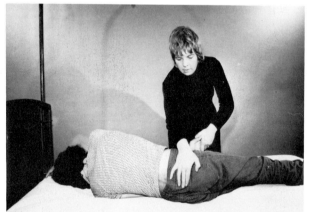

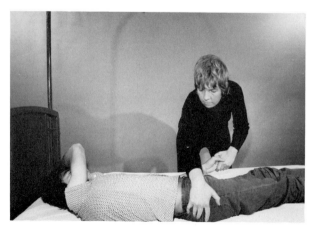

FIGURE 15-21

532

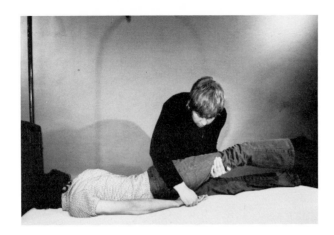
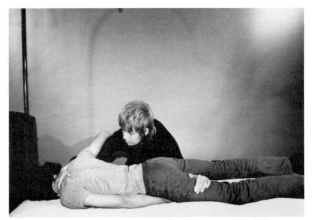

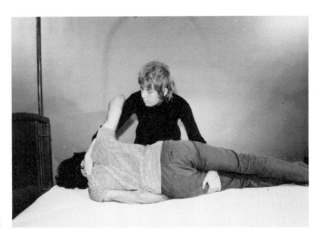
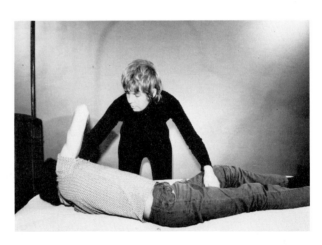

FIGURE 15-22

tucked palm up under him to midline. This arm must be straight, thus eliminating any blocking by a flexed elbow and ensuring that the arm will not be hurt. The helper near the head places one arm under the patient's axilla from the direction of

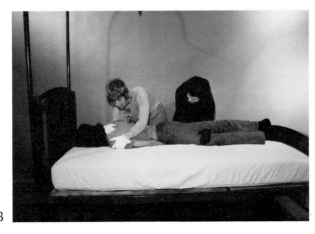
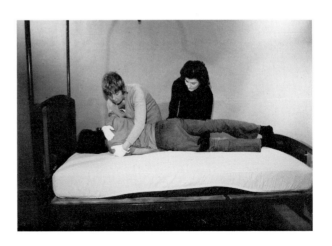

FIGURE 15-23

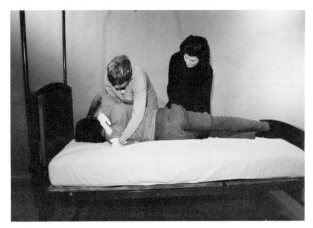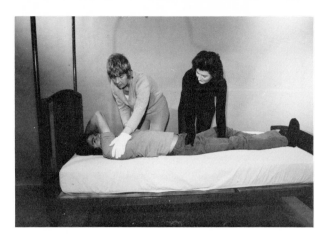

FIGURE 15-23 Continued

the foot of the bed. This arm is continued through over the back of the neck and onto the far shoulder. The other hand rests on the patient's far shoulder blade to tuck it under as he is levered over. The second helper places the hand nearer the head of the bed under the patient's hip, and the second hand is placed under the near leg and over the far leg at midthigh level. The helpers pull simultaneously, an action which will not only turn the patient, but also position him at any point wished on the bed.

Method 4: Turning Bed (Fig. 15-24).   If a patient is unable to turn independently, an electric hydraulic turning bed may be used, which can be activated by manual switch by the patient or an assistant; or the control can be programmed to turn the patient from side to side at regular intervals. Many patients will sleep through the night without noticing the turns. This turning can be a tremendous boon to a family, who may find it extremely tiring to get up during the night to turn the patient. An added advantage to this bed is the availability of an electric gatch to sit the patient up.

MOVING ACROSS THE BED

Method 1: Shoulder Hip Pull (Fig. 15-25).   The helper stands by the side of the bed farthest away from the patient. She grasps the slacks near the trochanter and the patient's upper arm near the axilla. The helper leans back with elbows extended to pull the patient over.

534

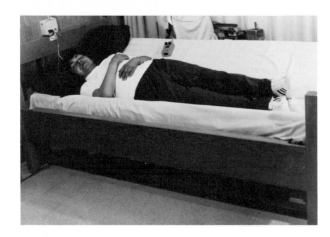
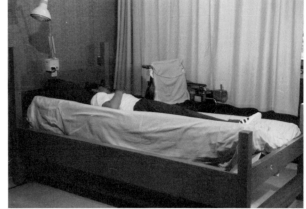

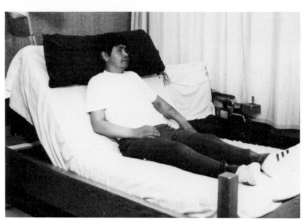

FIGURE 15-24

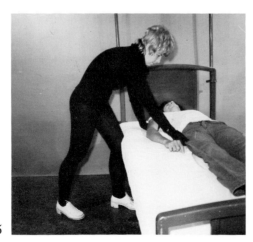

FIGURE 15-25

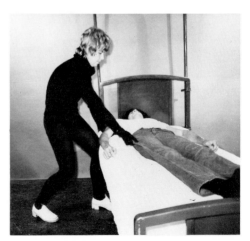

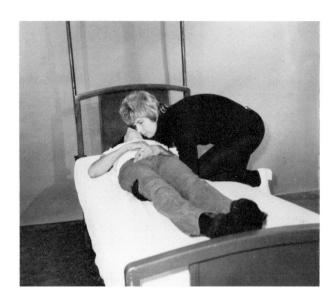 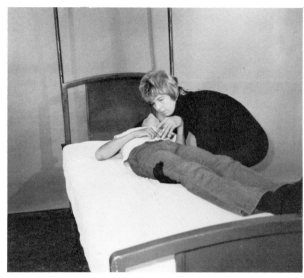

FIGURE 15-26

Method 2: Hands Under Pull.   The helper stands by the side of the bed farthest from the patient with a knee against the side of the bed or on the mattress. She slides one arm under the patient's upper thighs and one arm under the patient's shoulders. Cupping both hands, the helper leans back to slide the patient over (Fig. 15-26). This method may be used for a very heavy patient, moving first the shoulders, then the buttocks, and then the legs.

Method 3: Sitting Bounce.   Momentum can be used very effectively in moving the patient. The helper maintains the patient's sitting balance with one hand and grasps the slacks at the hip joint with the other hand. A rhythmical bouncing combined with a pull will allow the patient to be moved as his buttocks clear the mattress (Fig. 15-27).

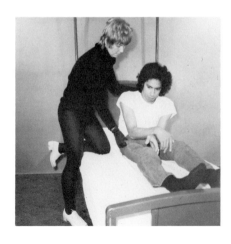 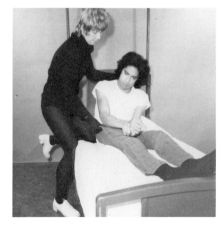

FIGURE 15-27

536

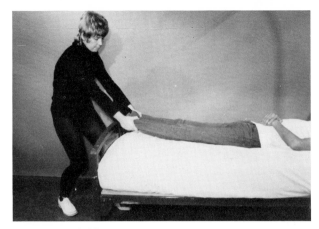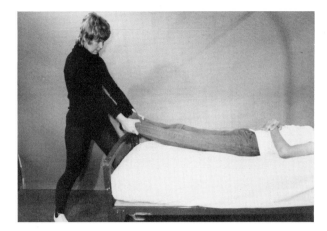

FIGURE 15-28

MOVING DOWN THE BED

Ankle Pull: The helper moves to the foot of the bed and grasps the patient's ankles, including the slacks. The helper leans back with one knee braced against the foot of the bed and pulls the patient into position, keeping her arms straight (Fig. 15-28).

MOVING UP THE BED

Method 1: Shoulder Pull (Fig. 15-29).   The helper moves to a position behind the head of the bed. Using a knee to stabilize herself against the head of the bed, the helper grasps the patient's upper arms and leans back to slide the patient up the bed.

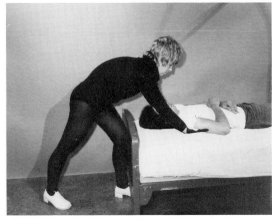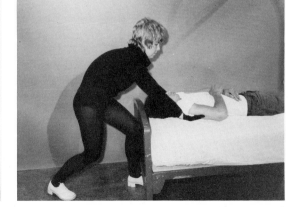

FIGURE 15-29

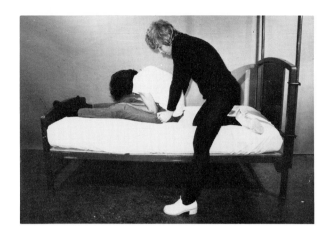
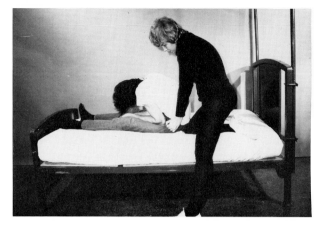

FIGURE 15-30

Method 2: Sitting Bounce (Fig. 15-30).   The patient is placed in long sitting on the bed and the helper kneels on one or both knees behind him. The slacks are grasped at the hips, or the hands are placed under the buttocks if no slacks are worn. In this position the patient is fully stabilized. The patient may be pressed down into the mattress, thus giving a bouncing assistance from the mattress springs. In rhythm with the bouncing the helper sits back on her heel, thus moving the patient back with a minimum of friction.

Method 3: Lever (Fig. 15-31).   The helper stands beside the bed facing the head and places a knee on the bed. She slides her hands palm down under the patient's axillae and then clenches her fingers. The patient is asked to adduct his arms. The helper rocks forward on her knee and flexes her wrists while pressing down into the mattress. The leverage obtained by this method moves the patient a short distance, but with relative ease.

Method 4: Two Person Lever (Fig. 15-32).   A method similar to Method 3 may be used by two helpers who place the hands nearest to the bed under the patient's axillae. The fingers are clenched and pressed into the mattress. The far hands are used to hold the patient's elbows to his sides. By flexing the wrists and rocking forward, the helpers will move the patient up the bed.

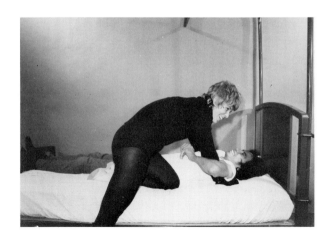
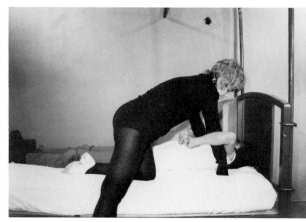

FIGURE 15-31

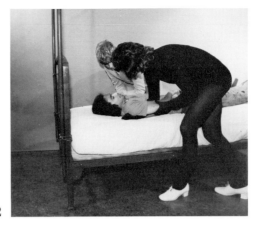

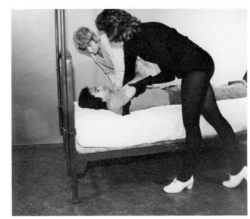

FIGURE 15-32

Method 5: Shear Leg Lever (Fig. 15-33).   The patient is placed in long sitting and the two helpers stand on either side facing the head of the bed. Each places one knee on the bed at the level of the patient's hips. The helpers' shoulders are placed under the patient's axillae with his arms resting on the helpers' backs.

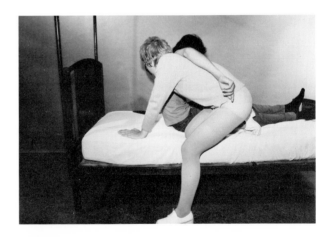

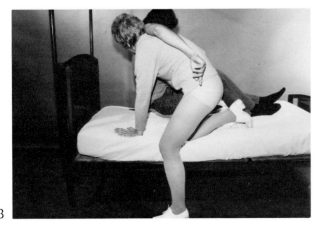

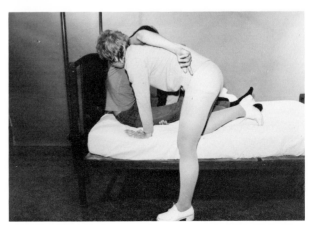

FIGURE 15-33

The helpers' outside hands are placed on the bed toward the head and with their elbows locked. The inside hands are placed under the patient's upper thighs from the medial sides. The helpers rock forward together onto their knees and locked arms, thus lifting the patient up the bed.

SITTING THE PATIENT UP IN BED

Method 1: Pull with Back Protected (Fig. 15-34).   To sit the patient on the edge of the bed the helper moves the patient's buttocks toward the side of the bed and then swings the patient's legs over the edge. Standing facing the patient, she then blocks the patient's knees with her own. Holding against an overhead bar to protect her back, she extends an arm to the patient to allow him to hook his wrists over her forearm to pull himself up. If the patient is unable to pull, this method should not be used, as weak shoulders can be injured.

Method 2: Rock Up (Fig. 15-35).   To sit the patient on the side of the bed, the helper stands by the bed, facing the patient with the knee nearest the head resting on the bed. The helper slides one hand under the patient's knees and flexes his knees and hips. She slides the other hand under the patient's far shoulder, supporting his head in the crook of her elbow. The patient is rocked back and then forward and is pivotted so that his feet are swung to the floor as he is placed in the sitting position.

Method 3: Lever Up (Fig. 15-36).   The helper stands by the patient's shoulders and slides the hand near the top of the bed under the patient's far shoulder. The patient's head rests in the crook of the helper's elbow. The helper leans forward to raise the patient's head and places a knee on the bed under the patient's

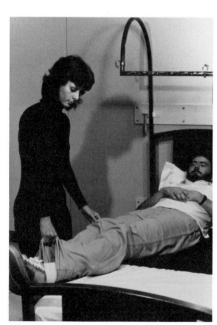
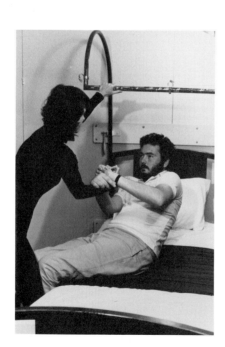
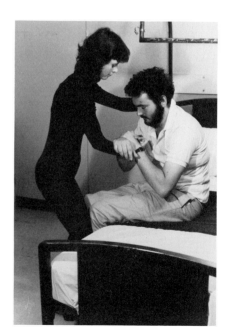

FIGURE 15-34

540

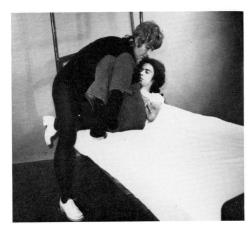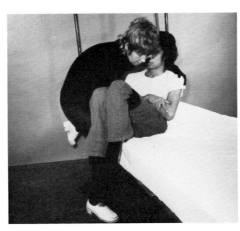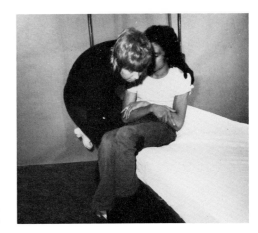

FIGURE 15-35

head. The helper's other hand is placed under the patient's other shoulder. By rocking forward the patient will be placed in a long-sitting position. As the patient nears the upright position the helper's hands are slid over the shoulders so that forward momentum can be controlled.

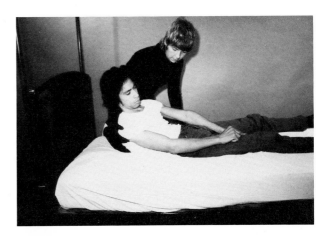

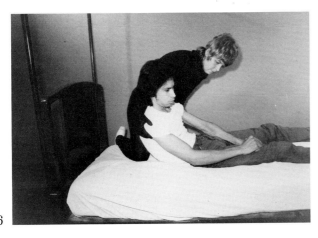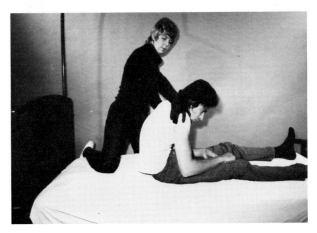

FIGURE 15-36

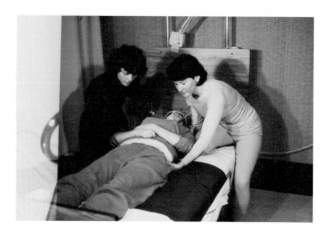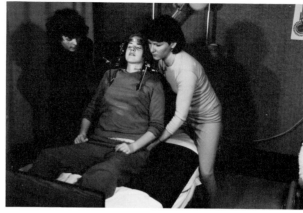

FIGURE 15-37

Method 4: Two Person Lever Up (Fig. 15-37).   Two people may be required to sit a very heavy or tall patient, or a patient in a halo thoracic brace. Each helper places one knee on the bed near the patient's shoulder. They each place a hand behind the patient's back using an arm to support the patient's head and neck. They both rock up onto a straight arm placed by the patient's hip, eliminating any strain on their backs.

TRANSFERRING ONTO THE BED FROM COMMODE
OR WHEELCHAIR

The bed should be equipped with a firm deck or plywood base, a firm mattress, and a nylon contour sheet. The compressed mattress should be the same height as the compressed wheelchair cushion. The wheelchair usually is positioned at 30° to the bed facing the foot. The front castors should be swung forward and locked to give maximum stability, and the brakes must be applied. The armrest by the bed should be removed. If a bridgeboard is necessary it should be positioned at this time. Talcum powder or silicone spray on the bridgeboard will facilitate sliding.

Method 1: Sling Swing Lift Transfer.   Some patients can take part of their weight by having their arms placed in an overhead strap (Fig. 15-38). The helper places one arm under the patient's knees and one by the trochanter while standing close to the patient. She pulls the patient forward, thus clearing his buttocks from the chair seat, and swings him onto the bed. The hand by the trochanter guides the direction of travel.

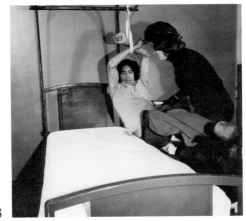
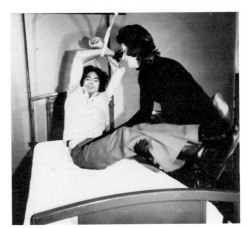

FIGURE 15-38

Method 2: Sling Pull Slide Transfer (Fig. 15-39).   The patient's buttocks are pulled forward in the chair and his legs are lifted onto the bed. His forearms are placed in an overhead sling. The helper now moves to the other side of the bed. She puts one knee on the bed and grasps the belt or slacks. The other hand pushes on the bed while the patient is pulled across the bridgeboard towards the helper. Some helpers may have to kneel on the bed in order to reach the belt comfortably.

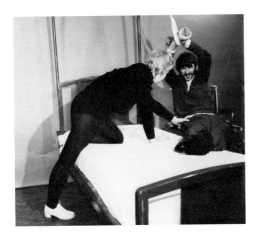
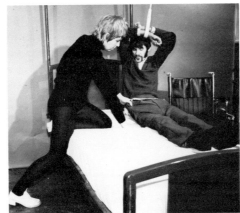
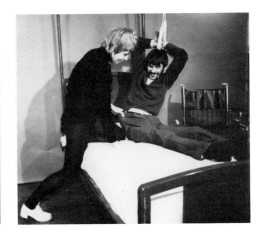

FIGURE 15-39

Method 3: Roll Transfer (Fig. 15-40). The area between the wheelchair cushion and the bed is padded with a pillow. The patient's buttocks are moved forward in the chair and his feet are placed on the bed, preferably with the outside leg crossed over. The helper moves to the rear of the chair and grasps the patient's slacks by the trochanter with her outside hand. She now steps close to the bed so that this arm rests across the patient's back. The other hand controls the shoulder nearest the bed. When the helper's outside arm is straightened and she pivots towards the bed, the patient is rolled onto the bed. The speed is controlled by her hand on the patient's shoulder. The patient may assist by swinging his arms towards the bed in synchronization with the helper's movement. A foot retainer board will be necessary if the patient's legs tend to slide off the bed during this transfer.

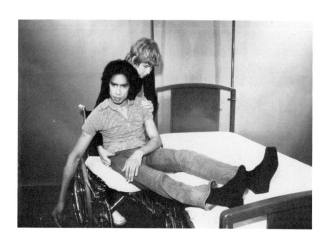

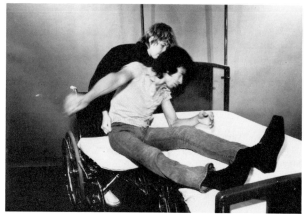

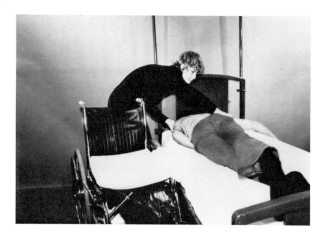

FIGURE 15-40

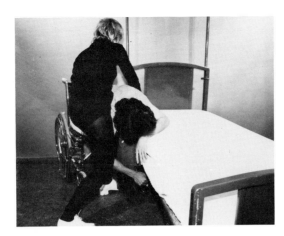
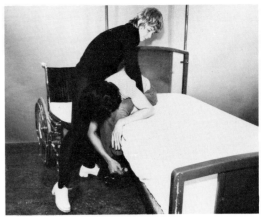
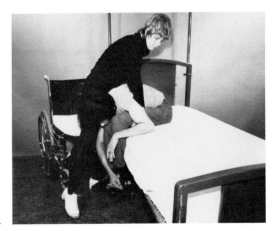

FIGURE 15-41

Method 4: Teeter Totter Pivot Lift Transfer (Fig. 15-41).   The helper moves the patient forward in the wheelchair and stands with one foot inside the footrests to stabilize the patient's thigh against her own. The patient's trunk is flexed far forward onto his knees. The helper reaches over and grasps the slacks in front of the hips. This places one arm against the patient's shoulder blade, thus adding an extra fulcrum. By rocking back and pivoting toward the bed the patient's buttocks are very easily levered onto the bed.

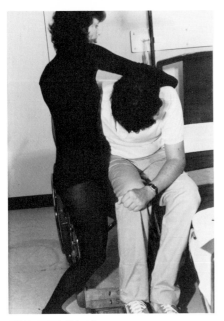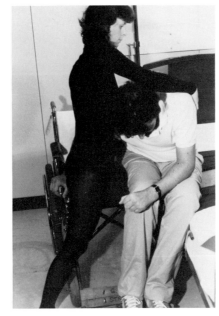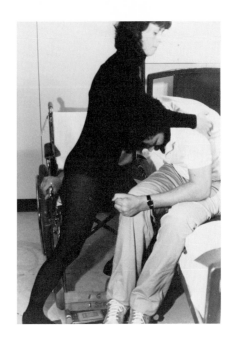

FIGURE 15-42

Method 5: Thigh Pivot Slide Transfer (Fig. 15-42).   This transfer is useful both for patients who can flex forward, and for those who cannot tolerate this. It is also useful because most of the pressure is against the patient's strong femur, and no strain is placed on his shoulders. This is a very easy transfer because it makes maximum use of first class levers.

The patient is pulled well forward in the wheelchair and his trunk is flexed forward. The helper stands facing the bed with the leg nearest the patient far forward, and under his thigh, close to the seat cushion. She reaches over to his far shoulder and pulls this shoulder down toward her. She synchronizes this action with a hand pushing against his hip and a push with her leg against his thigh. She should rise onto her toes as her leg moves forward so that he will be lifted onto the bed.

Method 6: Low Pivot Lift Transfer (Fig. 15-43).   The helper stands with the outside foot inside the footrests and stabilizes the patient's knees against her own. The helper places her palms on either side of the patient's rib cage and abducts her shoulders so that her elbows protrude. The patient places his arms over the helper's elbows and hugs strongly. The helper rocks back and pivots, thus raising the patient's buttocks and swinging him over onto the bed.

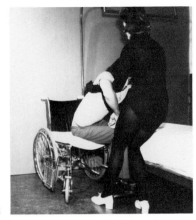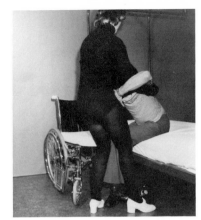

FIGURE 15-43

Towel Tucking—for Towel Lift Transfer (Fig. 15-44).   A towel can be used for transferring a patient if he is not dressed, if slacks are hard to grasp, or if the assistant needs to grasp higher or lower because of her height. The towel is most useful in a bare skin transfer to keep the buttocks together, preventing natal cleft tears. This is particularly important during toilet transfers, because as the patient's buttocks settle down into the toilet, they are pulled apart by the edges of the seat.

Placement of the towel far back under the buttocks is extremely important for good leverage, and so that the towel will remain in place during the transfer. The back edge of the towel is folded over the helper's hand, so that when the towel is pushed under the buttock the patient cannot be scratched. To insert the towel the patient's leg is lifted to allow the towel to be tucked well under. The towel is then held in position while the patient is pulled forward onto it.

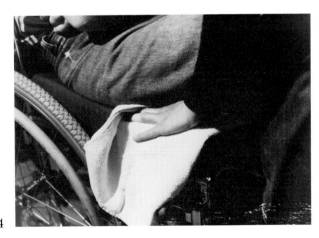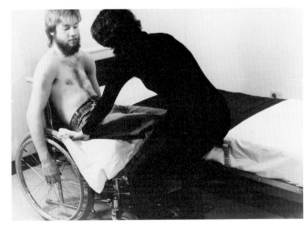

FIGURE 15-44

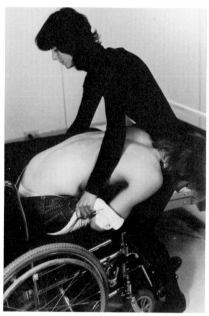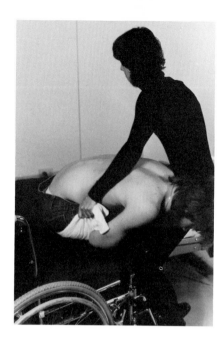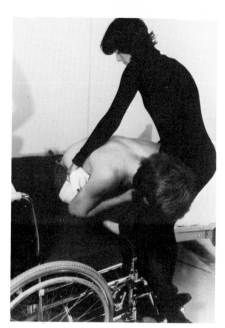

FIGURE 15-45

Method 7: Towel Lift Transfer (Fig. 15-45).   The patient's feet are placed on the footrest closest to the bed and the other footrest is swung away. The patient is now leaned forward with his head away from the bed. The helper places her outside foot forward and blocks the patient's outside knee. The foot nearer the bed is placed further back so that the pivot will not be impeded. The towel is gathered near the back to create a hammock, and with a straight back and straight arms, the patient is rocked in place to get the feel of the weight, and then the helper rocks back and pivots, thus using her body weight as a counterbalance.

Method 8: Two Person Towel Lift Transfer (Fig. 15-46).   A heavy patient may require two people to do a towel transfer. The front person does exactly the same transfer as in the previous method. The person at the rear stands as close to the bed as possible, either straddling the wheel, or with one bent knee on the bed. The helper at the rear also grasps the ends of the towel, and at the count of three, the patient's buttocks are pivoted towards the bed.

Method 9: Front Approach Slide Transfer (Fig. 15-47).   The patient is placed facing the bed and his feet are lifted onto the mattress. The leg rests are swung away and then the chair is pushed up to the bed, leaving no gap between bed and cushion. The brakes are now applied. The helper goes to the opposite side of the bed facing the patient. The helper abducts the patient's legs to provide lateral stability and grasps the patient's wrists, pulling his trunk forward into flexion. The patient's hands are placed on his ankles. The helper grasps the patient's hands and ankles together, and placing one knee on the bed she rocks back, thus pulling the patient onto the bed. The patient is placed lengthwise on the bed by swinging his feet towards the foot of the bed.

548

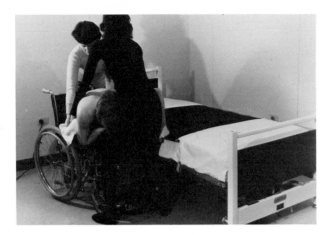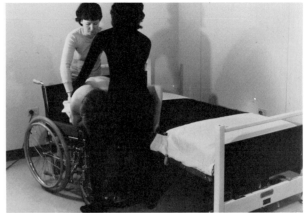

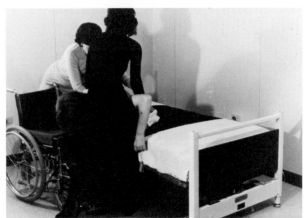

FIGURE 15-46

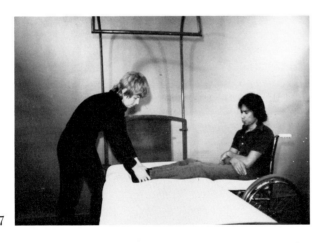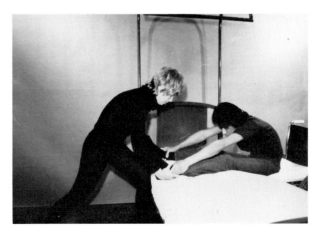

FIGURE 15-47

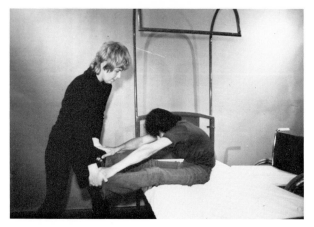 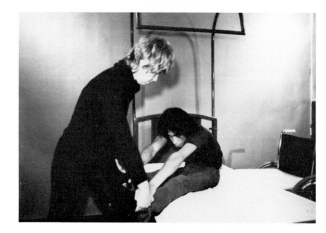

FIGURE 15-47 Continued

Method 10: Rear Approach Lift Transfer (Fig. 15-48). The chair is wheeled backward to contact the bed about two thirds of the way up. The brakes should *not* be applied. The patient's head must be supported while the wheelchair is tipped back. The hips are grasped and lifted towards the bed. The feet are now placed on a leg strap before lifting the hips again. Just before the patient's buttocks are free of the wheelchair back, his feet are moved to the seat. The helper now moves to the other side of the bed to pull him further back, holding under one arm, and supporting his head. The patient's knees are lifted into flexion, releasing the chair and allowing it to fall onto four wheels. The helper's arm nearest the foot of the bed is slipped right under the patient's knees, and the other arm still supports the patient's head while holding the shoulder. He is now easily swivelled into position.

Halo Brace. The halo brace may be used to stabilize the spine while allowing the patient some mobility. This brace, however, creates some problems when the patient is transferred, owing to the rigidity of the patient, the many projections of the brace, and the need for caution when moving the patient during the early stages.

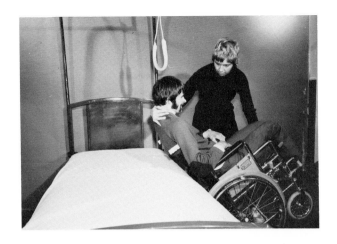
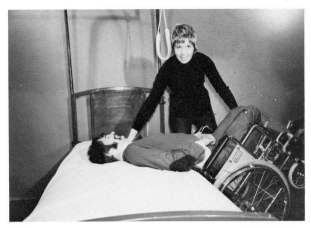

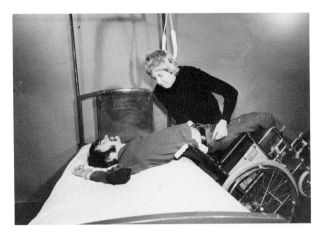
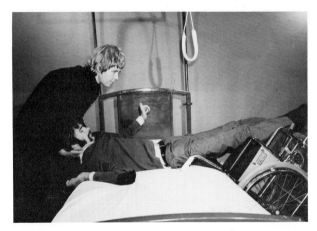

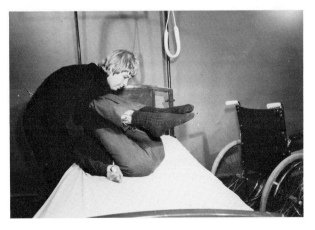

FIGURE 15-48

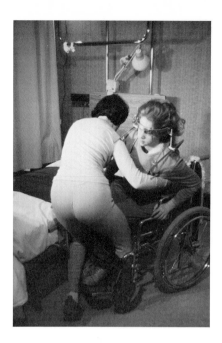

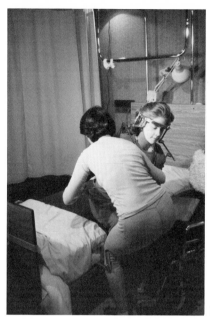

FIGURE 15-49

Method 11: Halo Slide Transfer (Fig. 15-49).   The assistant places the transfer board in position and leans the patient away from the bed, supporting the patient's trunk over her arm. She grasps the patient's slacks at the hip and pivots the patient's buttocks towards the bed. This is a useful transfer for someone who cannot bend forward.

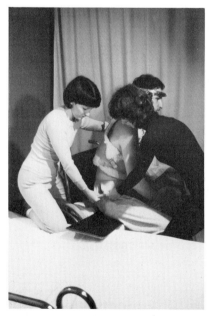

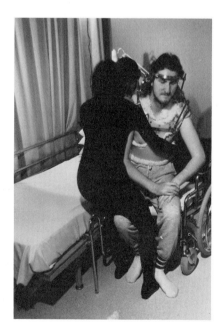

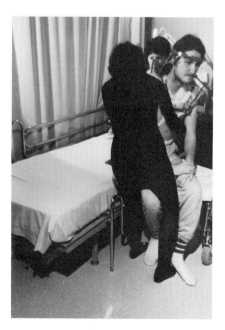

FIGURE 15-50

552

Method 12: Two Person Halo Slide Transfer (Fig. 15-50).   A patient who must stay upright can be moved most easily if he is leaned away from the direction of travel. This is particularly convenient when a person in a halo thoracic brace is moved because the helper is thus in a position to avoid the projections on the brace. The front helper leans the patient away from the bed while the transfer board is inserted. The helper's hand near the bed is used to hold the slacks at the hip while she supports the patient over her other arm under the brace and blocks his knee. He is leaned, turned, and flexed forward away from the bed. The helper at the back places one knee on the bed, uses one arm to support the patient's shoulders and the other to hold the slacks. As the patient is leaned further away his buttocks are pivoted onto the bed. The person at the back then controls the shoulders while the front helper lifts the patient's legs onto the bed.

Method 13: High Bed Two Person Lever Lift Transfer (Fig. 15-51).   On occasion it may be necessary to transfer a patient onto a high bed. The patient is slid forward in the wheelchair and the arm rest may be removed. The patient's feet are placed on the bed and one footrest is swung away. The front helper squats with her legs astride the outside wheelchair front upright. She places her arm nearest the foot of the bed under the patient's thighs as close as possible to his buttocks,

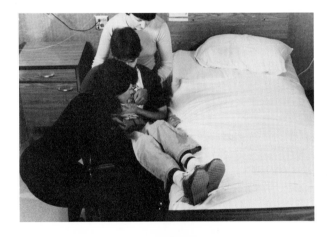
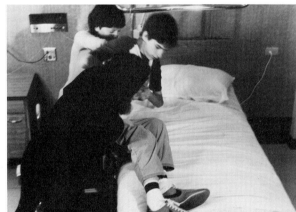
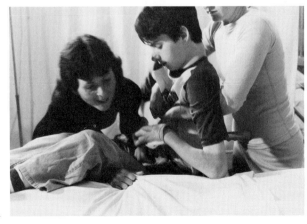
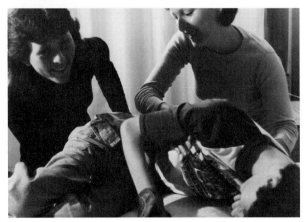

FIGURE 15-51

553

and grasps the bedding on top of the bed. Her other hand is placed flat against the patient's lower back. The back helper straddles the wheel by the bed and places her hands under the patient's axillae to guide him onto the bed. On a count of three, the front helper stands, so that one arm becomes a lever and the other arm pushes him across this lever onto the bed. The back helper takes very little weight, but must control the patient's shoulders.

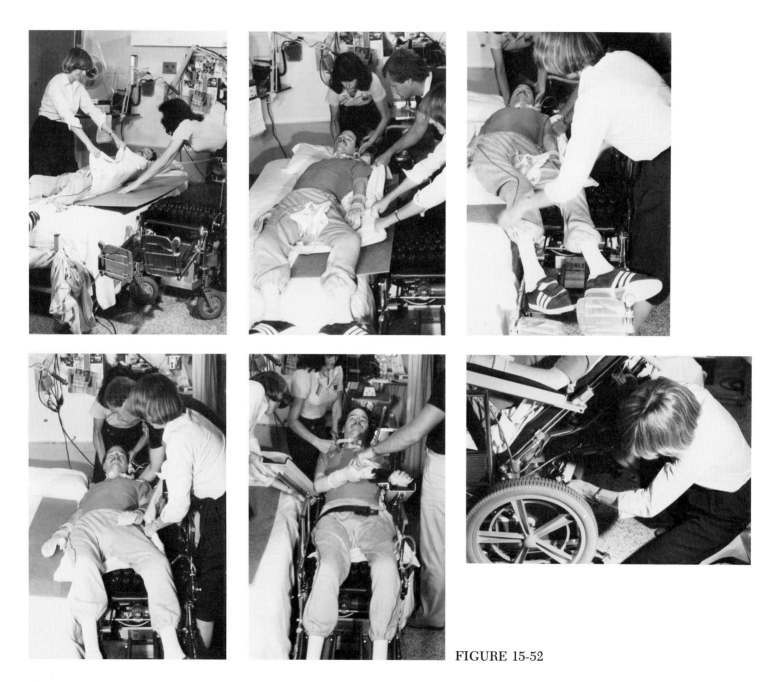

FIGURE 15-52

A person with tight hamstrings may be transferred using this method, but without lifting the feet onto the bed first.

Method 14: Two or Three Person Horizontal Slide Transfer (Fig. 15-52).   The fully reclined wheelchair is placed alongside the bed, and the bed is lowered so that both are at the same height.

One helper on the far side of the bed grasps the edge of the transfer sheet by the wheelchair and pulls to half roll the patient onto his side. This enables another helper to insert a transfer board under him. This transfer board reaches from the patient's knees to his shoulders.

Two helpers move to the wheelchair side of the bed, and one moves to the head of the bed to support the patient's head and ensure that his airway is not interfered with during the transfer. The patient's urinal collecting bag is placed so that it will move with him.

The two helpers grasp the transfer sheet, and in unison with the person at the head, they slide the patient towards the wheelchair. One helper moves the patient's legs over onto the legrests before they complete the slide into the wheelchair.

The controls are now placed so that the patient can operate the wheelchair, and he uses them to raise the wheelchair back. For respirator-dependent patients this allows room to place the respirator in position on the tray at the back of the wheelchair. It is most important that the wheelchair battery is not used to power the respirator or vice-versa. The respirator power source is switched from the wall source to external battery, and the patient is now mobile.

This transfer can be used to move a patient back to bed, or to a stretcher for bathing.

Method 15: Three Person Horizontal Lift (Fig. 15-53).   The wheelchair is placed so that the head of the wheelchair is at the foot of the bed and at right angles to it so that a minimum of movement is required.

The patient is prepared for the lift; her hands are placed so that they cannot fall, her urinal apparatus, if not worn on the leg, is unhooked from the wheelchair, and the wheelchair is put into the horizontal position. Since this girl can

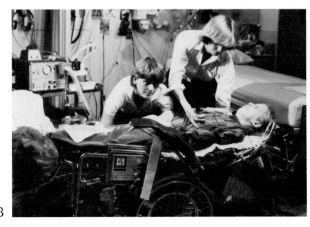 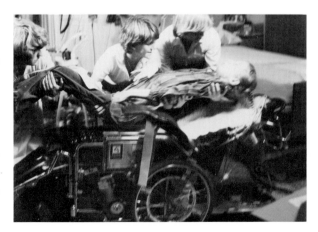

FIGURE 15-53

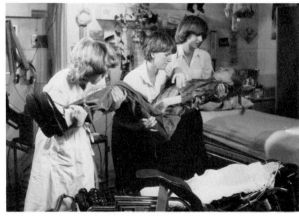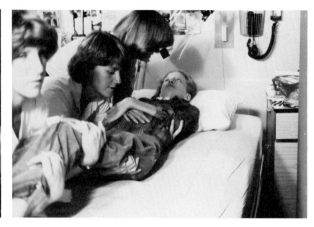

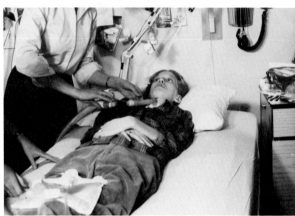

FIGURE 15-53 Continued

breathe on her own for short periods, all apparatus is prepared so that she can be disconnected from the respirator at the last moment, and reconnected quickly when the transfer is complete.

The three helpers stand on one side of the wheelchair; the helper near the patient's head is prepared to disconnect the respirator with one hand while she holds the patient's head and shoulders with the other. The other two helpers bend their knees and place their arms well under the patient. The helper near the head now disconnects the respirator, and places this hand under the patient giving the count of one, two, three; for all three to lift in unison. The patient is pulled in towards the helpers before they straighten their legs to lift. If the patient could tolerate it, she would be rolled in tight to the helpers' chests to reduce the weight on their arms.

The helpers walk to the raised bed and lower the patient, again keeping their backs straight and using their legs as much as possible. The respirator is now reconnected by the person at the head end.

This lift can be used for transfer back to the wheelchair, or to a stretcher for bathing.

556

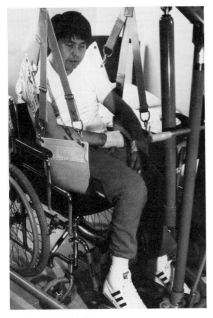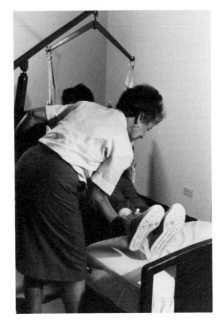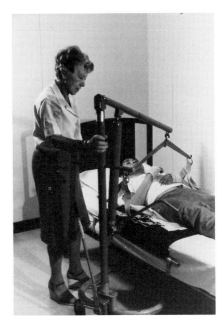

FIGURE 15-54

Method 16: Two Sling Hoist Lift Transfer (Fig. 15-54). If a hoist is used, a one-piece sling may be left in the wheelchair under the cushion. The edges and back can be rolled down out of the way until they are required. The patient and his cushion are lifted out of the wheelchair together. Two slings are required so that the sling in the wheelchair can be positioned before he is lifted into the wheelchair again. Fine adjustment of the sling straps are best done while the patient is in the wheelchair, so that the angle of tilt will be secure, and still allow him to be reseated in the chair easily. The adjusted position should be marked.

Method 17: Two Part Sling Hoist Lift Transfer. A track may be attached to an overhead bar, an A frame, or to the ceiling and used in conjunction with a mechanical hoist or block and tackle. Slings (see Appendix), one under the thighs and one behind the back, are attached to one another near the hips by means of an adjustable strap and hooks (Fig. 15-55A). The four ends of the slings are equipped with snap hooks and the hooks are clipped onto chains, which are held apart above head level by means of a spreader bar. The center of the spreader bar is attached to the lifting mechanism (Fig. 15-55B).

The sling at the back may be stiffened so that when the patient is flexed forward in the wheelchair it may be dropped into position without collapsing behind him. The other sling may be placed in position well under his thighs by lifting his legs one at a time to allow the sling to be pushed far back. This sling is hooked to the back sling at each side, thus ensuring that the back and base slings do not slide apart. The slings are now hooked onto the suspended chains so that when the lifting mechanism is operated, the patient is in a comfortable sitting position. When the patient's buttocks are clear of all obstacles the mechanism may

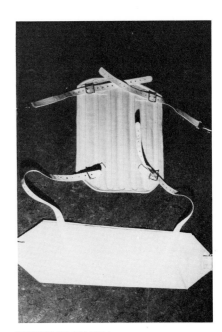

FIGURE 15-55A

557

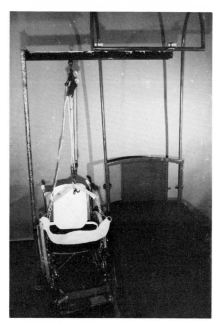

FIGURE 15-55B

be moved along the track and the patient lowered to the bed (Fig. 15-56). This sling can be positioned without lifting the patient, and is easily adjustable to the individual patient. These mechanisms are versatile in that they may be moved to another track, that is, in the bathroom.

TRANSFERRING FROM THE BED

Method 1: Sling Swing Lift Transfer (Fig. 15-57).   The patient's forearms are placed in an overhead sling. The helper stands beside the patient and lifts his legs with one arm under his thighs. The other hand is placed behind and under one buttock to guide and swing him forward from the bed and back onto the chair. The patient who can hold his weight will maintain and perhaps improve his strength; therefore, this method is used sometimes for preparing patients for learning independent transfers.

Method 2: Sling Pull Slide Transfer (Fig. 15-58).   The patient's forearms are placed in an overhead strap so that he can take some of his weight. The helper holds him by the belt or pants by the trochanter to swing and slide him into the chair over a bridgeboard.

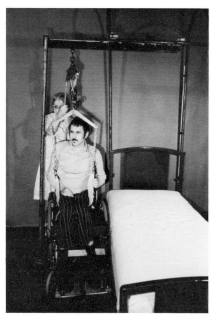

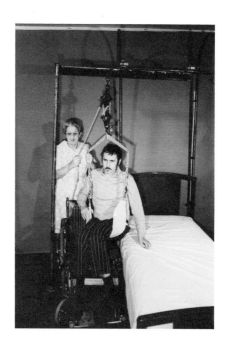

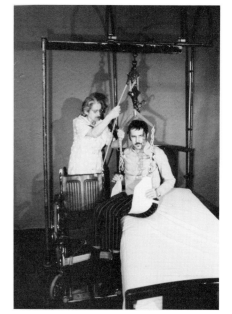

FIGURE 15-56

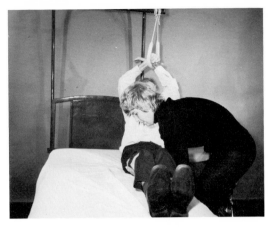

FIGURE 15-57

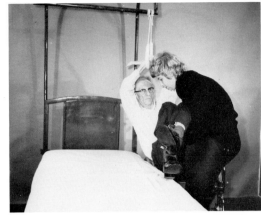

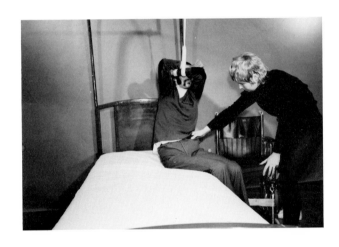

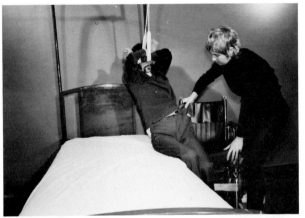

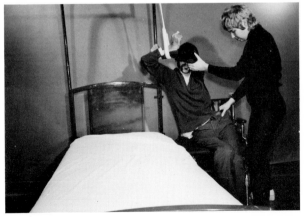

FIGURE 15-58

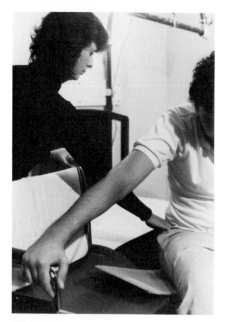
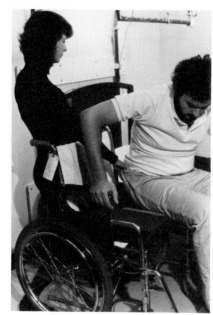
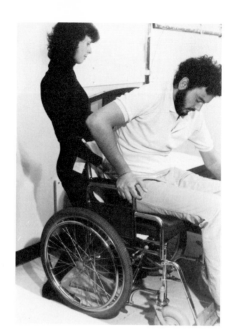

FIGURE 15-59

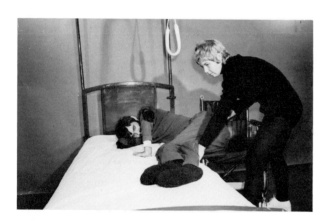
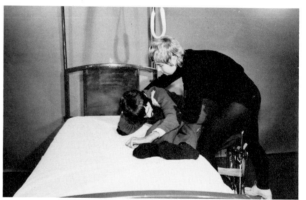

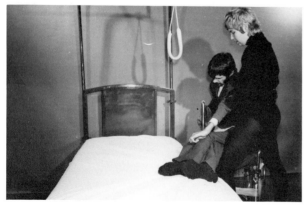

FIGURE 15-60

560

Method 3: Pull Slide Transfer (Fig. 15-59).   The patient's feet are positioned on the footrests, and if he can, he helps to maintain his balance with an arm on the wheelchair. The helper stands behind the wheelchair and stabilizes herself to protect her back by holding the pushing handle of the wheelchair with the arm nearest the bed. She uses the other hand to grasp the patient's slacks by the hip, and pulls him diagonally across the wheelchair seat into the back corner. The helper may alternatively stand on the outside of the wheelchair, but she must switch hands so that the patient is still pulled into the back corner of the wheelchair.

Method 4: Roll Up Transfer (Fig. 15-60).   The patient is in side-lying facing away from the chair, in a jack-knife position. The patient's belt is grasped to lift and slide his buttocks into the chair seat. The helper's knee is placed against the bed to hold the patient's legs in position and to provide a fulcrum when rolling the patient up to sit.

Method 5: Teeter-Totter Pivot Lift Transfer (Fig. 15-61).   The helper places the patient's feet on the footrests so they are free to turn as he is pivoted. She now flexes the patient's trunk forward so that his trunk rests on his thighs. The helper places one foot beside the footrest on the outside to block the chair and to position

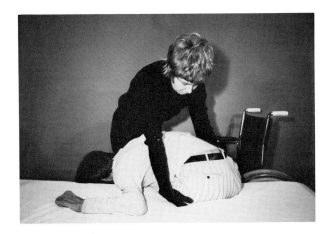

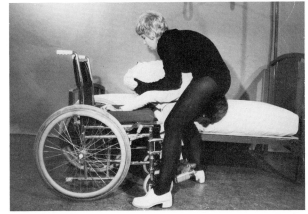

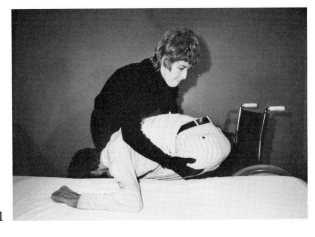

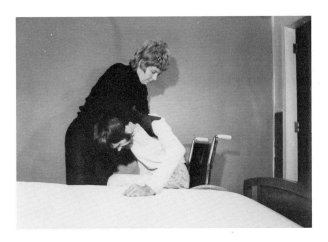

FIGURE 15-61

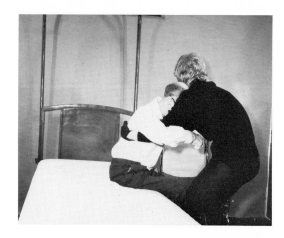

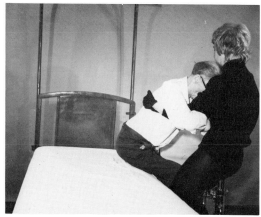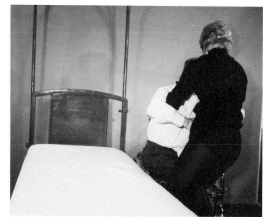

FIGURE 15-62

herself correctly. The patient's thigh is blocked and controlled by the helper's inside knee as the patient is rocked onto the chair.

As in all transfers when the patient's weight is transmitted to the footrests, castors must be turned forward and locked.

Method 5: Low Pivot Lift Transfer (Fig. 15-62).　The helper stands in front of the patient and blocks the patient's knees with her own. She places her palms on either side of the patient's rib cage and holds her elbows out. The patient puts his arms on the helper's elbows and hugs to assist holding. The helper rocks back to pivot the patient onto the chair.

Method 6: Towel Lift Transfer (Fig. 15-63).　The towel is placed in position while the patient is lying down. He is then sat up with his feet in position on the footrests. The assistant stands with the patient's knee blocked and with her leg nearest the bed slightly back, in a comfortable position. She bends his trunk down with his head and shoulders away from the wheelchair and gathers up the towel so that it is well back, creating a hammock under the patient's buttocks. She then rocks back with straight arms and back, and pivots on her feet to place him in the wheelchair.

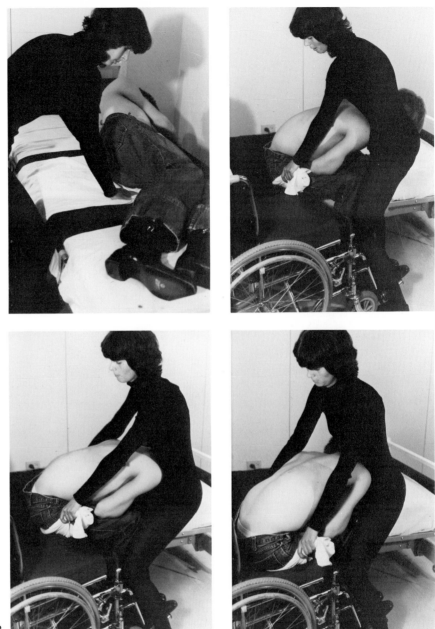

FIGURE 15-63

Method 7: Two Person Towel Lift Transfer (Fig. 15-64). A heavier person may require two people to assist him. The front person does not vary her technique, as described in the previous method. The second helper stands close to the bed either straddling the wheel near the bed, or with one knee on the bed. Both helpers grasp the towel, and on the count of three, the patient is pivoted over onto the wheelchair.

Method 8: Front Approach Slide Transfer (Fig. 15-65). The helper swings the footrests back and butts the chair against the bed facing it. The patient is sat up, and his trunk is flexed forward. The helper holds the patient under the upper thigh and bounces the patient to shift him back into the chair. This is an excellent method for the very flaccid patient who can lie forward on his legs.

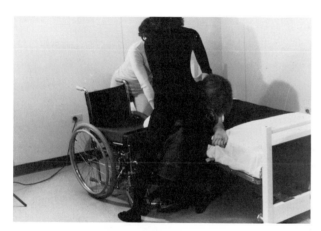
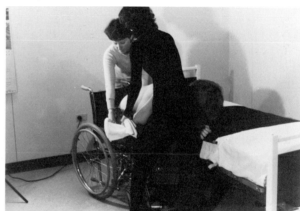
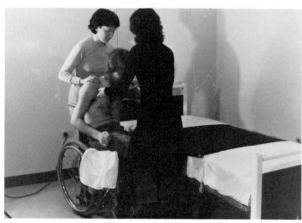

FIGURE 15-64

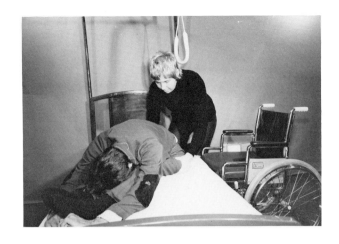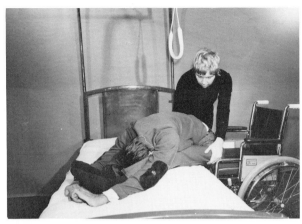

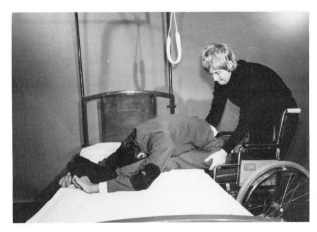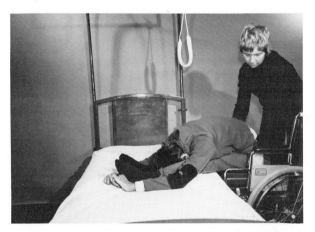

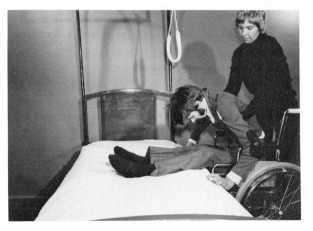

FIGURE 15-65

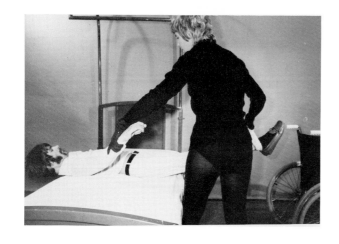

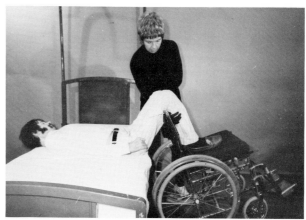

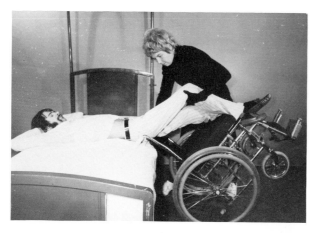

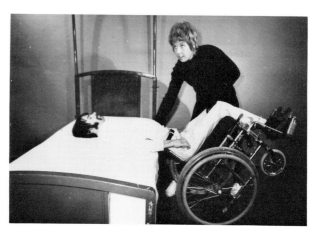

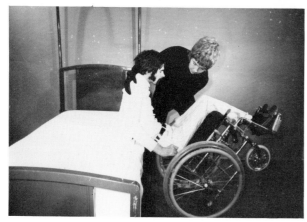

FIGURE 15-66

566

Method 9: Rear Approach Lift Transfer (Fig. 15-66).   The helper holds the patient's far wrist and his slacks at the ankles. She synchronizes her pull on the arm and swing of the legs to pivot the patient on his buttocks. She now hooks the patient's legs over the back of the chair. The helper pushes the wheelchair handles down onto the mattress and straightens the patient's legs to rest over the edge of the seat. She pulls the patient's legs forward alternately to pull his buttocks into the chair. As the patient slides into the chair the slacks are pulled to ensure that they are not tight at the groin. The helper slips an arm under the patient's neck to the far shoulder and sits him up while controlling the chair position with her hand on the pushing handle. Throughout this transfer, the wheelchair brakes are not applied, so that the wheelchair can be tipped. The pushing handles digging into the mattress will stabilize the wheelchair when there is weight in the chair.

Halo Brace. The halo brace may be used to stabilize the spine while allowing the patient some mobility. This brace, however, creates some problems when the patient is transferred, owing to the rigidity of the patient, the many projections of the brace, and the need for caution when moving the patient during the early stages.

Method 10: Halo Slide Transfer (Fig. 15-67).   The helper blocks the patient's knee and then the patient is leaned away from the wheelchair over the helper's arm, which supports the patient's trunk. A pull on the patient's slacks at the hip will pivot the buttocks into the wheelchair. Most of the force to move his buttocks is derived from the patient's head and shoulders, as he is leaned and turned away from the direction of travel.

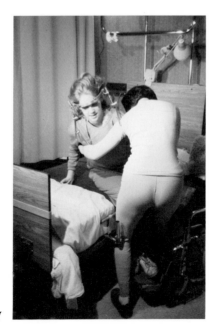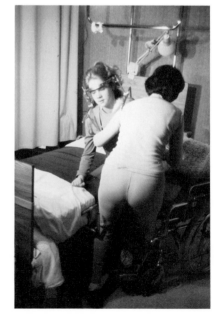

FIGURE 15-67

Method 11: Two Person Halo Slide Transfer (Fig. 15-68).   The front assistant uses the same technique as in the previous method. The assistant at the rear supports the patient's shoulders as he is leaned away from the direction of travel. Her other hand grasps the slacks at the hip and assists to pivot him into the wheelchair on the count of three.

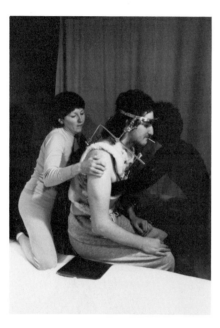
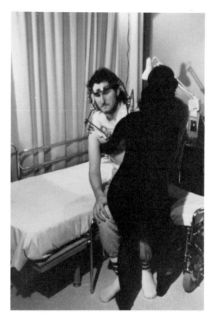
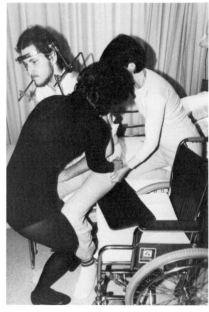
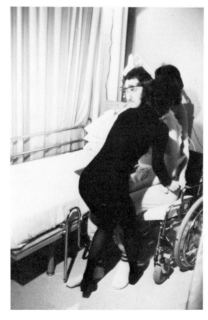

FIGURE 15-68

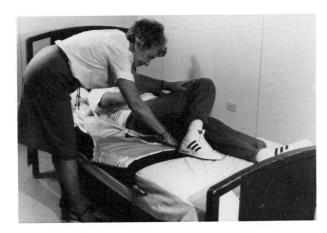
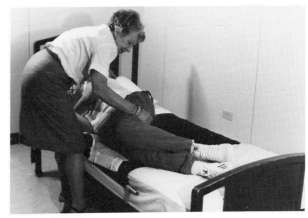
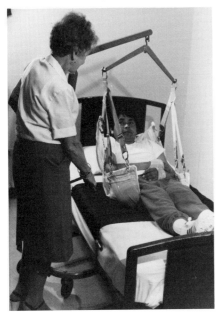
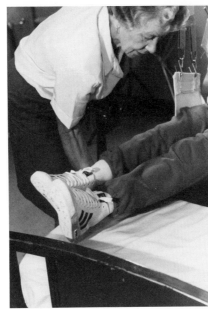
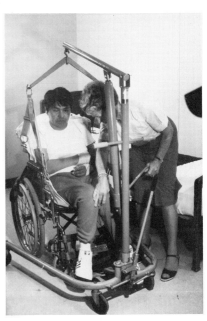

FIGURE 15-69

Method 12: Two Slings Hoist Lift Transfer (Fig. 15-69).   A sling is placed under the cushion of the wheelchair with the sides and back neatly rolled down beside the cushion. The helper rolls the patient to one side, bending his knee and using it as a lever to roll him and hold him in position. She uses her other hand to tuck the second sling, half rolled up, under the patient's back. The patient is rolled to the other side in the same way so that the sling can be unrolled and pulled out on the other side. The hoist is hooked on, and the patient is lifted to a sitting position just clear of the bed before his feet are swung off the bed. The hoist is wheeled to the wheelchair, taking care that the base is spread and that the patient is controlled so that he does not swing and overbalance. As the patient is lowered into the wheelchair, a push against his knees will ensure that he is seated well

569

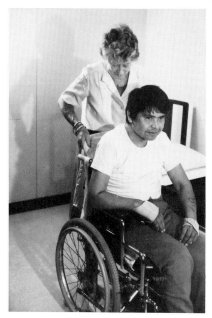

FIGURE 15-69 Continued

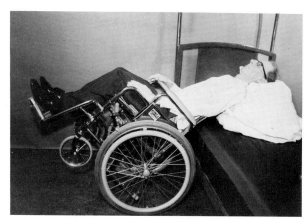

FIGURE 15-70

back. The sling is now removed by pulling it up the back, leaving the first sling in position in the wheelchair under the cushion.

Resting Position. There is a quick method of semi-reclining a patient in his chair without transferring him to a bed. Pillows are placed halfway down the bed. Then the chair is backed to the bed and tipped so that the patient's head rests on the pillows and the pushing handles rest on the mattress (Fig. 15-70). The brakes may now be applied for additional safety. This method should only be used when the bed is immobile. This resting position can be very useful when the patient is becoming conditioned to the upright position. It is also useful to relieve the weight from the patient's buttocks.

FLOOR TO WHEELCHAIR

Method 1: Chair Roll Up (Fig. 15-71). The chair is tipped back with the pushing handles on the floor by the patient's feet. The patient's legs are lifted and the chair is slid towards the patient's buttocks until his ankles rest on the edge of the chair seat. The helper now moves around to the front of the chair and grasps the patient's ankles and slacks together. The helper also places one knee on the cross bars to block the chair and keep the chair open. By leaning back with straight arms, the patient's buttocks are lifted and pulled into the chair. His feet may now be placed on the footrests. The helper now moves to the rear of the chair. She squats by the patient's head and places one hand under his neck and one under the pushing handle. The chair is righted as the helper stands. As the chair nears the upright position, the helper's hand is moved from the patient's neck to the front of his shoulder in order to steady him.

570

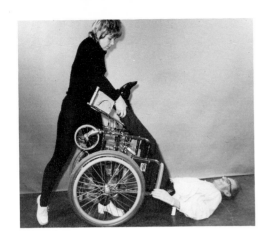
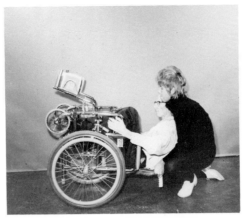
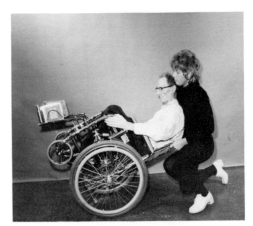

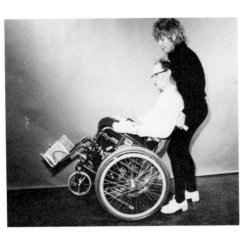
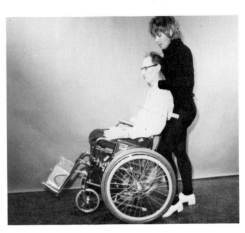

FIGURE 15-71

Method 2: Two-Person Chair Roll-Up (Fig. 15-72).   Method 1 is easier with two helpers, one on either side of the patient, working as a synchronized team. In this case, the patient's head is supported with the helpers' inside arms, while the outside hands lift the pushing handle.

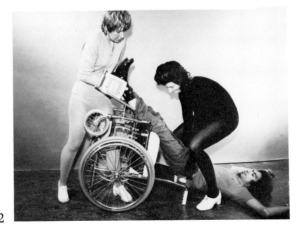
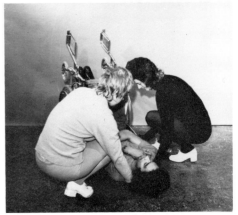

FIGURE 15-72

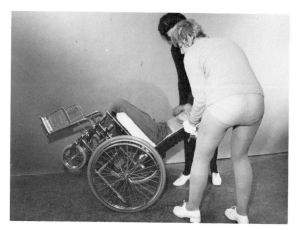
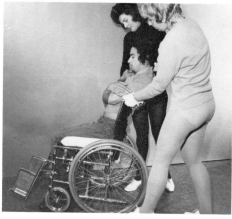

FIGURE 15-72 Continued

Method 3: Quad Lift (Fig. 15-73).   This lift is particularly useful because the patient's body weight is always close to the assistants', and because there is no strain on the patient's shoulders. The patient is brought to a sitting position. The assistants then face in the opposite direction to the patient and place one hand under his thigh from the inside. This is usually comfortable for the lifters at about midthigh level. The other hand grasps the slacks at the back, using the belt. If the person is unclothed, a towel may be used as a hammock under the buttocks. The patient's trunk is bent forward until his shoulders rest against the helpers' arms, a position which is secure for the patient. On the count of three, both helpers stand with their backs straight and the weight taken at full arm length. In this position, each helper has good control and cannot easily be knocked off balance by the other when moving the patient.

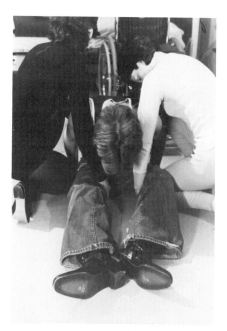
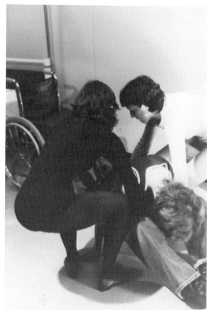
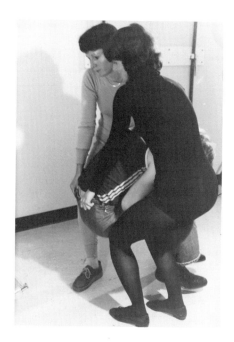

FIGURE 15-73

572

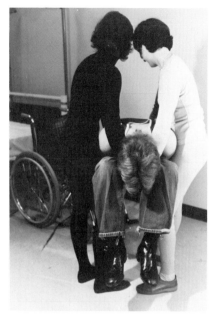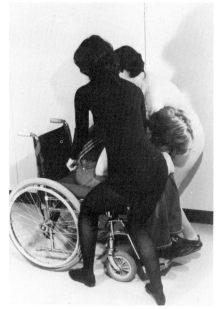

FIGURE 15-73 Continued

Method 4: Forearm Lift (Fig. 15-74).   The helpers squat, one on each side of the patient, facing his feet, and bring the patient to the sitting position. The hand closest to the patient is placed underneath the patient's axilla from behind and over the patient's forearm near the elbow. This is a flat handhold with the thumb aligned with the fingers. The other hand is placed under the patient's thigh near his knees. Both assistants stand to lift, keeping their arms straight. This method permits each helper to maintain balance even though movements may not be in perfect unison.

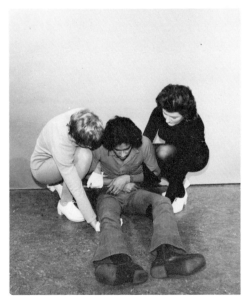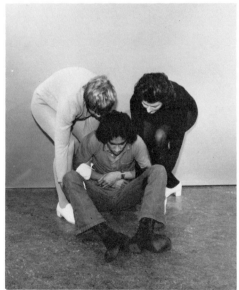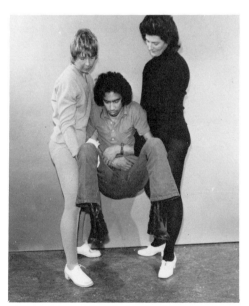

FIGURE 15-74

The chair should be backed in alongside the toilet at approximately 40°. This angle may be increased to 90° if the size of the room demands this approach. A toilet seat raised to the height of the compressed wheelchair cushion top, and a footstool to compensate for this increased height will facilitate transfer. For all transfers, the arm of the chair near the toilet is removed and the brakes are locked. The castors are turned forward and locked.

Method 1: Sling Swing Lift Transfer. Some patients can lift part of their own weight by having their arms placed in an overhead strap centered over the toilet (Fig. 15-75). Standing close to the patient, the helper places one arm under the patient's knees and one by a hip. She pulls the patient forward, thus clearing his buttocks from the chair seat, and swings him onto the toilet. The patient who cannot lift as he reaches the toilet must be lifted slightly by the helper to avoid grazing the buttocks against the toilet seat.

Method 2: Teeter-Totter Pivot Lift Transfer (Fig. 15-76). The helper stands with the foot furthest from the toilet inside the footrests and stabilizes the patient's knees between her own. The patient's trunk is flexed far forward onto his thighs and away from the direction of travel. The helper reaches over and slides her hands, palm up, under the upper thigh just below the crease of the patient's buttocks. The helper rocks back and pivots towards the toilet to position the patient. Care must be taken to ensure that the buttocks are not parted during this maneuver to prevent the possibility of a natal cleft split.

Note that one castor was not turned forward. This is not serious in this case because the patient is tall and his feet can be placed on the floor for the transfer.

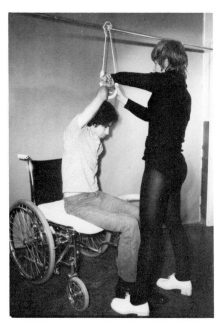
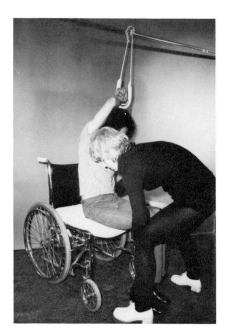
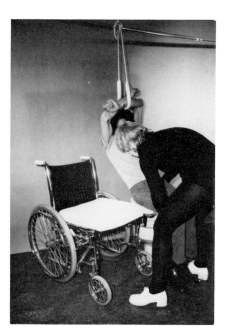

FIGURE 15-75

574

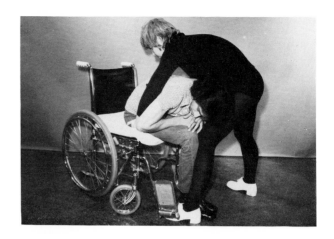

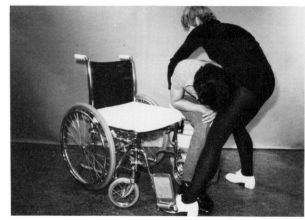

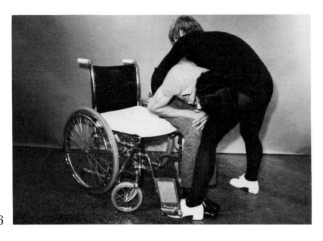

FIGURE 15-76

Method 3: Thigh Pivot Slide Transfer (Fig. 15-77).   This transfer is useful both for patients who can be bent forward and for those who cannot tolerate this. It is also useful because most of the pressure is against the patient's strong femur, and no strain is placed on the shoulders. It also requires only minimal effort by the

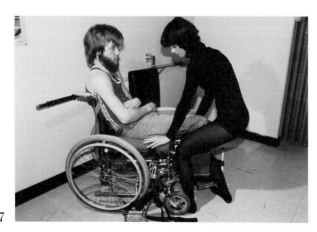

FIGURE 15-77

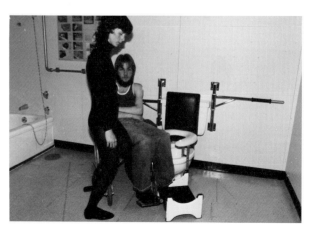

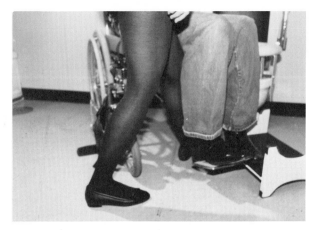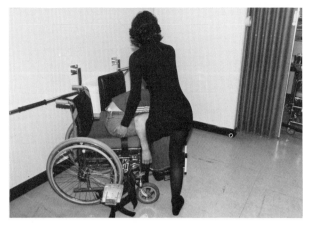

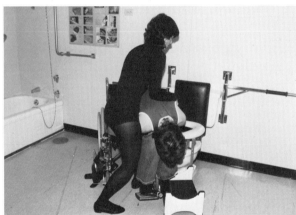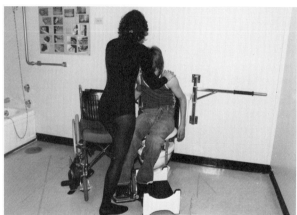

FIGURE 15-77 Continued

helper. The patient is pulled well forward in the wheelchair, and one or both of his feet are placed on a footstool. The helper stands facing the toilet with the leg nearest the patient against the wheelchair and under the patient's thigh, with her foot as close to the toilet as possible, thus placing her thigh in position to act as a lever. She reaches over his flexed trunk, to his far shoulder, ready to pull his trunk down and towards her. Her other hand pushes against his hip. As she pulls his shoulder down and in, and pushes on his hip, she levers him towards the toilet with her leg, rising up onto her toes to gain lift. This movement must be synchronized, and when the movement is smooth it is one of the easiest pivot transfer methods.

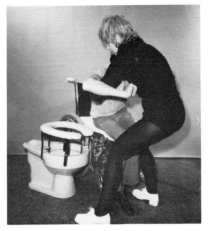 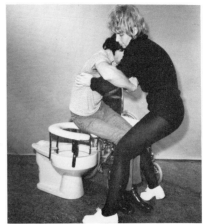

FIGURE 15-78

Method 4: Low Pivot Lift Transfer (Fig. 15-78).   The helper stands with the outside foot inside the footrests and stabilizes the patient's knees between her own. The helper places her palms on either side of the patient's rib cage and abducts her shoulders so that her elbows protrude. The patient places his arms over the helper's elbows and hugs. The helper rocks back and pivots, placing the patient on the toilet. Any further positioning required may be obtained by repeating the procedure.

Towel Lift—Tucking the Towel Under (Fig. 15-79).   This is a particularly useful transfer for the toilet because the towel keeps the buttocks together, helping to prevent natal cleft splits as the patient sinks slightly into the toilet hole; if a heavy patient is lifted with hands on the bare buttocks, it is easy to part the cheeks even before they are further parted by the toilet seat. This transfer is also useful because the towel creates a handle in a situation where there is no clothing to be grasped.

Placement of the towel far back under the buttocks is extremely important for good leverage, and so that the towel will remain in place during the transfer. The back edge of the towel is folded over the helper's hand, so that when the towel is pushed under the buttock the patient cannot be scratched. To insert the towel the patient's leg is lifted to allow the towel to be tucked well under. The towel is then held in position while the patient is pulled forward onto it.

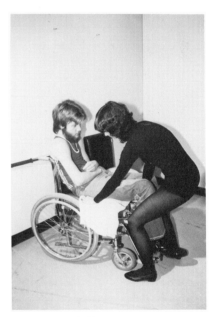

FIGURE 15-79

Method 5: Towel Lift Transfer (Fig. 15-80).   The patient's trunk is bent forward with his head away from the toilet. The assistant places her foot furthest from the toilet inside the footrest, and blocks the patient's knee with hers. She grasps the towel, which forms a hammock well back under the patient's buttocks. With straight arms and a straight back, she rocks back and pivots him to the toilet. In this lift, the helper's body counterbalances that of the patient, their knees forming the fulcrum.

Method 6: Two Person Towel Lift Transfer (Fig. 15-81).   When two people are required for a heavy patient, the second person stands behind, straddling the wheel by the toilet. Both helpers grasp the towel, and on the count of three, the front helper rocks back and pivots as before, while the back helper lifts and helps guide the patient over.

Method 7: Two Person Halo Slide Transfer (Fig. 15-82).   The front helper places the patient's feet on the floor, because this patient is very tall. A towel is placed well back under his buttocks. She grasps the towel end nearest the toilet and leans him forward and away from the direction of travel, supporting his trunk over her arm which is placed against his ribs, under the projections of the halo thoracic brace. The helper at the back straddles the wheel nearest the toilet, and

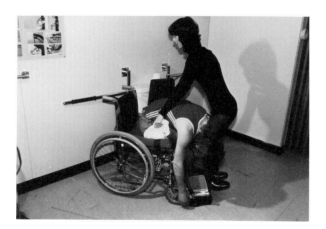
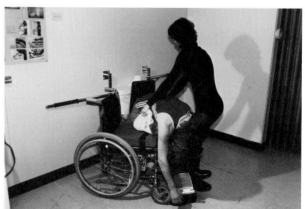
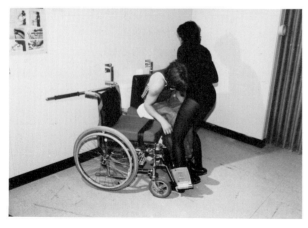

FIGURE 15-80

578

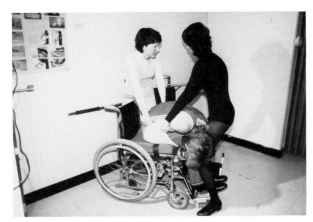
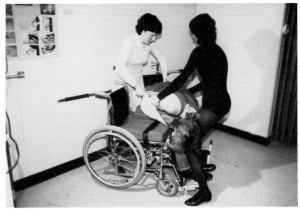
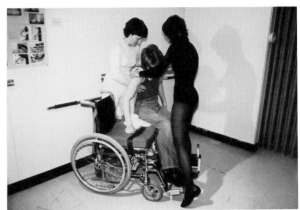

FIGURE 15-81

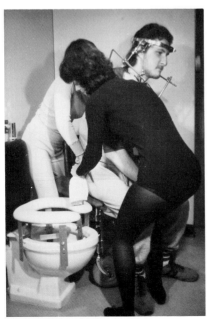
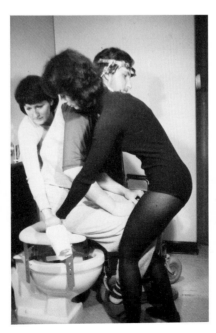
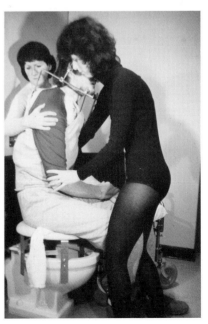

FIGURE 15-82

579

grasps both ends of the towel to help move and guide the patient's buttocks over. The front helper blocks his knee, and helps to move him over by rocking back and pivoting him towards the toilet. The back helper can now control his shoulders as he is brought to the upright.

FROM TOILET TO CHAIR

Method 1: Sling Swing Lift Transfer (Fig. 15-83).   The patient's forearms are placed in an overhead sling, which is then centered over the wheelchair seat. The helper stands in front of the patient and lifts his legs with one arm under his thighs. The other hand is placed behind and under one buttock to guide and swing him forward from the toilet and back onto the chair. This method is not useful if the patient's trunk elongates excessively when he holds his weight.

Method 2: Teeter-Totter Pivot Lift Transfer (Fig. 15-84).   The helper stands in front of the chair and blocks the patient's thighs with a knee. The patient is flexed far forward, thus transferring most of his weight to his feet. The helper slides both hands under the patient's thighs just forward of the hips. The patient is levered over as the helper rocks back and pivots. The helper's back and arms should remain straight as she pivots, only her legs should bend.

Method 3: Thigh Pivot Slide Transfer (Fig. 15-85).   In order to gain room for the helper to place her leg well under the patient's thigh, the wheelchair must be turned at right angles to the toilet.

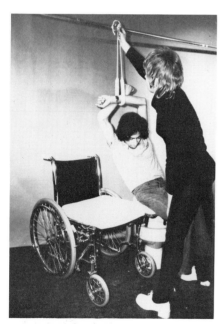 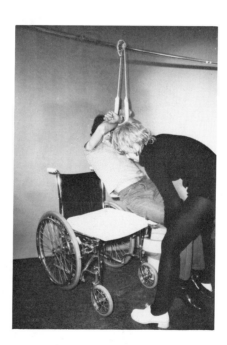 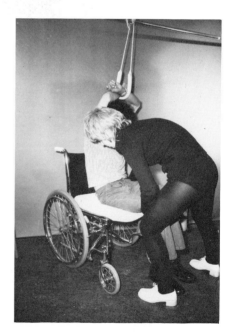

FIGURE 15-83

580

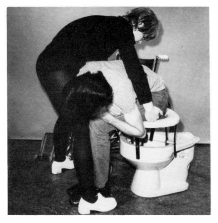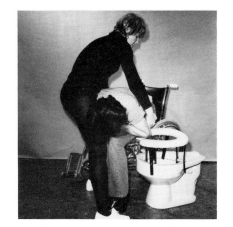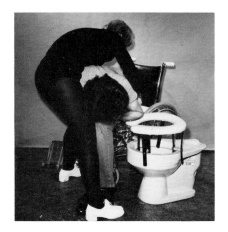

FIGURE 15-84

The helper moves the patient forward slightly on the toilet, and flexes his trunk forward. She places the foot nearest the patient far forward, with her leg remaining close to the toilet. She reaches over to his far shoulder and pulls this shoulder down and toward her in synchronized action, with a hand pushing on his buttocks and a push with her leg against his thigh. If she rises onto her toes as she levers him with her leg he will be lifted onto the wheelchair, while his body is spun around the fulcrum point of her thigh.

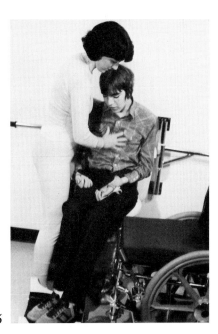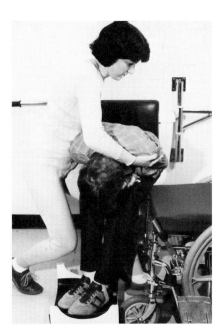

FIGURE 15-85

581

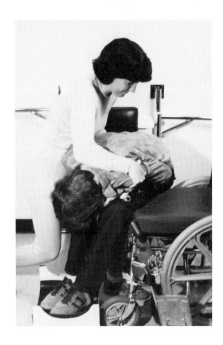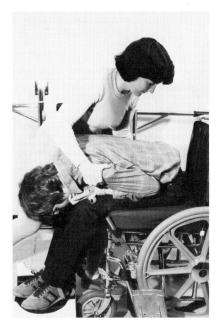

FIGURE 15-85 Continued

Method 4: Low Pivot Lift Transfer (Fig. 15-86). The helper stands in front of the patient and blocks the patient's knees with her own. She places her palms against the patient's rib cage on either side. The patient puts his arms over the helper's elbows and hugs to assist holding and the helper rocks back to pivot the patient onto the chair.

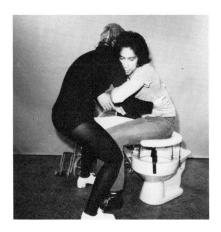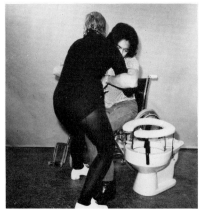

FIGURE 15-86

582

Method 5: Towel Lift Transfer (Fig. 15-87).   The helper places a towel well back under the patient's buttocks. This can be done fairly easily by rocking the patient's trunk to one side while the towel is slipped under the opposite buttock. Talcum powder may be used, but care must be taken not to get powder on the floor, as it is very slippery. The helper places both of the patient's feet on one footrest and blocks his knee with hers. She leans him forward as far as possible, with his head turned away from the direction of travel. She gathers the towel ends and holds them well back, and then rocking back with straight arms and back, she pivots him back into the wheelchair.

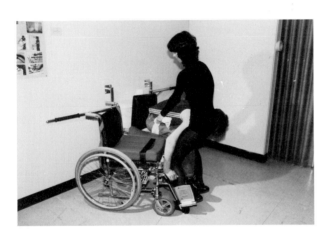
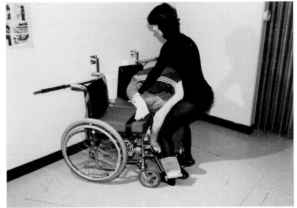
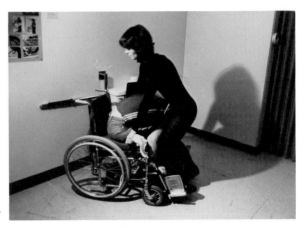

FIGURE 15-87

Method 6: Two person Towel Lift Transfer (Fig. 15-88). Where two people are required, the front helper uses the same techniques as described above. The helper at the back straddles the wheel near the toilet, and grasps the towel on either side. On the count of three, the front helper rocks back and pivots while the back helper assists.

Method 7: Halo Slide Transfer (Fig. 15-89). A towel is positioned under the patient's buttocks, and a very tall patient (as illustrated) will have his feet positioned on the floor. The front helper blocks the patient's knee with hers and holds the end of the towel nearest the wheelchair. The patient is leaned forward and away from the direction of travel, and is supported by the front helper's arm. The back helper straddles the wheel near the toilet, and grasps the towel on either side. On the count of three, the front helper pivots the patient over into the wheelchair while the back helper assists.

Method 8: Hoist Transfer (Fig. 15-90). Hoists used in conjunction with over-

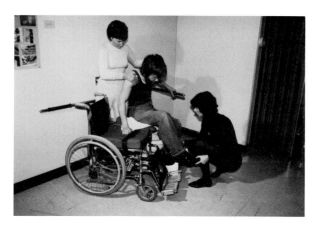

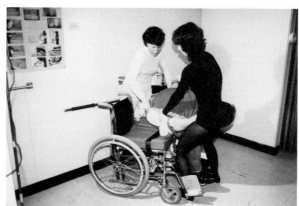

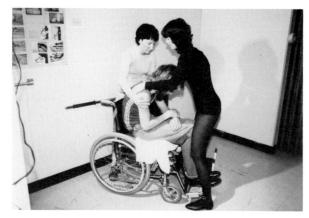

FIGURE 15-88

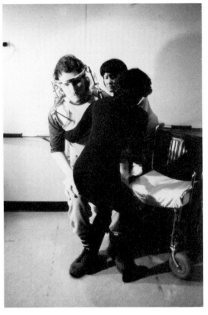
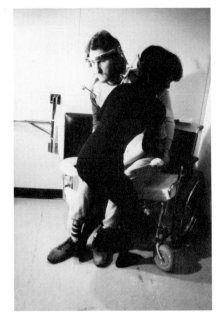
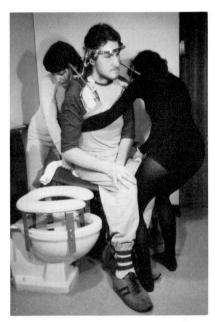

FIGURE 15-89

head tracks or commercial hydraulic hoists may be practical. The slings do not require a cutout, even for women, if the two-sling method is used. (See "Bed Transfer" for hoist information.)

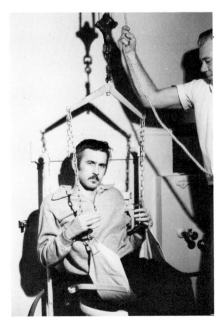
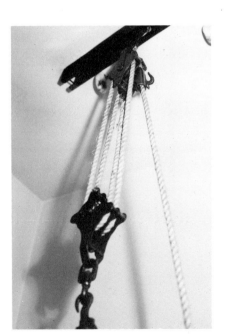
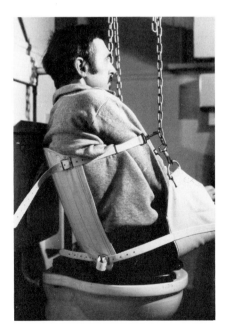

FIGURE 15-90

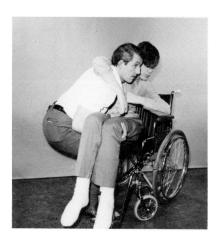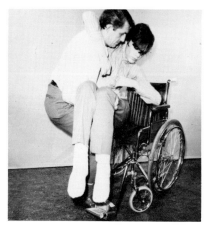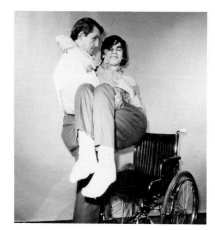

FIGURE 15-91

PICK UP AND CARRY BY ONE HELPER

This technique will be governed by the size of the patient and the strength and experience of the helper. The right-handed helper should stand on the patient's left side and remove the armrest. The patient's feet are moved to the far footrest, and the near footrest is folded up or swung away. The helper now places his right foot between the footrests with his knee close to the chair seat. The patient's right arm is placed over the helper's left shoulder, and the helper's left arm is slipped behind the patient to grasp his belt or slacks at the hip. The right arm is placed well under the patient's thighs. The patient is now pulled in toward the helper, thus allowing a direct lift (Fig. 15-91).

To lower the patient into the chair, the helper steps in very close before flexing his knees. A swinging motion is effective in placing the patient (Fig. 15-92). It should be noted that this technique is hard to learn and should be practiced with a lightweight person.

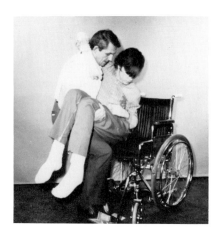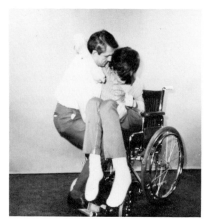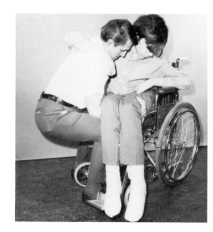

FIGURE 15-92

BATHING

Thorough cleanliness is essential for skin care. Because the dependent patient may be unable to check water temperature himself, the helper must be certain the temperature is safe.

A shower seat for the bathtub or shower has been described for the use of the independent patient in Chapter 5. This may also be used in the management of the dependent patient. A wheel-in shower, also described in Chapter 5, may be practical. The drive wheels are unnecessary, and a commode with castors will suffice, since help is readily available.

An overhead track hoist may be used. This can be installed over the toilet and tub so that the patient may be transferred directly from toilet to tub. Commercial hoists are available. These can be placed in a floor flange, which is purchased as an extra, especially for bathtub transfers.

Two strong people may lift a patient in and out of a bathtub (Fig. 15-93). The helper behind the patient places his hands under the patient's axillae and over his wrists using a flat hand hold. The front helper bends his knees to pick up the patient's legs, with one arm under both knees and the other at his ankles. The

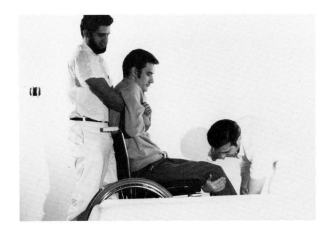
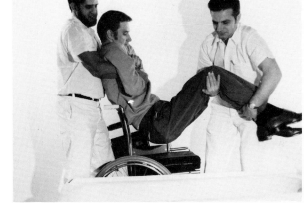
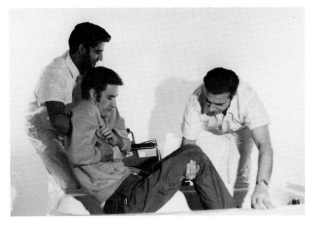
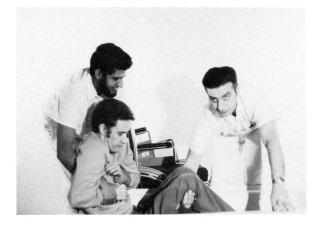

FIGURE 15-93

helper behind the patient swivels and holds while the helper in front swings the patient forward. This will lift the patient's buttocks up enough to clear the wheel and the bathtub edge. As the patient is lowered into the tub, the helper at the front supports his weight by placing a hand on the edge of the bathtub. This relieves any undue strain on his back. The rear helper must bend his knees to lower the patient into the tub. In this lift the rear helper holds most of the weight, but need not move a great deal. The front helper moves a good deal but takes less weight, thus protecting both helpers' backs.

The lift out of the tub is an exact reversal of the lift into the tub. For safety the patient should be towel dried before the lift is attempted.

Bedbaths may be a solution to the bathing problem.

CAR TRANSFERS

Wheelchair To Car

The car seat is moved as far back as possible before the patient's buttocks are pulled forward in the chair and his feet are placed inside the car. The chair is now pushed forward close to the car seat and at an angle so that the rear wheel is not in the way (Fig. 15-94). The patient's knees should now be in flexion. The bridge-board is positioned under the patient's buttocks, bridging the gap from the chair to the car. Any of the following methods may be used to transfer him to the car.

Method 1: Slide Transfer—Assistant Inside (Fig. 15-95).   The helper gets into the car on the driver's side. She may kneel on the seat facing the patient, kneel with one knee on the seat and one foot braced on the floor, or sit facing the

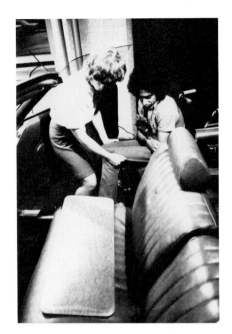

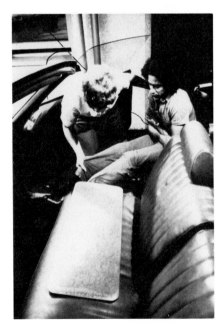
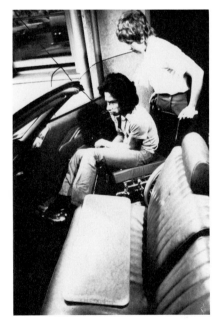
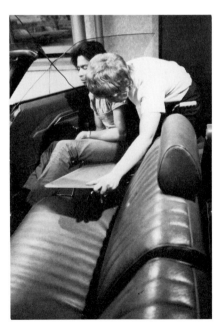

FIGURE 15-94

588

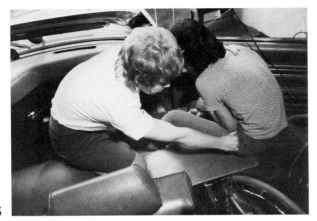
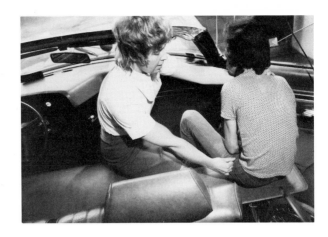

FIGURE 15-95

patient. The helper checks that the patient's knees are still flexed, or his legs will lock and prevent the patient from moving. She now grasps the patient by the shoulder and flexes the patient's upper trunk forward and away from the direction of travel. She grasps the belt or slacks with the other hand and leans back, pulling the patient across the bridgeboard and into the car. His feet are now repositioned for comfort and stability. This transfer method can be used by a small helper to move quite a heavy person with very little back stress.

Method 2: Slide Transfer—Assistant Outside (Fig. 15-96). The helper remains behind the chair and flexes the patient's trunk forward. She holds the patient's slacks by the hips and slides him over the bridgeboard by pulling with the arm near the car, and pushing with the other.

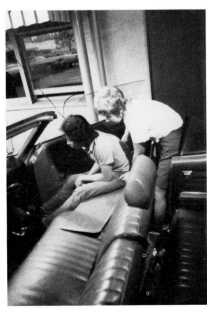
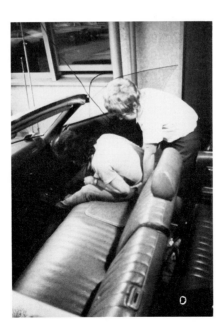
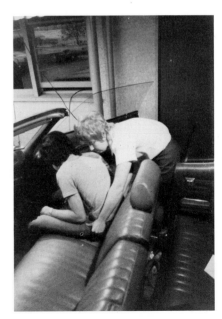

FIGURE 15-96

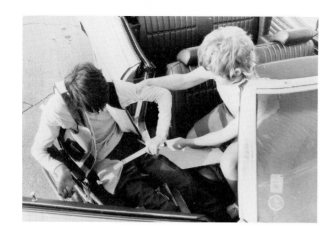

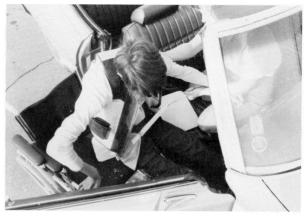

FIGURE 15-97

Method 3: Sliding Belt Transfer (Fig. 15-97).   The patient sits on a soft wide canvas belt with nylon sewn underneath to provide a good sliding surface. A buckle and strap are sewn to the ends of the belt so that it may be fastened around

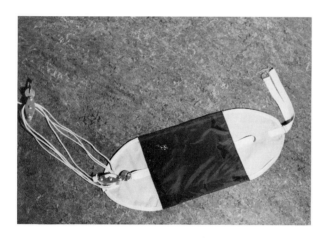

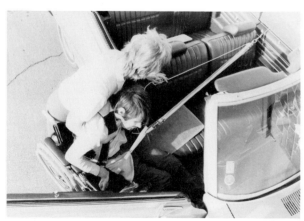

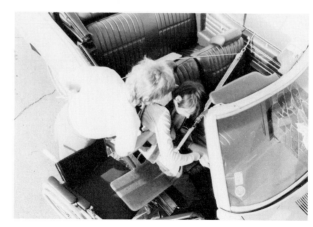

FIGURE 15-98

his hips. Webbing straps may be slipped through D-rings sewn to the belt near the patient's trochanters, providing a convenient hand hold. The patient may be pulled into the car over a bridgeboard.

Method 4: Pulley Transfer.   The patient is positioned as in the previous methods. He sits on the wide canvas belt with nylon sewn to the underside (Fig. 15-98A) and a pulley or block and tackle is added instead of the handle loop. The pulley is attached to the inside of the driver's door and one end of the rope is hooked to the D-ring on the canvas sling. The helper stands beside the patient and guides the patient by the shoulder as she pulls on the rope (Fig. 15-98B). At the same time the helper flexes the patient's trunk forward and away from the direction of travel. Very little effort is required to slide the patient over the bridgeboard into the car.

Method 5: Halo Transfer (Fig. 15-99).   Two people may assist a heavy patient, a tall patient with poor balance, or a patient wearing a halo thoracic brace. One or both of the patient's feet are placed in the car before the wheelchair is finally positioned. The brakes are then applied, and the transfer board is positioned well under the patient's buttocks. To do this, the inside helper positions the board while the helper outside leans the patient away from the car. The helper outside, standing behind the wheelchair, supports the patient and turns his trunk slightly away from the car. The helper inside grasps the patient's slacks near the hip with one hand, and may support her back by placing one hand on the car seat while she steers the patient into the car. The helper at the back must guide the patient's head under the car door as his buttocks are slid over. The very tall patient may need to be slid a long way into the car before his head will clear the door. The tall patient's legs may need to be moved over during the transfer.

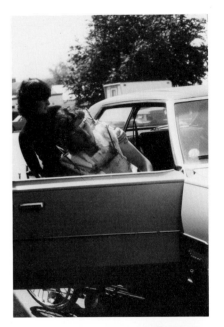

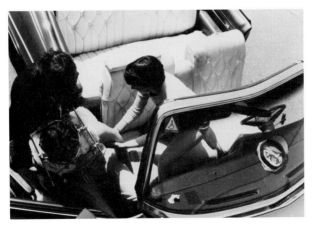

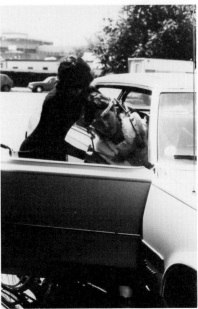

FIGURE 15-99

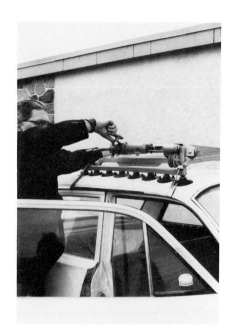 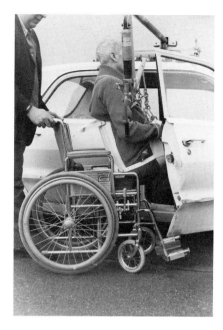

FIGURE 15-100

Method 6: Hoist Transfer. A commercial hydraulic car top hoist may be utilized (Fig. 15-100). Other commercial hoists are mounted just inside the car and may be used to load the patient and then the wheelchair.

CAR TO WHEELCHAIR

Method 1: Slide Transfer (Fig. 15-101). The helper places the sliding board well under the patient's buttocks and uses one hand to hold the patient's shoulders and lean him away from the direction of travel. He is pulled over onto the chair by his belt.

Method 2: Sliding Belt Transfer (Fig. 15-102.) The patient is pulled into the chair over a bridgeboard by pulling on a strap threaded through a D-ring on a canvas and nylon belt. Balance is maintained by the helper's other hand holding the upper arm under the patient's axilla.

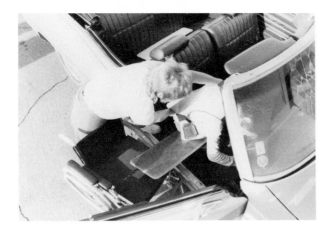

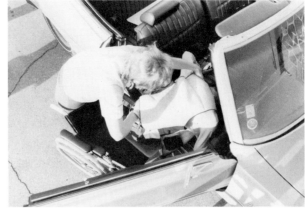

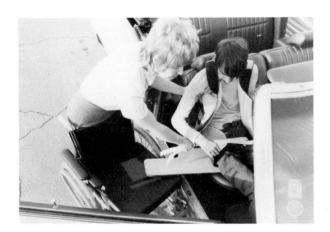

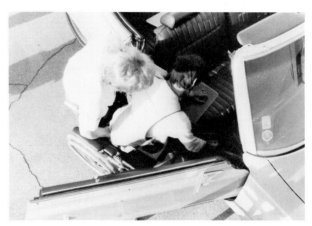

FIGURE 15-101

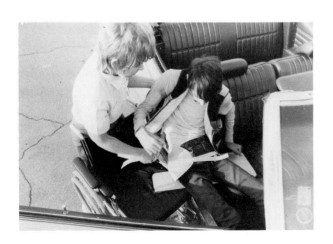

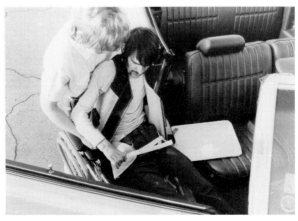

FIGURE 15-102

593

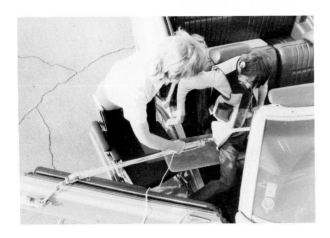
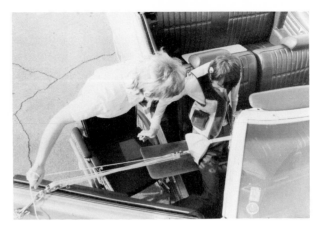
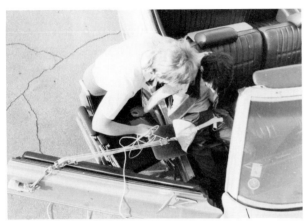

FIGURE 15-103

Method 3: Pulley Transfer (Fig. 15-103).   The pulley system may be used to slide a heavy patient out of the car. The pulley may be hooked to a ring on the car door or to the door handle and the other end is hooked to the D-ring on the canvas belt. It may be necessary to maintain the patient's balance with one hand.

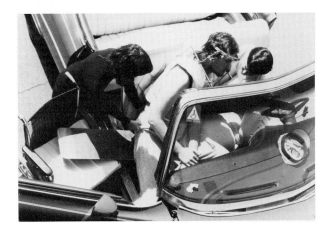

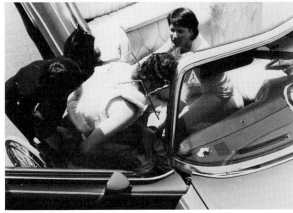

Method 4: Halo Transfer (Fig. 15-104).   Two people may be required to move a patient out of a car. The patient's feet are positioned so that his legs will not impede him as he is moved over. The wheelchair is positioned and the transfer board is inserted. The helper on the inside of the car supports the patient's shoulders, turning his trunk slightly towards her. The helper on the outside grasps the patient's belt, or his slacks, and slides him part way across the transfer board. Both helpers now reposition themselves, and possibly also reposition the patient's feet. The helper outside the car slides the patient into the wheelchair, while supporting her own back with a hand on the car. The inside helper now guides the patient's head out under the top of the door opening and the person outside then takes over the support of the patient's shoulders.

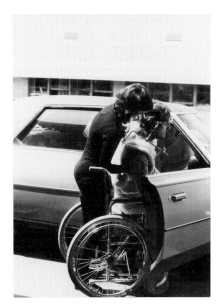

FIGURE 15-104

Manual Methods

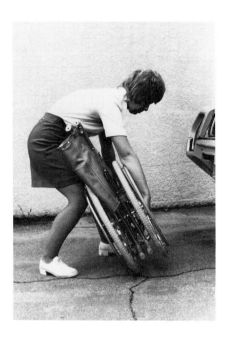

Method 1. (Fig. 15-105)   The helper folds the chair, applies the brakes, and tips the chair so she can reach over and grasp the spokes below the axle and the front of the chair. Rocking back using a thigh as a fulcrum, the helper pulls the chair in tightly so the armrests are against her body and the chair is swung up and placed in the trunk. The trunk well may be raised with plywood so that the chair is easier to lift out.

Method 2. (Fig. 15-106)   The chair may be loaded behind the front seats. The chair is folded, but the brakes are not applied. The chair is tipped back and the castors are placed over the doorsill. The chair is rolled into the car, but as the castors approach the transmission tunnel, the chair is tipped back with the castors high and the pushing handled resting on the car floor.

Method 3.   The area in the car between the doorsill and the transmission tunnel may be filled in with plywood or hardboard, leaving a half-inch ledge to prevent the chair from moving too much. The chair is rolled straight in and can remain with all four wheels on the floor (Fig. 15-107).

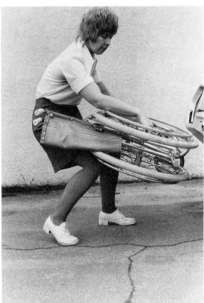
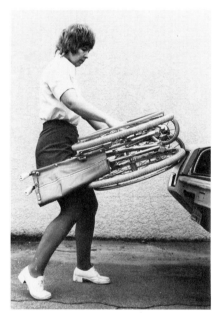
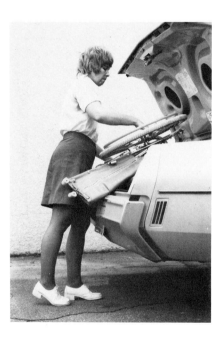

FIGURE 15-105

596

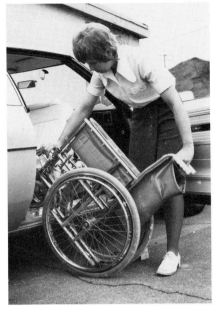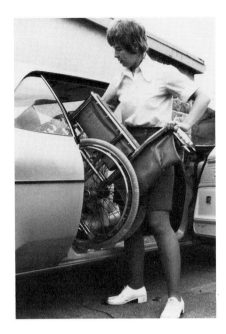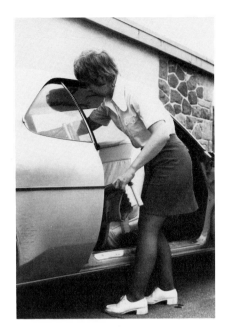

FIGURE 15-106

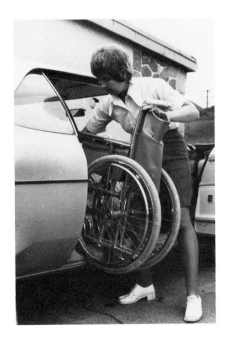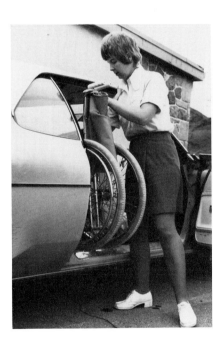

FIGURE 15-107

597

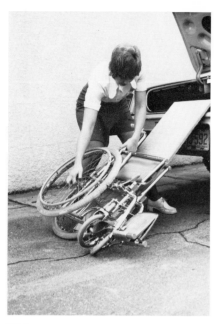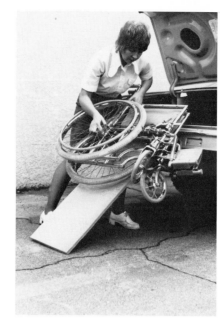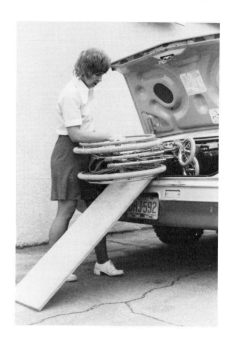

FIGURE 15-108

Method 4. (Fig. 15-108)   A ramp may be made from plywood with padded angle brackets attached to hook over the edge of the trunk so that the chair may be slid up and into the trunk.

Method 5.   A chair loader may be made from metal tubing. The bottom of the loader is bent to about 100° to form a lip to accommodate the folded wheelchair. The lip stays flat on the ground when the loader is leaned against the car so that the chair can be rolled over it easily. A handle is attached to the tubing at the bottom center of the lip (Fig. 15-109A). The top ends are bent to provide both a holding fulcrum and legs. The lengths of the legs are determined by the depth of the trunk. The legs have small fixed wheels at the ends, which will roll along the floor of the trunk. The loader illustrated was homemade from parts from a personal shopping cart. The folded chair is rolled onto the loader and the brakes are applied. One chair wheel and the handle are grasped together and raised until the loader wheels touch the trunk floor (Fig. 15-109B). The chair is now pushed into the trunk and left in position on the loader, ready for use when unloading.

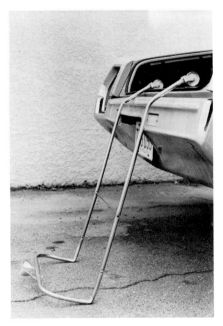

FIGURE 15-109A

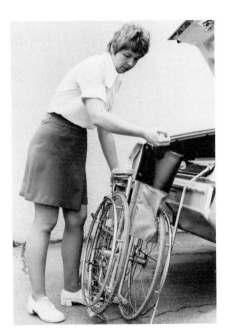

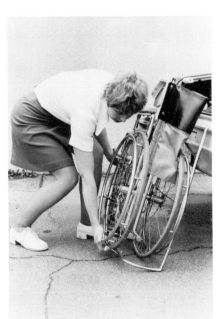

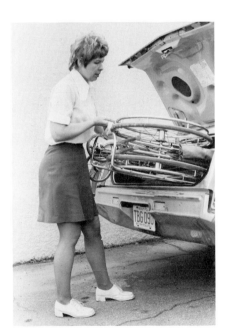

FIGURE 15-109B

Mechanical Assistance

There is a wide range of apparatus which can assist the helper to load the wheelchair into or onto a car.

Method 6. Very little effort is required for a helper to load a wheelchair onto a tilting carrier attached to the trailer hitch on a car (Fig. 15-110). The carrier can be folded when not in use, so that it doesn't protrude so far. As the unit cannot be seen, care must be taken when parking or backing up.

Method 7. (Fig. 15-111) A hoist is available to place the wheelchair in a box on top of the car; there is also a powered unit to put a wheelchair into the area behind the front seat.

Many of these hoists will be useful and consideration should be given to the

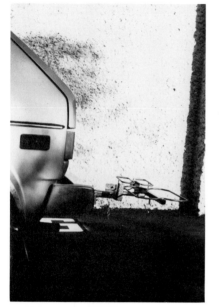

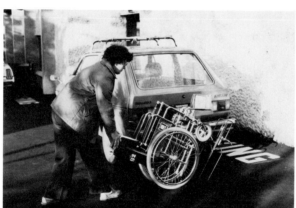

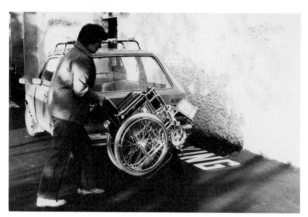

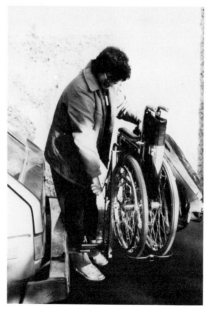

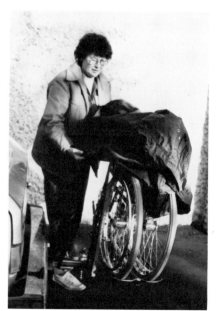

FIGURE 15-110

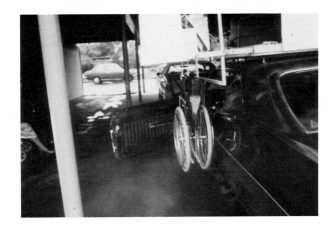
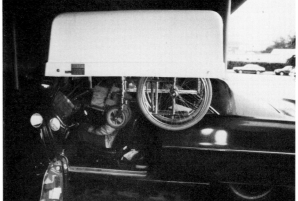

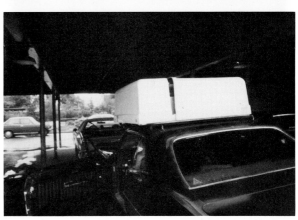

FIGURE 15-111

time required for loading, the reduction of space in the car, the power required, and the care of the wheelchair (it may become dirty if carried uncovered on the back of the car).

USING A VAN

The simplest possible method must be worked out for getting a patient in and out of a vehicle, even if this involves considerable expense for commercial hoists or lifts. Frequently a family will forego short expeditions, or leave the patient at home if transfers are difficult. Freedom of movement is of the utmost psychologic benefit to the patient and the family unit.

Use of a van is often the most practical method of transport because it eliminates the need to transfer the patient from the chair and the need to load the chair separately. The wheelchair should be fixed to the floor when loaded and the patient secured with a floor safety belt. A crossover safety belt attached to the ceiling is also recommended.

Three of the simplest mechanical hoists are illustrated here. These hoists are equipped with limit switches, so that when the hoist is in position, the motor cuts off. For safety, the mechanism locks if there is a power failure. These hoists may be self-operated or operated by an assistant.

A powered ramp may be self-operated by some patients, using a joystick or

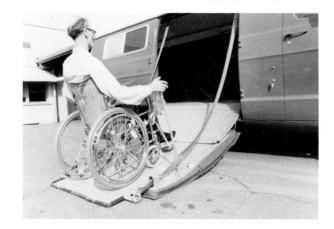
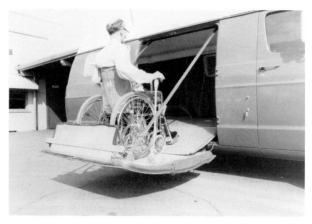
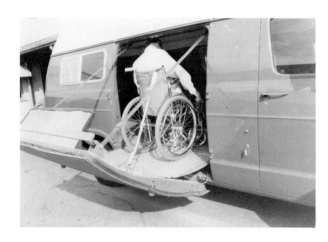
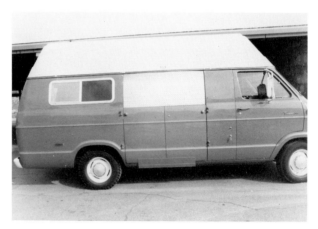
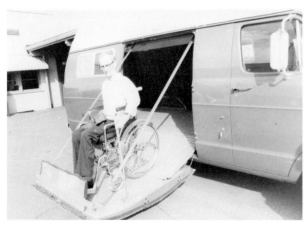

FIGURE 15-112

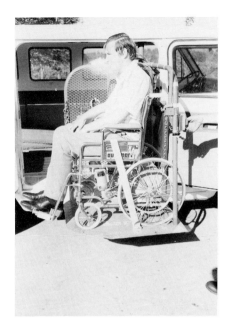
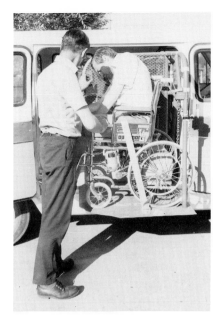
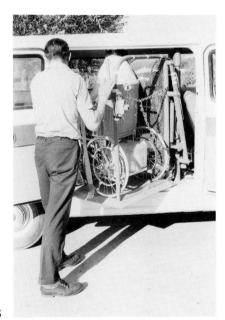
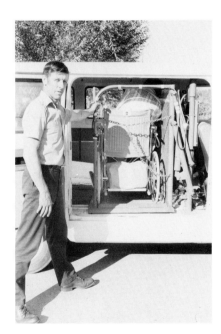

FIGURE 15-113

button control (Fig. 15-112). The patient wheels over the leading edge onto the apron. When activated, the ramp will raise the patient and roll the chair into the van, allowing the chair to remain horizontal.

A powered elevator, which can be swivelled into place, requires very few moves from the helper. The chair is secured to the elevator floor, then the elevator is raised and swivelled into the van (Fig. 15-113).

603

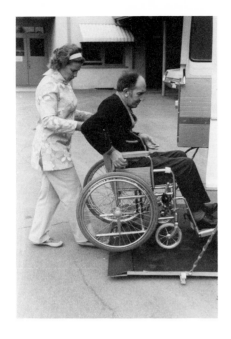
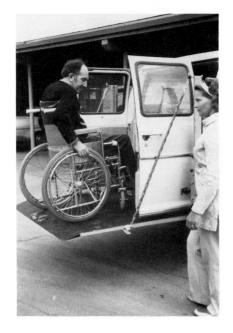

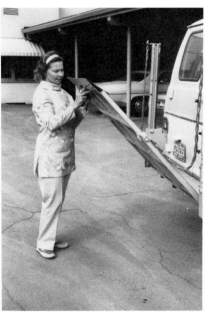
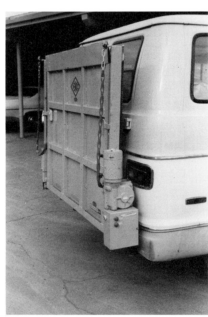

FIGURE 15-114

Another type of powered elevator is usually installed at the rear of the van. Once the elevator reaches the van floor height the patient must be pushed in, secured, the doors closed, and the elevator folded (Fig. 15-114). These tasks are not difficult but they are time consuming.

604

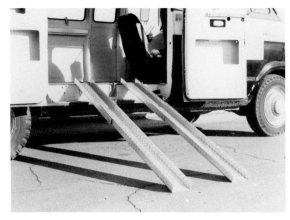

FIGURE 15-115

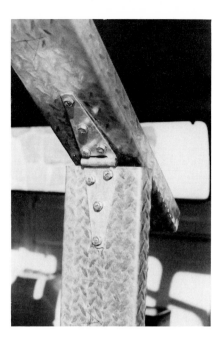

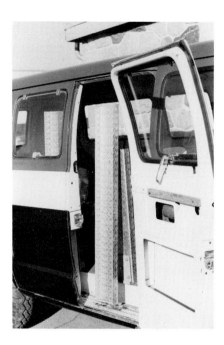

A metal ramp may be used if the helper is capable of pushing the chair up the grade safely. This model is attached to the floor of the van and can be folded to allow the door to be shut (Fig. 15-115). One ramp is on a slide so that the width can be adjusted (Fig. 15-116).

PUBLIC TRANSPORT

In some areas, public transport is wheelchair accessible, in other areas special transport for the disabled is available.

Taxis, converted for the special needs of the wheelchair user, and also used for the general public, are extremely useful for the traveler or for those who do not drive (Fig. 15-117).

Transport for the disabled is one of their top priorities, and this taxi service answers many of the wheelchair user's concerns, giving him equal opportunity with the able-bodied customer.

Moving The Patient By Wheelchair

Each patient must be prepared to instruct an inexperienced helper in easy and safe methods of controlling a chair. He will be wise to ask the helper to give him time to hook an elbow around the pushing handle first for extra safety. If an experienced helper is pushing the chair, she must warn the patient before tipping the chair back.

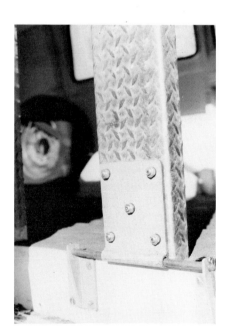

FIGURE 15-116

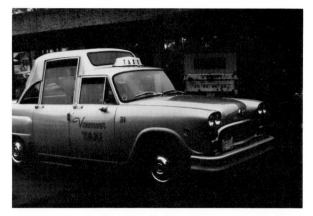

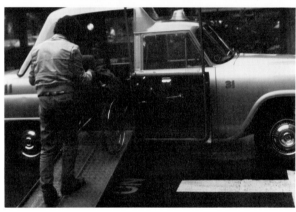

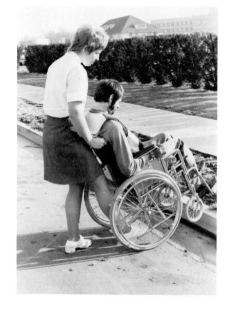

FIGURE 15-117

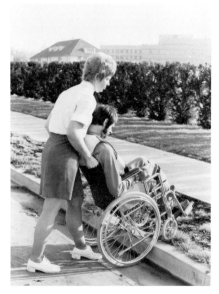

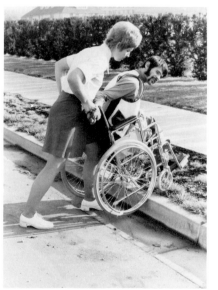

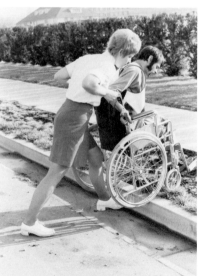

FIGURE 15-118

Mounting Curbs

Curbs may be mounted from a direct forward approach or from the rear. In the forward approach (Fig. 15-118), the chair is tilted back by stepping on the tipping lever, and the front castors are placed on the sidewalk. The wheelchair is lifted and pushed to roll the rear wheels up over the curb. If the patient is able to lean forward once the castors are on the sidewalk, this will considerably reduce the weight on the back wheels.

When the chair is backed towards the curb and the rear wheels touch the curb, the chair is tipped back. The helper leans back to pull the chair up the curb (Fig. 15-119). She wheels the chair back so that the front castors will be on the sidewalk when she lowers the chair.

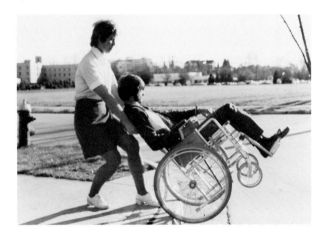

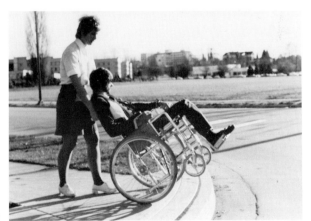

FIGURE 15-119

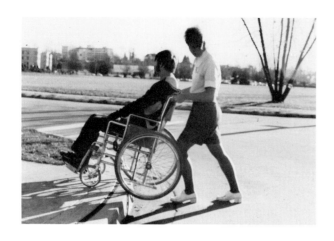

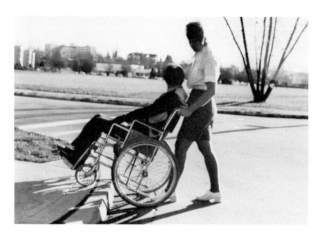
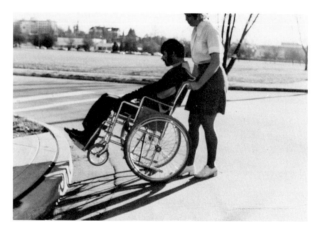

FIGURE 15-120

Descending Curbs

Again, there are two methods for descending a curb. In one instance, the chair is turned on the sidewalk so that it faces away from the road (Fig. 15-120). The helper steps backwards off the curb and, pulling the chair towards her, lowers the back wheels onto the road. The chair is balanced on the back wheels and wheeled back far enough so that the footrests do not hit the curb. The chair is lowered onto the front castors; the helper uses a foot on the tipping lever to give control. It may be necessary to place a hand over the patient's shoulder while lowering the chair to prevent him from falling forward.

In the forward method, the chair faces the roadway and is tipped back using its tipping lever and balanced on its back wheels. The chair is rolled over the curb edge and pushed forward before lowering it onto its front castors (Fig. 15-121). It may be convenient to maintain the chair in a tipped position while crossing the road to avoid tipping the chair again at the next curb.

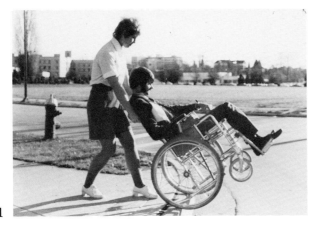
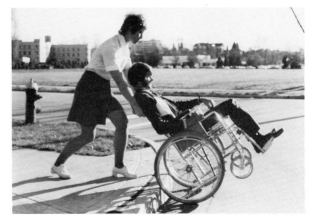

FIGURE 15-121

Wheeling Over Rough Ground

The chair should be tipped onto the rear wheels by stepping on the tipping lever. It may be pushed in this balanced position when the ground is rough or soft. If the terrain is very difficult it will be easier to pull the chair backwards in the tipped position.

Wheeling Down Slopes

When a steep slope is descended, the chair should be reversed and brought down backwards with the castors on the ground (Fig. 15-122). This ensures that the patient does not fall forward and leaves the helper free to control the chair.

The chair may be pushed forward if the slope is minor. It may be necessary to place one hand over the patient's shoulder to maintain the patient's balance (Fig. 15-123). If the slope levels abruptly, care must be taken not to snag the footrests when wheeling forwards.

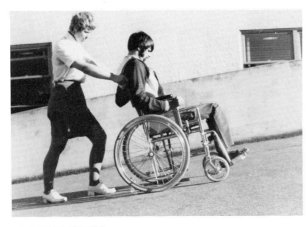
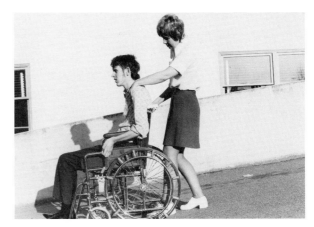

FIGURE 15-122   FIGURE 15-123

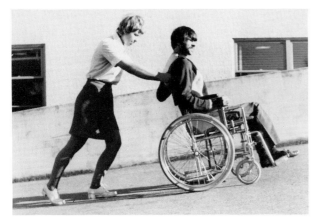

FIGURE 15-124

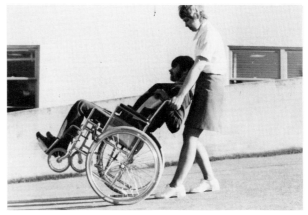

FIGURE 15-125

Wheeling Up Slopes

When ascending a slope the chair may be pushed forward in the normal manner (Fig. 15-124).

The helper may reverse the chair and tip it back onto the rear wheels on steep slopes. By leaning back to pull and keeping the elbows straight while holding the pushing handles, the helper will gain a considerable amount of mechanical advantage (Fig. 15-125).

On short steep slopes, the chair may be tipped well back (Fig. 15-126) and the chair pushed quickly up the slope to gain momentum, much like pushing a loaded wheelbarrow.

Ascending Stairs

With practice, one person can ascend stairs with the patient in the wheelchair (Fig. 15-27). This is, of course, dependent on the weight of the patient and

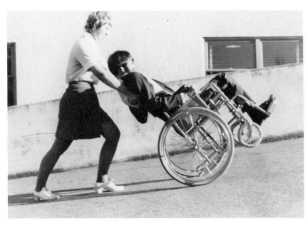

FIGURE 15-126

610

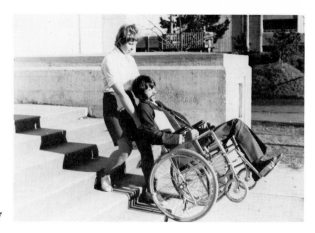

FIGURE 15-127

the strength of the assistant. The wheelchair is reversed and tipped back. The chair is then pulled to the stairs. The assistant mounts the stairs keeping one foot on the first step and one on the second. She pulls the chair up the first step keeping her elbows straight; then she moves her feet to the next step before proceeding. Any attempt to assist by lifting from the front will throw the helper at the rear off balance. If a second helper is available he may remain in front, prepared to hold the chair if necessary.

It may be necessary to carry the chair up the stairs if there are curves or corners in the stairway. The chair is faced away from the stairs and the rear assistant grasps the pushing handles and tips the chair back. The front assistant grasps the chair footrest supports and lifts the chair free of the stair. Both assistants proceed up the stairs in unison. When inexperienced persons are assisting they should be instructed to grasp parts of the chair that will not come loose. Removable arms, adjustable legrests and wheels are frequently grasped by the inexperienced. If the stairs width permits, four persons may carry a chair, one at each corner. This is less fatiguing if large numbers of chairs are to be moved.

Descending Stairs

The same positions used in ascending the stairs are used in descending the stairs.

Useful References and Aids

Caruth, F and Thompson, F: 1-2-3-Lift, Evergreen Press Ltd., Transfer Manual, P.O. Box 1341, Postal Station A, Vancouver, Canada V6C2T2

Duckworth, B: Dependent Transfers. 1 Man Towel Transfer, 2 Man Towel Transfer, Slide Transfer. Slide tapes, 10 mins. each approximately. Obtainable from Medical Library, G.F. Strong Rehabilitation Centre, 4255 Laurel Street, Vancouver, BC, Canada V52 2G9.

FORD, J: Transfer Techniques Parts I and II. Video tape ³/₄″ color, 27 mins. Jack Ford. Obtainable from U.B.C. Biomedical Communications, Vancouver, BC, Canada V52 2G9.

USEFUL REFERENCES: GENERAL

BEDBROOK, GM: Spinal injuries with tetraplegia and paraplegia. The Journal of Bone and Joint Surgery. Vol. 610B, No. 3, August 1979. (Overview of history, treatment, and recommendations for the future for spinal cord injured. Rich bibliography.)

BURKE, DC AND MURRY, DD: Handbook of Spinal Cord Medicine, Macmillan Press Ltd. 1975.

CORBETT, B: Changes. Color film, 16 mm. 28 mins. Access Incorporated, 177 S. Lookout Mountain Road, Golder, Colorado 80401, 1973. (Realistic and sensitive film. People with recent spinal cord injury.)

DeTROYER, A, ET AL: Mechanism of active expiration in tetraplegic subjects. New England Journal of Medicine 314(12), March 20, 1986.

Equipment for the Disabled: 2 Foredown Drive, Portslade, Sussex, BN42BB, England, 1978.

FALLON, B: So You're Paralysed. The Spinal Injuries Association, 126 Albert Street, London N.W. 17, NF, England, 1975.

GROSS, D, ET AL: The effect of training and endurance of the diaphragm in quadriplegics. The American Journal of Medicine, Vol. 68, June 1980.

GUTTMANN, L: Spinal Cord Injuries, Comprehensive Management and Research, Blackwell Scientific Publications, 1973, 76.

HALE, G: The Source Book for the Disabled, London, Paddington Press, 1979. (Many useful equipment ideas.)

KING, R ET AL, Eds: Rehabilitation Guide, Medical Rehabilitation Research and Training Center. No. 20. Chicago, Northwest University and Rehabilitation Institute of Chicago.

LATHEM, PA ET AL: High level quadriplegia: An occupational therapy challenge. The American Journal of Occupational Therapy. 39(11). Nov. 1985. (Functional activities leading to improved quality of life.)

LIFCHEZ, R AND WINSLOW, B: Design for Independent Living, Watson-Guptil Publications, New York, 1979. (Sensitive and informative about many aspects of disability, including architectural needs.)

Lowman, EW and Klinger, JL: Aids to Independent Living. McGraw Hill, 1969.

Lowman, EW and Sell, GH: Spinal Cord Injury, A Guide for Care, Revised Primer for Spinal Cord Injured. New York Spinal Cord Injury Center, Institute of Rehabilitation Medicine, 400 East 34th Street, New York, New York, 10016, 1979.

Pinkerton, AC, Griffin, ML: Rehabilitation outcomes in females with spinal cord injury. A follow-up Study. Paper presented at the Annual Scientific meeting of the International Medical Society of Paraplegia, Athens, Greece, 1982.

Phillips, RJ and Weiss, MS (editors): Spinal Cord Injury: Home Care Manual. Santa Clara Medical Center, Norman B Nelson Rehabilitation Center, San Jose, California, March, 1983.

Rogers, JC, and Figone, JJ: Psychosocial parameters in treating the person with quadriplegia. American Journal of Occupational Therapy 33(7): 432-439, 1979.

Sargent, JV: An Easier Way, Handbook for the Elderly and Handicapped. Iowa State University Press, Ames, Iowa, 1981. (Aids and Equipment, some will be useful for quadriplegic people)

GF Strong Rehabilitation Centre: Rehabilitation Manual, Spinal Cord Injury. GF Strong Rehabilitation Centre, 4255 Laurel Street, Vancouver, British Columbia, Canada, V5Z 2G9, 1984.

Trieschman, RB: Spinal Cord Injury, Psychological, Social and Vocational Adjustment. Pergamon Press, 1980.

I

Appendix

LESION LEVELS ASSOCIATED WITH FUNCTION

Therapists who are new to working with people with spinal cord injury often ask what functional transfers can be expected from a person with a certain level of injury. The following examples may help to clarify some of the reasons why one person with a certain lesion level may find it easier to move than another with a similar lesion level, and why certain transfers may be easier for one patient than for another. The muscle charts are shown with each person, and these show how difficult it is to divide people neatly into lesion level categories, partly because it would be highly unusual to have a horizontal lesion at an exact segmental level. The lesion level guide to the key muscles for function shows what sparing could be expected at different levels (Table A-1).

INFLUENCING FACTORS

Sparing may or may not be useful; for instance, strong isolated movement in a big toe is not functional, whereas weak movement in the trunk may be a great asset in balancing.

Breathing capacity is also very important; low vital capacity can seriously affect endurance, and also motivation and drive. A training valve used daily for a short period of time to increase breathing endurance can be most valuable. This apparatus provides for graduated resisted inspiration and unresisted expiration.

Spasticity may or may not be useful, depending upon the degree and type. Severe spasticity may prevent a person from transferring, but if the spasticity can be reduced by appropriate treatment, he may transfer with ease. Mild spasticity will help to maintain circulation and skin tone, and slight spasticity may make it easier for a movement in one area of the body to have mechanical effect on another area.

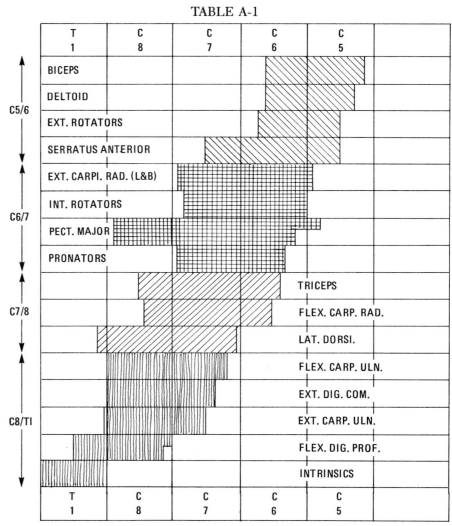

SHADED BOXES REPRESENT THE PRIMARY INNERVATION OF THE MUSCLES/MUSCLE GROUPS LISTED.

An example of individual variation in innervation can be demonstrated in the pectoralis muscle, a key muscle for the quadriplegic person. Some people have the clavicular and a large part of the sternal portion of the muscle innervated at the C $^{5/6}$ level, and others with the same lesion level have only a small portion of the clavicular head innervated.

RULES OF THUMB

There are certain rules of thumb that can be used as approximate guidelines to possible levels of function. The person with only weak active wrist extension may learn to do transfers, but often finds this too tiring and does not persist. The person with no active wrist movement is most unlikely to do a functional transfer.

A person lacking pectorals will find it difficult to do the "hugging" movement so necessary for easy transfers, for pushing a hand under a knee, and for locking the elbows; this person may not continue with independent transfers if he achieves them.

A person does not have to have triceps to do a good transfer; elbows can be "locked" using the anterior deltoid and the pectorals with the wrist extended and the arm externally rotated. Some people consider that the fingers will be over-stretched if the hand is flat on the bed; but generally the patient cannot control his finger position, which may be flexed or extended. Whichever position they fall into, the time in this position will be short and the long finger flexors are unlikely to be overstretched. The person who lacks pronation when he extends his wrist will find it more difficult to pick up his legs because of the extra distance he has to lean forward to keep his arm under the knee.

INFLUENCE OF BODY BUILD

Three examples of people with greatly differing body builds but with much the same lesion level and muscle power, showed widely differing function:

Example 1: One man had a very long trunk and short arms and legs. When he leaned forward, he would tip out of the wheelchair because so much of his trunk was forward of his knee. He was also unable to fling his arm around the pushing handle to pull himself up while leaning forward on his knees. Doing a push up was difficult when he was sitting.

Example 2: A young woman of normal build found transfers difficult because she had heavier hips and weaker shoulders than a comparable man. Women will often perform functionally like a man who has a higher lesion level.

Example 3: A young man who was short and light, with relatively long arms, and who was an athlete before his injury, learned transfers surprisingly fast and had very little difficulty with any of the moves required.

TEACHING TIPS

When teaching transfers, or any other skill, some success must be expected by the therapist. Muscle strengthening and improvement in balance can be gained through exercise, games, and weight lifting before the patient is introduced to selfcare tasks. It should be obvious from watching the person's performance and the weight he can lift or pull whether he will be able to succeed in a task. It is disheartening for a patient if he is asked to lift his fifteen-pound leg when he cannot lift a five-pound weight, and is doomed to failure. It might be better to have him lift a foot onto a leg strap, or to add a few ounces daily to his pulleys so that he can see his progress, until he is ready to lift the leg. Before asking a patient to do a bed transfer, the patient should be able to shift his buttocks and change his position in the wheelchair.

STANDING IN (SPOTTING) AND ASSISTANCE

Before the start of the transfer the helper can ask the patient to work out the mechanics required; which way, for instance, he should move his head and shoul-

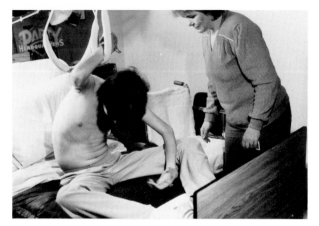

FIGURE A-1

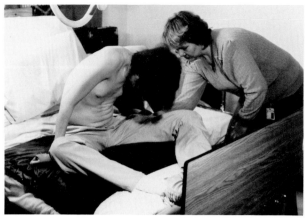

FIGURE A-2

ders to force his buttocks over. Some patients work better if they are told which mechanics will work for them. The choice of teaching method depends upon the needs of the patient.

When the patient is learning to maneuver, the helper must anticipate any fall or loss of balance, and hold herself ready to catch. The part of the patient she is going to hold and her own possible position must be anticipated so that neither she nor the patient will be hurt (Fig. A-1).

The helper is shown pulling steadily on the patient's pants at hip level. The sustained assisting pull will complement any effort he makes to move correctly, and will give him feedback; this encourages him to repeat the correct moves. The patient should always be informed when he is being assisted (Fig. A-2).

When doing a more difficult balance activity, such as when placing a hand behind the wheelchair arm upright, the helper may have to hold him in the balanced position, and help him place his hand, or make sure that his hand is secure (Fig. A-3).

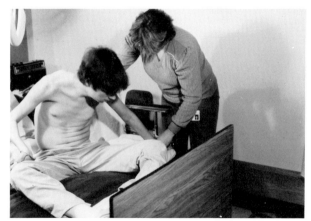

FIGURE A-3

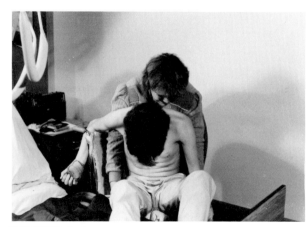

FIGURE A-4

When the patient changes direction and attempts to move backward, the helper moves to the back of the wheelchair so that she is pulling straight towards herself so that her own back is protected. Once again, the steady pull may be used to give the patient feedback when he moves correctly (Fig. A-4).

It is essential that the patient have full confidence that the helper will catch him if he loses balance. This particular patient became independent in his transfer a day or two after the series was photographed. He had learned to work up a rhythmical bounce using the spring of the mattress, and to put greater effort into his moves.

MUSCLE CHARTS AND EXAMPLES

Example 1 (Fig. A-5). This nineteen-year-old was six foot one inch (1.85 m) with relatively long arms and legs and a fairly short trunk. He weighed 141 pounds (63.96 kg). His breathing capacity was estimated at 52 percent of normal. He was athletic and well coordinated. He was able to transfer quickly and easily, and because of his ability to lift he did not require slippery surfaces or exactly level

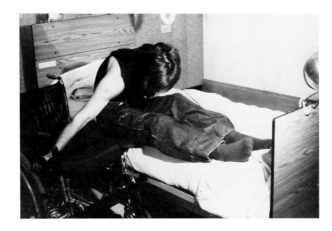
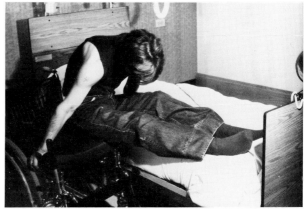
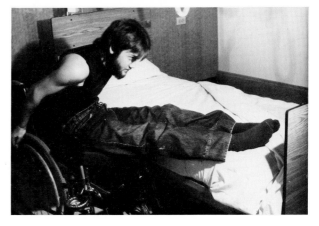

FIGURE A-5

619

surfaces. Even though he lacked triceps in his left arm he was able to lock it using his external rotators and his shoulder flexors (Table A-2).

Example 2 (Fig. A-6). This thirty-eight-year-old man was five foot nine inches tall (1.75 m) and weighed 166 pounds (75 kg). He was well proportioned,

LEFT				RIGHT
4	SCAPULA	Abductor	Serratus anterior	5
5	SHOULDER	Flexor	Anterior deltoid	5
0		Extensors	Latissimus dorsi	0
5		Abductor	Middle deltoid	5
5		Horizontal abd.	Posterior deltoid	5
3		Adductor	Clavicular	4
0		Pectoralis major	Sternal	3
4		External rotators		5
3		Internal rotators		4
5	ELBOW	Flexors	Biceps	5
5			Brachioradialis	5
1		Extensor	Triceps	2
5	FOREARM	Supinators		5
3		Pronators		4
0	WRIST	Flexors	Flex. carpi. rad.	2
0			Flex. carpi. uln.	0
4		Extensors	Ext. carpi. rad. l. & br.	4
0			Ext. carpi. uln.	0
0	FINGERS	Flexors		1
0		Extensors		1
0		Intrinsics		0

TABLE A-2

KEY:

0 Zero
1 Palpable contraction.
2 Movement with gravity eliminated.
3 Complete range of movement against gravity.
4 Complete range of movement against gravity with considerable resistance.
5 Apparently normal.

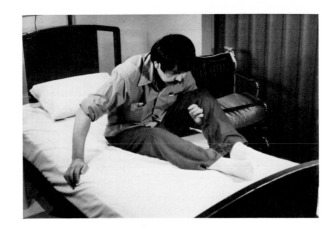 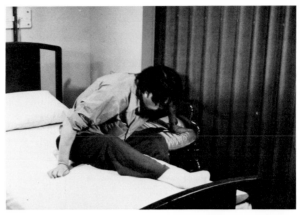

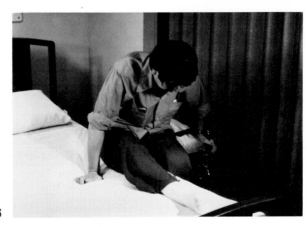

FIGURE A-6

with an average length of trunk and limbs. His estimated breathing capacity was 50 percent of normal. He had a great deal of flexor spasticity of his legs, which prevented him from doing independent transfers until his spasticity was reduced.

Though from the muscle chart it would appear that he should transfer almost as easily as Example 1, this was not so, partly due to spasm, weight, and age, and also because he was inclined to move in a slower and more deliberate fashion, having to rely on muscle power rather than momentum. He was independent in all transfers on discharge (Table A-3).

LEFT				RIGHT
5	SCAPULA	Abductor	Serratus anterior	5
5	SHOULDER	Flexor	Anterior deltoid	4
4		Extensors	Latissimus dorsi	3
4		Abductor	Middle deltoid	4
4		Horizontal abd.	Posterior deltoid	4
5		Adductor	Clavicular	4
5		Pectoralis major	Sternal	3
4		External rotators		3
4		Internal rotators		4
5	ELBOW	Flexors	Biceps	4
5			Brachioradialis	4
4		Extensor	Triceps	3
4	FOREARM	Supinators		4
4		Pronators		4
4	WRIST	Flexors	Flex. carpi. rad.	3
0			Flex. carpi. uln.	0
4		Extensors	Ext. carpi. rad. l. & br.	4
0			Ext. carpi. uln.	0
0	FINGERS	Flexors		0
1		Extensors		1
0		Intrinsics		0

KEY:

0 Zero
1 Palpable contraction.
2 Movement with gravity eliminated.
3 Complete range of movement against gravity.
4 Complete range of movement against gravity with considerable resistance.
5 Apparently normal.

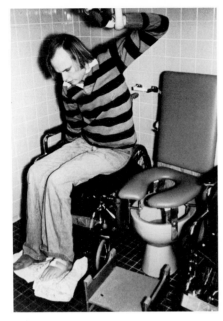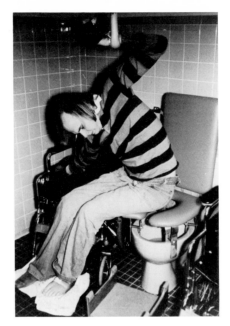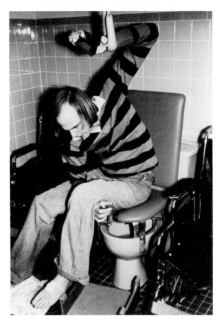

FIGURE A-7

Example 3 (Fig. A-7). This young man was five foot eleven inches tall (1.80 m), with short arms and legs, and a long trunk. He weighed 134 pounds (60.78 kg), was relatively flaccid and had poor balance, particularly when he was not in long sitting. Though he attempted to do his transfers by a push-up method, he had poor results. With the overhead method he learned quickly, and was able to retain his balance during a lift. This overhead method can be particularly useful for those with short arms or poor balance (Table A-4).

Example 4 (Fig. A-8). This man had some nonfunctional sparing on one side, and considerable spasticity. He was six foot three inches (1.90 m) tall, and was heavy, 189 pounds (86 kg). Breathing (vital capacity) was estimated at 43 percent of normal.

Because of his spasticity he had difficulty in coming to sitting while his legs were in extension, and for this reason he used the overhead bars to pivot his rigid, spastic body around on his buttocks until his legs were over the edge of the bed. He then had to wait for his knees to relax into flexion before he was able to pull his trunk into flexion.

When he sat up to dress in bed, he had to use a bed with a head gatch that also flexed his knees; and even so, at first he required an extra loop from the foot of the bed to pull himself forward.

623

LEFT				RIGHT
4	SCAPULA	Abductor	Serratus anterior	5
4	SHOULDER	Flexor	Anterior deltoid	4
2		Extensors	Latissimus dorsi	3
4		Abductor	Middle deltoid	4
5		Horizontal abd.	Posterior deltoid	4
4		Adductor	Clavicular	4
2		Pectoralis major	Sternal	2
4		External rotators		4
4		Internal rotators		4
5	ELBOW	Flexors	Biceps	5
5			Brachioradialis	5
0		Extensor	Triceps	0
5	FOREARM	Supinators		5
0		Pronators		0
0	WRIST	Flexors	Flex. carpi. rad.	0
0			Flex. carpi. uln.	0
4		Extensors	Ext. carpi. rad. l. & br.	4
0			Ext. carpi. uln.	0
0	FINGERS	Flexors		0
0		Extensors		0
0		Intrinsics		0

KEY:

0 Zero
1 Palpable contraction.
2 Movement with gravity eliminated.
3 Complete range of movement against gravity.
4 Complete range of movement against gravity with considerable resistance.
5 Apparently normal.

His main difficulty was in learning to lift his legs onto the bed. This was partly because he had heavy and spastic legs, and because he had weak pectorals so that it was difficult for him to thrust his arm under his knee, and weak pronators, so that he could not use his wrist extension to keep his arm in place.

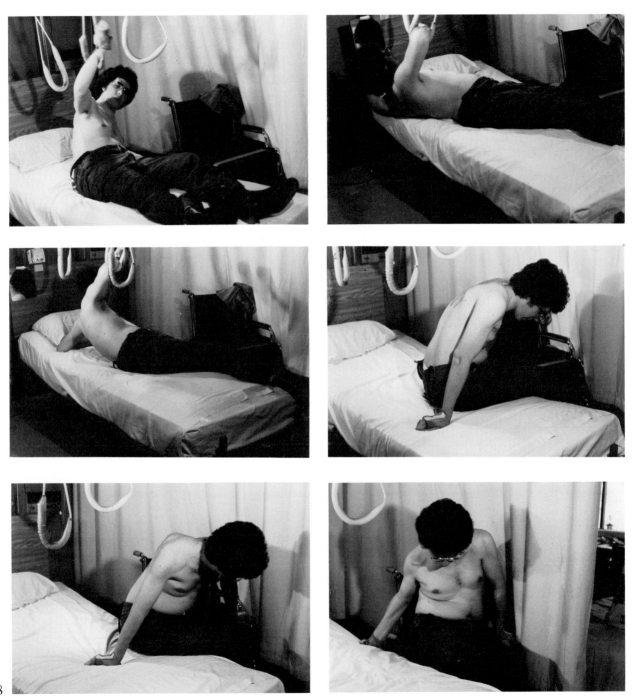

FIGURE A-8

This man was independent on discharge, except for some minimal help in personal care which would be required only for a short time (Table A-5).

LEFT				RIGHT
			TABLE A-5	
5	SCAPULA	Abductor	Serratus anterior	5
5	SHOULDER	Flexor	Anterior deltoid	5
1		Extensors	Latissimus dorsi	0
5		Abductor	Middle deltoid	5
4		Horizontal abd.	Posterior deltoid	4
2		Adductor	Clavicular	3
1		Pectoralis major	Sternal	0
4		External rotators		4
5		Internal rotators		5
5	ELBOW	Flexors	Biceps	5
5			Brachioradialis	5
2		Extensor	Triceps	2
5	FOREARM	Supinators		5
1		Pronators		2
0	WRIST	Flexors	Flex. carpi. rad.	0
0			Flex. carpi. uln.	0
4		Extensors	Ext. carpi. rad. l. & br.	4
0			Ext. carpi. uln.	0
1	FINGERS	Flexors		0
1		Extensors		0
1		Intrinsics		0
S1	TRUNK	Flexors		1S
S1		Extensors		1S
S1	HIP	Flexors		0
S1		Extensors		0
2		Abductors		0
S2		Adductors		0

LEFT				RIGHT
1	KNEE	Flexors		**0**
S2		Extensors		**0**
S1	ANKLE	Plantar Flexors		**0**
1		Dorsi Flexors		**0**
2	TOES	Flexors		**0**
2		Extensors		**0**

KEY:

0 Zero
1 Palpable contraction.
2 Movement with gravity eliminated.
3 Complete range of movement against gravity.
4 Complete range of movement against gravity with considerable resistance.
5 Apparently normal.
S Spasm

Example 5 (Fig. A-9). This man was tall, 6 foot 2 inches (1.88 m), and thin, weighing 147 pounds (66.5 kg), with a long trunk, and poor balance owing to his flaccidity. He also had elbow flexion contractures bilaterally and poor breathing capacity (estimated 17 percent of normal). He had excellent sense of movement and could use momentum extremely well, provided that all surfaces were level and slippery. He used a pulling action, developed mainly by his strong biceps and deltoids, which was very effective once his hand was locked behind the upright post.

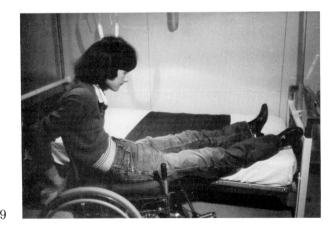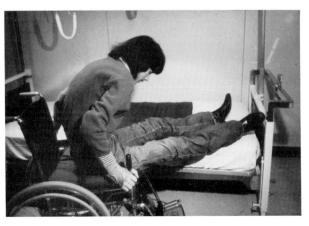

FIGURE A-9

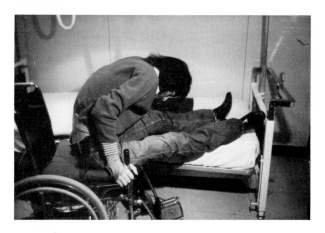 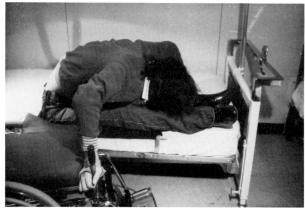

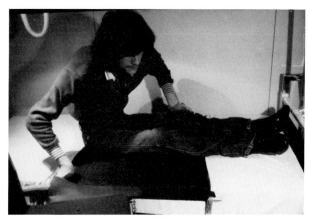

FIGURE A-9 Continued

This man was independent in transfers on discharge. Since discharge, he accepts some minimal assistance in transfers since a helper is present for other requirements (Table A-6).

628

LEFT				RIGHT
4	SCAPULA	Abductor	Serratus anterior	3
5	SHOULDER	Flexor	Anterior deltoid	4
0		Extensors	Latissimus dorsi	0
5		Abductor	Middle deltoid	4
4		Horizontal abd.	Posterior deltoid	4
2		Adductor	Clavicular	0
0		Pectoralis major	Sternal	0
5		External rotators		4
4		Internal rotators		4
4	ELBOW	Flexors	Biceps	4
4			Brachioradialis	4
0		Extensor	Triceps	0
4	FOREARM	Supinators		4
1		Pronators		1
0	WRIST	Flexors	Flex. carpi. rad.	0
0			Flex. carpi. uln.	0
4		Extensors	Ext. carpi. rad. l. & br.	4
0			Ext. carpi. uln.	0
0	FINGERS	Flexors		0
0		Extensors		0
0		Intrinsics		0

KEY:

0 Zero
1 Palpable contraction.
2 Movement with gravity eliminated.
3 Complete range of movement against gravity.
4--Complete range of movement against gravity with slight resistance.
4 Complete range of movement against gravity with considerable resistance.
5 Apparently normal.

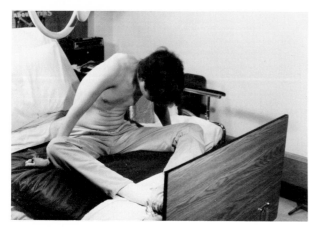
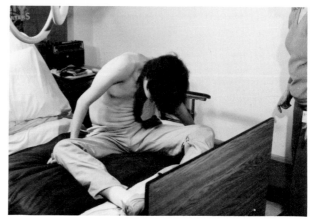
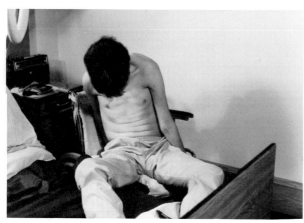

FIGURE A-10

Example 6 (Fig. A-10). This young man has an estimated 21 percent of normal breathing capacity. He has some spasticity in his legs, and has long arms compared with the length of his trunk. He requires level surfaces, a spring filled mattress, and nylon covered surfaces on both bed and pants. He can transfer independently out of bed, using momentum from throwing his head and shoulders forward, but is not yet independent in getting into bed or lifting his legs into bed, though he is close to reaching this goal. With his muscle power, he may find that the effort of transferring uses up too much energy, and he may not persevere later. A person with the same muscle power, who was not as athletic, and not of a similar build probably would not succeed in transferring at all (Table A-7).

USEFUL REFERENCE

Gross, D et al: The effect of training on strength and endurance of the diaphragm in quadriplegics. The American Journal of Medicine, Vol 68, June 1980.

LEFT				RIGHT
2	SCAPULA	Abductor	Serratus anterior	2
4	SHOULDER	Flexor	Anterior deltoid	4
0		Extensors	Latissimus dorsi	0
4		Abductor	Middle deltoid	4
3		Horizontal abd.	Posterior deltoid	4
0		Adductor	Clavicular	1
0		Pectoralis major	Sternal	0
2		External rotators		4
2		Internal rotators		2
4	ELBOW	Flexors	Biceps	4
3			Brachioradialis	4
0		Extensor	Triceps	0
4	FOREARM	Supinators		4
1		Pronators		1
0	WRIST	Flexors	Flex. carpi. rad.	0
0			Flex. carpi. uln.	0
1		Extensors	Ext. carpi. rad. l. & br.	4
0			Ext. carpi. uln.	0
0	FINGERS	Flexors		0
0		Extensors		0
0		Intrinsics		0

KEY:

0 Zero
1 Palpable contraction.
2 Movement with gravity eliminated.
3 Complete range of movement against gravity.
4 Complete range of movement against gravity with considerable resistance.
5 Apparently normal.

II

Appendix

SAMPLE BATHROOM PLANS

Diagonal Small Bathroom With Wheel-in Shower

Design B is very small and should only be used if no further room is available. Neither design is good if a helper is required beside the toilet. This bathroom should be enlarged, if possible, by moving the wall opposite the sink out 6 inches (15.24 cm) to 12 inches (30.48 cm), as in Design A. This will allow the door to be moved over and widened and the counter to be enlarged slightly. The angle of the toilet may be changed slightly to keep it parallel with the new angle of the counter. In the larger bathroom the toilet may have more room left between it and the counter if desired, but if the toilet is moved far from the counter along the angled wall, the back wall must be moved back to allow room for the wheelchair.

Commodes

A person who uses the commode for toileting will not require the cutback on the back wall behind the toilet, and the wall behind the toilet may be continued in a straight line until it meets the back wall of the bathroom.

Transfers

Those who transfer to the toilet from the side require a cutback to allow the chair wheels to move back far enough so that the transfer is possible. Toilets that do not normally extend 2 feet 7 inches (78.74 cm) from the wall will require to be moved forward to accommodate the wheelchair transfer. Persons with a deeper

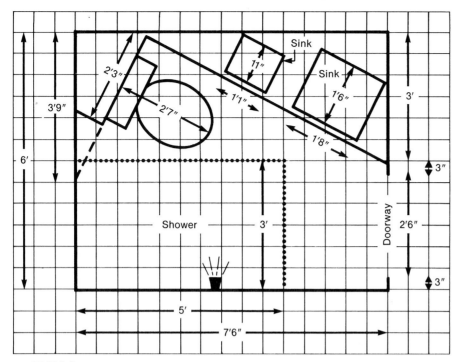

DESIGN A

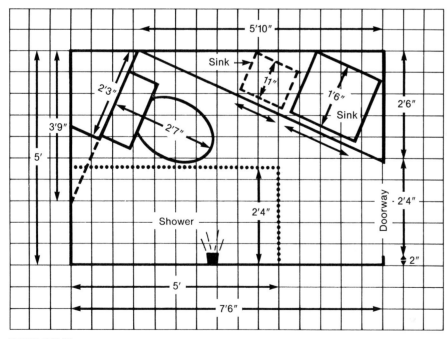

DESIGN B

634

wheelchair will require the wall behind the wheelchair to be moved back. If the toilet were moved forward instead, inadequate maneuvering space would be left.

Counters

If the counter is at a good height for a person transferring, grab bars may be attached to the front edge. Because the counters are open underneath, there is adequate room for turning, particularly in the normal size bathroom, though the "turning circle" is an elipse rather than a circle, even in this design. Even in this small area, a larger sink, and a smaller one for urinary apparatus can be installed if required.

Shower

The shower area—shown by dotted lines—should be level, with a sunken area beneath. Cedar slats, or expanded metal flooring level with the floor must be used, since most people will be unable to manage the amount of slope required to drain this small area, if it is tiled. Curtains may be installed if desired, but they are not a necessity and do take extra room.

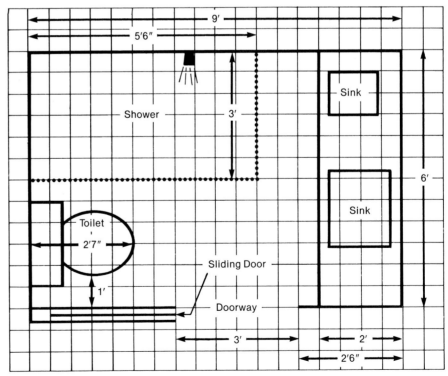

SMALL BATHROOM: DESIGN C

Mirror

A mirror down to the counter top will be convenient for grooming. The larger the mirror, the larger the room will seem.

Doors

Doors must swing outward, or a sliding door must be installed. Some extra door width may be gained by angling the doorway, but turning room will be lost, and the wheelchair will have to be backed in. Storage space can be added if the bathroom is enlarged.

STRAIGHT DESIGN FOR SMALL BATHROOM WITH WHEEL-IN SHOWER

Design C is not large, and many people will wish to have more room. Design D is for a minimal size bathroom, and should be larger if possible.

Shower

The small shower area in these designs must be level with the floor, using cedar or plastic slats with narrow gaps between so that a wheel will not catch, and

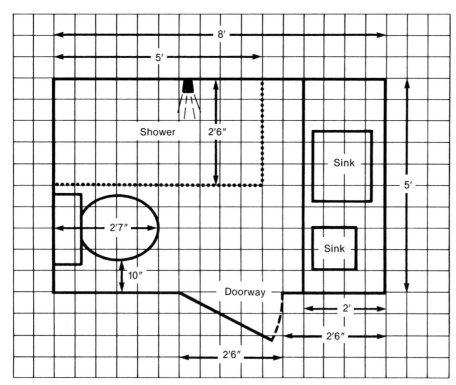

EXTRA-SMALL BATHROOM: DESIGN D

with a sunken area and a drain beneath. In a larger area, tiles may be used, with the drain set in a corner so that the slope to the drain will be minimal. This is more suited to a commode wheelchair since a person may have trouble transferring from a wheelchair if it is on a slope.

Toilets

The toilet must be standard height to allow a commode over it, and the tanks must be high or narrow enough to allow the wheels to go back.

If a toilet without a tank is used, the toilet should still extend 2 feet 7 inches (79 cm) into the room so that the person does not have to transfer moving back onto the toilet, over the chair wheel.

Counters

These should open underneath, except for drawers in the corners if desired, which will not impinge on the turning circle. Storage may also be installed over the counter in one or both corners. Two sinks may be desired by some who need to soak and wash GU apparatus.

Mirrors

A mirror to counter level will be convenient, and will make the small room seem larger.

Doors

Doors must swing outward, or a sliding door must be installed. If the corridor outside is narrow, the door must be wider.

SAMPLE KITCHEN PLANS

Design A is the floorplan of the kitchen illustrated in Fig. 11-16, page 421. This kitchen is used as a training kitchen and also as a basic kitchen design so that the homemaker can adapt her own kitchen design to her own and her family's requirements.

A person who has worked in a wheelchair kitchen will find it very much easier to decide on features that are desirable for her own kitchen, and which features would be best changed or adapted for her circumstances, such as physical needs, size of family, and cooking preferences.

The kitchen illustrated has a short refrigerator with a freezer above, a side-opening-type oven and drawers where possible in the counter top. A pantry would be required by most users.

Design B is the floor plan of the kitchen illustrated in Figure 11-2, page 413, and has been used for many years by a single man in a very small apartment. The design was adapted for the smaller area from the training kitchen in Design A. The user found the design very satisfactory.

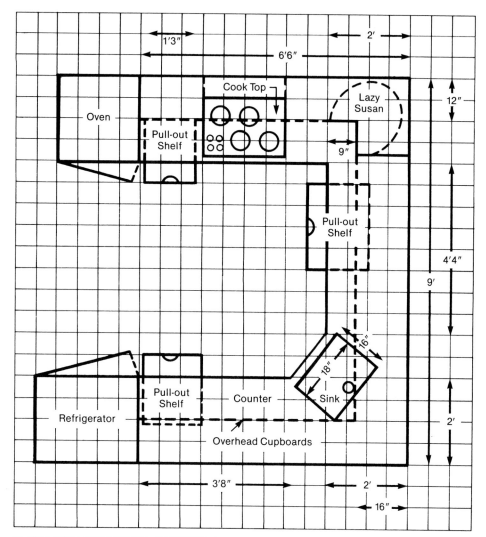

U-SHAPED KITCHEN: DESIGN A

HEIGHT FROM COUNTER TO UNDERSIDE OF OVERHEAD CUPBOARDS 14″ (35.36 cm) (INCREASE FOR MICROWAVE OVEN)

COUNTER DEPTH, INCLUDING DRAWERS, PULLOUT SHELVES, SINK, AND COOK-TOP 6″ (15.25 cm)

FLOOR TO UNDERSIDE OF COUNTER 27″ (64.8 cm)

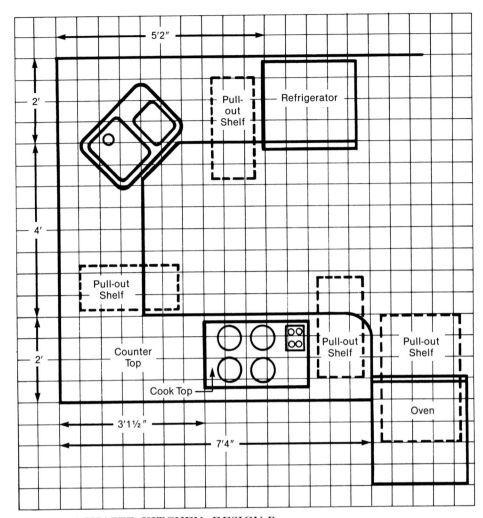

SMALL U-SHAPED KITCHEN: DESIGN B

PUSHER MITTS

Pusher mitts can be made of cowhide and velcro. The hand is placed palm down on a piece of paper to make a pattern. The outline of the hand is traced and the knuckle line and the wrist extension skin crease are sketched in. The hand is turned over, keeping the ulnar border on the paper. The outline of the hand is traced again and the palmar crease and the wrist flexion crease are drawn in. The pattern follows inside these lines with an overlap for fastening. Care must be taken not to overlap the wrist flexion and extension creases; an abrasion can develop very quickly if the edge of the pusher mitt should rub against the skin.

The thumb hole should be as small as possible because the pushing area is often close to the thumb. It is simple to enlarge the hole if necessary. The thumb loop should be low around the metacarpal below the metacarpophalangeal joint, or it will tend to pull the thumb into hyperextension. The leather loop should be

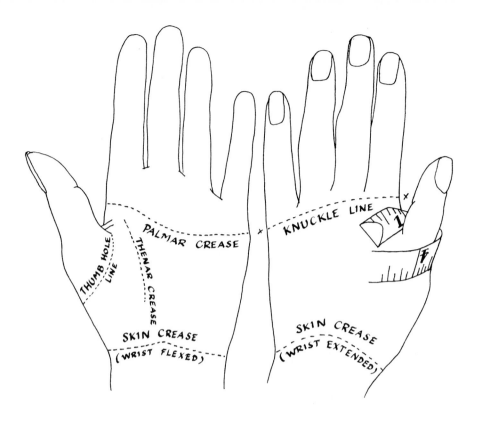

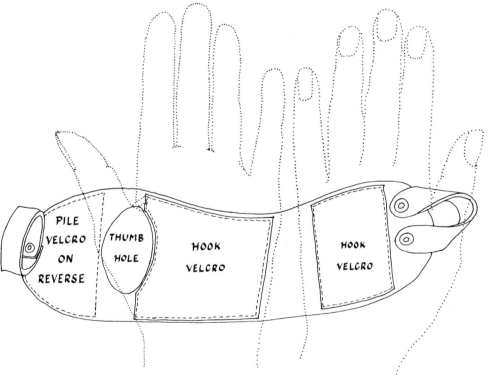

PUSHER MITTS

640

twisted so that it is in contact with the skin all around the thumb. The fastening loop must provide room for the insertion of a finger or thumb.

Velcro is stitched to the cowhide. It may be replaced when it loses its friction value. The mitt may be made symmetrical so that it can fit either hand, thus prolonging the life of the pushing surface.

Other pusher mitts may be adapted from shingle mill workers protective gloves. These normally have a thumb web protector, which must be sewn down on one side if used as a pusher mitt. Velcro closure must be added. Because these mitts are commercially available they are cheaper, but fit only larger hands.

CONSTRUCTION OF PADDED TRANSFER BOARD A

A plywood base is cut according to the pattern with the grain running along the length. The edges are slightly rounded and the underside of the wheel cutout is beveled. The floor flange is cut, filed, and positioned. The T-nut holes are drilled and the T-nuts are inserted from the top of the board. A wide U-shaped leather gusset is cut and stapled at the bevel line under the board by the wheel cutout so that it bulges through to about 2 inches (5.08 cm) above the board, allowing the curve of the wheel to be accommodated.

Foam is glued over the board and around all edges before upholstering with slippery material such as nylon taffeta, or naugahyde sprayed with silicone. A gusset will be required at the right angle by the floor flange. Care must be taken to maintain the height of the covering over the wheel cutout when the upholstery is pulled tight.

The floor flange is now bolted on. A 3½-inch (8.89 cm) tube is made of ½-

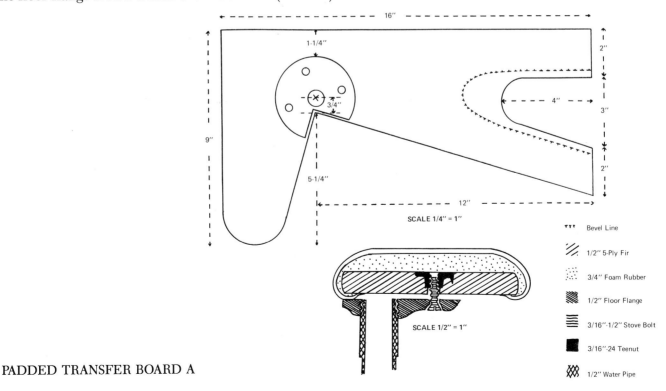

PADDED TRANSFER BOARD A

641

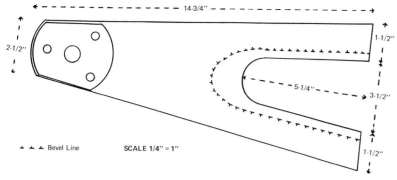

14-3/4"

2-1/2"

1-1/2"

5-1/4"

3-1/2"

1-1/2"

Bevel Line   SCALE 1/4" = 1"

PADDED TRANSFER BOARD B

inch (1.27 cm) water pipe which is threaded at one end, and turned down on a lathe for 2 inches (5.08 cm) at the other end to fit the front wheelchair arm socket. The measurement from collar to flange is usually 1 inch (2.54 cm), but may require adjustment so that the bridgeboard is the same height as the compressed wheelchair cushion. A tridon clamp may be used as an adjustable collar instead of the turned collar.

The pattern shows the underside of a board to fit on the left of the wheelchair. It should be reversed for a right transfer.

This pattern fits a standard active duty lightweight wheelchair. Modifications will be required for other models.

CONSTRUCTION OF PADDED TRANSFER BOARD B

If a patient does not require the tongue, which extends the sliding surface between the front of the wheelchair seat and the bed, a smaller version may be used. Advantages are that right or left transfers may be made using the same board, and it may be more useful for toilet transfers.

The construction of Transfer Board B is similar to A, except that an extra hole must be drilled at the front of the flange, since two holes are eliminated when the sides of the flange are cut off. If 2-hole flanges can be obtained, they should be used instead of the 4-hole type.

CONSTRUCTION OF DELTA WING TOILET SEAT

In the pattern, the bracket lines and the locking ledge positions are shown on one side only for clarity. The seat is made of 3/4-inch (1.91 cm) plywood, and the edges and corners are rounded. The four brackets are placed on the toilet bowl and are adjusted until they are on the bracket lines as drawn on the pattern. The positions are marked so that the T-nuts can be fixed in the top of the seat. The T-nuts are also positioned for the floor flanges and the hinges.

The seat is padded with 1-inch (2.54 cm) foam carried down to cover all edges and upholstered with naugahyde. The naugahyde must be brought well under the seat at the hole. The underside is now covered. A back 18 × 12 inches (45.72 × 30.48 cm) of 3/4-inch (1.91 cm) plywood is cut and the T-nuts are placed for the hinges before it is upholstered. Cadmium plated 8-inch (20.32 cm) strap

642

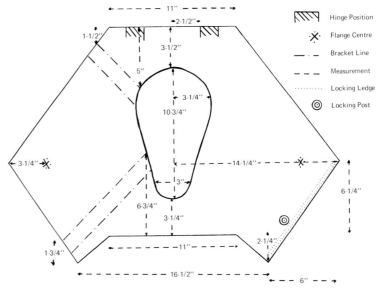

DELTA WING TOILET SEAT

SCALE 1/8" = 1"

Hinge Position
Flange Centre
Bracket Line
Measurement
Locking Ledge
Locking Post

hinges are used, and both leaves are offset at right angles 1¹/₄-inch (3.18 cm) from the hinge center to allow the top to fold flat on the seat for easy transportation. Two ³/₄-inch (1.91 cm) floor flanges to fit ³/₄-inch (1.91 cm) water pipe are bolted to the underside, and two metal locking edges ¹/₂-inch (1.27 cm) square and about 5 inches (1.27 cm) long are screwed to the underside of the seat under the edges of the wings.

A single leg is made of ³/₄-inch (1.91 cm) water pipe threaded on one end, ready to be screwed into one of the flanges on the underside of the seat. The leg should be approximately 20¹/₂ inches (52.07 cm) long but this should be checked before final cutting. Allowance must be made for the extra length of the crutch tip, which is slipped over the pipe to protect the floor. A locking post is made of ¹/₂-inch (1.27 cm) water pipe turned on a lathe for 1-inch (2.54 cm) of its length to fit into the front arm socket of the wheelchair. The protruding pipe is measured, so that with the addition of a crutch tip, the pipe will fit under the seat and catch behind the locking edge. When in use, the leg is screwed into the flange on the side furthest from the patient. This seat is very useful for training purposes since it can be adjusted to transfer from either side.

CONSTRUCTION OF RAISED TOILET SEAT
AND DELTA WING TOILET SEAT BRACKET

The brackets are made of ¹/₈ × 1-inch (0.32 × 2.54 cm) rolled steel or aluminum alloy. The bolt is a ⁵/₁₆-inch (0.79 cm) carriage bolt. A piece of I.V. tubing may be sleeved onto the bolt to protect the toilet bowl. The projecting ends may also be covered. Adjustment holes are ³/₄-inch (1.91 cm) apart, center to center. Two holes should be drilled in the top for screwing to the underside of the toilet seat with a ⁵/₁₆-inch (0.79 cm) bolt protruding through. The bolt fits through the hole at the bracket top and is fastened with a wing nut. This model allows the brackets to be swiveled slightly to adapt to different makes of toilet bowl.

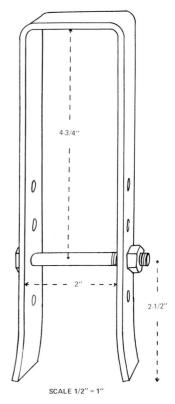

SCALE 1/2" = 1"

TOILET SEAT BRACKET

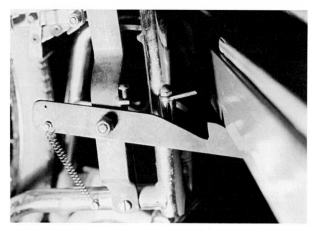

FRONT APPROACH BED HOOK

FRONT-APPROACH BED HOOK

This hook is used to lock the front upright of the wheelchair to the bed during a front-approach transfer. A right hook is shown from above. The drawing is reversed for the left hook, which must be used at the same time on the left upright of the chair.

The S-shaped hook is made of $^1/_8 \times ^1/_2$-inch (0.32 × 1.27 cm) rolled steel and a $^5/_{16}$-inch (0.79 cm) bolt is brazed to it vertically near one end. A $1^1/_2$-inch (3.81 cm) length of $^1/_8 \times ^1/_2$-inch (0.32 × 1.27 cm) cold rolled steel is brazed to the tip of the S and gently curved so that when the wheelchair front makes contact, it will cause the hook to swing back in position to spring in to lock around the chair front uprights. The bracket, which is bolted to the bed frame, is made of $^1/_8 \times 1^1/_2 \times 2^1/_2$ inches (0.32 × 3.81 × 6.35 cm) of cold rolled steel. A U-shaped tongue is brazed to the bottom edge of the plate. A bushing is brazed to the underside of the

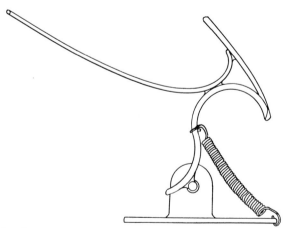

FRONT APPROACH CHAIR BED HOOK

644

tongue and a $5/16$-inch (0.79 cm) hole drilled through the tongue using the bushing as a guide. Small holes are drilled for attaching a light spring. About 8 inches (20.32 cm) of $3/16$-inch (0.48 cm) welding rod is brazed to the hook and bent so that it can be reached and used to release the hook.

FRONT-APPROACH CHAIR BED HOOK

These hooks are permanently attached to the wheelchair and are ready for use when the leg rests are swung away. Brackets are placed vertically and bolted to the top and bottom tubing of the chair frame so they do not interfere with folding. The hook is set in position so that when the chair is wheeled against the bed, the hooks will engage under the bed frame. A stop is placed on the vertical bracket to prevent the hook from swinging past the horizontal. The springs at the rear of the hook rocker arms must be heavy enough to keep the chair locked to the bed during transfers. A light chain, cable, or nylon cord may be fastened to the back of the hook rocker arm and led to a position that allows the patient to reach and pull to release the hook.

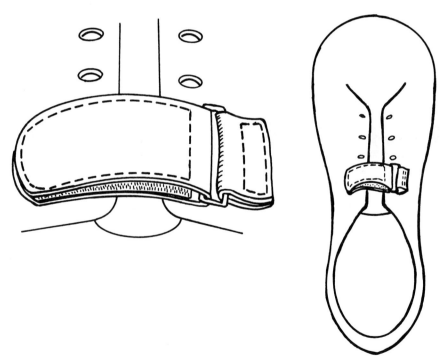

SHOE FASTENING FOR PERSON PULLING TO THE LEFT
Made from leather and velcro. A thumb loop probably will be required.

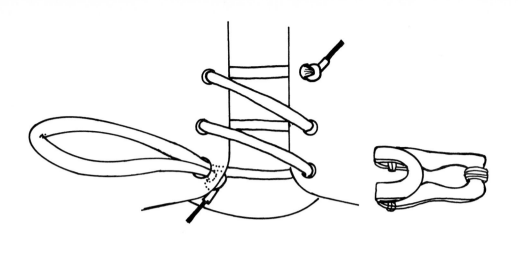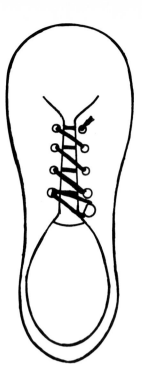

SHOE FASTENING FOR PERSON PULLING TO THE RIGHT

Elastic laces may be used. An additional finger loop or simulated bow may be added.

HOME ACCESSIBILITY EVALUATION

NAME _____ DATE _____ Wheelchair _____

ADDRESS_____ Ambulatory _____

THERAPIST _____ HOME VISIT BY _____

Household members, available help: _____

Type of home — split level, 2 storey, etc. _____

— apartment — size, location of suite _____

HOME PLAN: If necessary, include access and relevant measurements. Draw suggested changes in another colour.

✓	Accessible
✓E	Accessible with equipment
X	Inaccessible

N/A	Not applicable
3.5m	Measurement - Example
✓H	Accessible with available help

HOUSE LOCATION	KEY	COMMENTS
Terrain: Flat/Hilly		
Roads Paved: Ramped sidewalks		
Accessibility — to stores, banks		
Accessibility to other houses		
Type of transportation		
HOUSE ENTRY		
Access: Car to building		
Front Entrance: stairs, number, height		
Building Entrance: rails —		
— height/side		
— open/close, lock		
— sill height		
— width		
Back Entrance: stairs, number, height		
rails — height, side		
door — open/close, lock		
— sill height		
— width		
Apartment: suite entrance		
elevator — access		
— controls		
corridor — flooring		
— width		
— rails		
— fire doors		
— sills		
fire exit		
access to other suites		
access to mailbox		
Other:		
MOBILITY IN HOUSE		
Stairs: number, height, width		
rail, height		
Corridor: width		
rail		
Rooms: all accessible		
Floors: type		
Carpets: depth of pile		
Furniture: allows mobility		
wheelchair space		
Dining: wheelchair space		
height of table		
Other:		

RECOMMENDATIONS

BATHROOM PLAN with relevant measurements: Draw suggested changes in another colour.

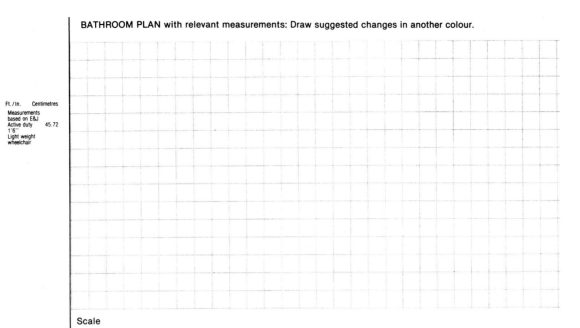

In.   Ft./In.   Centimetres

Measurements
based on E&J
18''   Active duty   45.72
     1'6''
     Light weight
     wheelchair

Room beside
toilet, side
transfer - slight
or large angle
32'' — 35''
2'8'' — 2'11''
81.28 — 88.9cm

Average
33''   2'9''   83.82

27''   2'3''   68.58

Scale

BATHROOM	KEY	COMMENTS
Access: Room to turn to doorway		
Doorway width		
Toilet: Access		
Height		
Type		
Position of studs for grab bars		
Wash Basin: Access		
Height of counter top		
Knee room under		
Drain insulated		
Taps within reach, on/off		
Plug within reach, on/off		
Mirror usable		
Storage accessible		
Tub: Access		
Height		
Taps within reach, on/off		
Plug within reach, on/off		
Position of studs for grab bar		
Shower: Type of wall		
Wheel-in Shower: Access		
Duck board or tile sloped to drain		
No lip		
Width, length		
Shower control within reach, on/off		
Type of shower head		
Thermostat for water		
Other:		

RECOMMENDATIONS

BEDROOM PLAN with relevant measurements: Draw suggested changes in another colour.

Scale

BEDROOM	KEY	COMMENTS
Door Width		
Bed: accessible		
type		
bars, rails		
frame height		
Mattress: compressed height		
soft/hard		
type		
width		
Light Switches		
Intercom		
Night Table		
Dresser, open drawers		
Closet, access, rod height		
Mobility in room		
Windows		
Other:		

RECOMMENDATIONS

650

KITCHEN PLAN with relevant measurements: Draw suggested changes in another colour.

In. Ft./In. Centimetres

Measurements
based on E&J
18'' Active duty 45.72
1'6''
Light weight
wheelchair

Scale

KITCHEN	KEY	COMMENTS
Mobility: access to kitchen		
manoeuverability within room		
Counters: Height		
Depth of shelves		
Distance counter/cupboards		
Knee space under counter		
Sink: Access for wheelchair		
Height to underside of sink		
Taps on/off, type		
Drain insulated		
Burners: Type (gas/electric, countertop)		
Height		
Control placement		
Control type, on/off		
Access to fan/light switches		
Oven: Type (gas/electric, wall/floor)		
Height		
Control placement		
Control type, on/off		
Type of door opening		
Fridge: Access to		
Freezer: Access to		
Wall plugs: Access to		
Flooring: Type		
Other:		

60'' Circle 5' 152.4

33'' Average 2'9'' 83.82
24'' Average 2' 60.96

27'' Average 2'3'' 68.58

NOTE:
SOME CONTROLS REQUIRE
PRESSURE BEFORE TURN-
ING

RECOMMENDATIONS

651

Household Evaluation

Name: _____ Therapist: _____

Disability: _____ Person available to help: _____

Code:

✔	Independent	
✗	Standby	
A –	Minor assistance	
A +	Major assistance	
X	Fully dependent	

N/A	Not applicable
H	Help available
E	Equipment required

		Dates		Method and/or Equipment
		Code		
MENU PLANNING	Plan nutritional menus: daily			
	weekly			
	Plan grocery list			
	Budgeting			
MARKETING	Transportation			
	Shopping			
	Payment			
	Carry and put away groceries			
MEAL PREPARATION	Hygiene			
	Organize activity			
	Remove food from fridge			
	Reach into low cupboards			
	Reach into high cupboards			
	Turn taps			
	Open packaged goods			
	Use can opener			
	Peel vegetables			
	Cut vegetables			
	Prepare meat			
	Handle sharp tools safely			
	Break an egg			
	Measure ingredients			
	Stir			
	Use egg beater			
	Pour batter in pan			
	Roll dough			
	Turn on stove			
	Pour hot liquids safely			
	Move hot dish, oven to table			
	Handle small appliances			
	Handle milk container			
	Work safely			
	Tidiness during preparation			

		Dates		Method and/or Equipment
			Code	
MEAL SERVICE AND CLEAN-UP	Set table/select dishes & cutlery			
	Carry meal to table			
	Dish out meal			
	Remove, scrape and stack dishes			
	Wash dishes			
	Wash pots and pans			
	Clean up stove and work areas			
	Wring out dish cloth			
	Use dishwasher			
	Dry dishes/put away			
COMPETENCY LEVEL	Able to make	breakfast		
		lunch		
	☐ for self	dinner		
	☐ for family	snacks		
		total daily menu		
		total weekly menus		
LAUNDRY	Hand wash/wring out			
	Use washing machine			
	Use clothes dryer			
	Hang clothes on line			
	Hang clothes on rack			
	Iron clothes			
	Fold clothes			
	Put clothes away			
SEWING	Thread needle and knot			
	Use scissors			
	Sew on buttons			
	Mend tear			
	Use sewing machine			
ROUTINE HOUSEKEEPING TASKS	Tidy			
	Dust			
	Use dust pan and broom			
	Wipe spills on floor			
	Make bed			
	Change bedding			
	Clean bathroom			
	Take out garbage			
	Organize housecleaning: self			
	delegated			

		Dates		Method and/or Equipment
		Code		
INFREQUENT HOUSEHOLD TASKS	Use vacuum			
	Mop floor			
	Clean refrigerator			
	Clean oven			
	Wash windows			
	Change light bulb			
	Maintain furniture/drapes/carpets			
	Maintain outside area			
CHILD CARE				

ORGANIZATIONAL SKILLS

Organize food preparation and clean up, (include planning, sequencing and timing:)

Organize daily schedule:

Organize weekly schedule:

SAFETY AWARENESS & PROBLEM SOLVING

Aware of safety precautions/hazards

Identify problems, eg. plugged sink, fuse

Able to deal with emergency procedures, eg. fire

Able to organize household maintenance

654

Glossary

Abduction. Moving limb away from midline.

Adduction. Moving limb toward midline.

A-Frame. A track or bar running between the top of two A-supports.

Anesthesia. Lack of sensation.

Anterior. In front.

Autonomic dysreflexia (hyperreflexia). An unopposed sympathetic reflex in a patient with a lesion above T-6 which causes a swift rise in blood pressure.

Axilla (ae). Armpit/armpits.

Balkan beam. Bar over the bed running from head to foot.

Ball-bearing support. Commercially available mobile arm support that requires little effort to operate but needs a considerable amount of individual fitting.

Bridgeboard. Board to bridge a gap so that the patient can cross it. Also known as a transfer or sliding board.

Bumper. Rubber-tipped furniture guard at front of chair.

Cock-up splint. Splint to immobilize wrist in some extension.

Condom. Prophylactic rubber sheath worn on the penis, used in collection of urine.

Cord lesion level. Level where the cord is damaged; not necessarily where the vertebrae are broken or displaced.

Depression of shoulder. Pulling shoulder down.

D.I.P. joint. Distal interphalangeal joint. Last finger joint.

Distal. Far, away from trunk. Opposite to proximal.

Dorsum. Back, i.e., dorsum of hand—back of hand.

Drive rims. Small rims outside wheelchair wheels, used for pushing.

Elevation of shoulder. Pulling shoulder up.

Extension. Straightening (usually). Opposite to flexion.

External rotation. Turn outward, i.e., external rotation of hip—leg and foot are turned out.

Extremities. Upper—arms. Lower—legs.

Fixed strap (sling). A strong loop of webbing or leather taped or bolted to a bar.

Flaccid. Lack of muscle tone, lack of spasticity, loose.

Flexion. Bending. Opposite to extension.

Flexor-hinge splint. A lively splint that causes the fingers to meet the thumb when the wrist is extended.

Floating strap (sling). A strong loop of webbing or leather that moves freely on a bar.

Front bumper. Rubber-tipped furniture guard at front of chair.

Gatch frame. Bed frame that is divided into independent movable sections. May be used for raising a patient to a sitting position, etc.

Genitourinary apparatus. Tubing, bag, etc., for urine collection. Also known as genitourinary system and G.U. apparatus or system.

Grab bar. A bar, firmly fastened to a wall or floor, used as a handhold.

Hamstrings. Muscles at back of thigh. They bend the knee and extend the hip.

Hanger. Fixture on wheel of wheelchair for fastening the drive rim.

Hyperextended. Extended beyond the normal position, i.e., extended beyond 180° at the elbow.

Ileostomy bag. An ileal bladder bag placed over the opening of a diversion from kidney to abdominal wall used to collect urine.

Iliac crest. Bony ridges at sides of abdomen. Outer portion of pelvis on either side.

Internal rotation. Turn inward, i.e., internal rotation of shoulder—back of hand placed on small of back.

Intrinsic muscles. Small muscles of the hand, (or foot).

Ischial tuberosity. Bony protrusion under the buttock region.

I.V. tubing. Intravenous tubing.

Joint D.I.P. Distal interphalangeal joint, last finger joint.

Joint M.P. Metacarpophalangeal joint, joint at base of finger.

Joint P.I.P. Proximal interphalangeal joint, middle finger joint.

Lateral. Outside, away from midline. Opposite to medial.

Limit switch. Switch that cuts off automatically at predetermined point.

Long sitting. Sitting with legs straight on a flat surface.

Medial. Inside, near midline. Opposite to lateral.

M.P. joint. Metacarpophalangeal joint, joint at base of finger.

Natal cleft. Crease between the buttocks.

Palmar. Front, palm side of the hand.

Pentaplegic. A person who has some degree of impairment of all four limbs and of breathing.

Perineal crease. Crease formed where the buttocks meet the legs.

Phalanx (Phalanges). Bone (bones) of the finger (fingers)

P.I.P. joint. Proximal interphalangeal joint, middle finger joint.

Posterior. Behind, the back of.

Postural hypotension. Rapid drop in blood pressure when the patient comes to the upright position.

Prone, pronated. Face down, palm down. Opposite to supine.

Protraction. Pulled forward, i.e., protraction of shoulder—the scapula moved forward on the chest wall.

Proximal. Near, close to trunk. Opposite to distal.

Pubis symphysis. Bony part at the base of the abdomen.

Quadriplegia. Some degree of impairment in all four limbs. Also known as tetraplegia.

Reflex. Movement that is not controlled voluntarily. Involuntary muscle response to nerve stimulation.

Retraction of shoulder. Draw shoulders back, i.e., retraction of shoulder—shoulder blades together.

Sacrum. Bony part at base of back.

Scapula. Shoulder blade.

Shoulder depressors. Muscles that pull the shoulder down.

Shoulder elevators. Muscles that pull the shoulder up.

Shoulder girdle. Collar bone, shoulder, shoulder blade, and the muscles that stabilize and move them.

Shoulder protractors. Muscles that pull the shoulders forward around the chest wall.

Shoulder retractors. Muscles that pull the shoulders back.

Sliding board. Bridgeboard, transfer board.

Sling. Usually a canvas support for use with hoists, etc.

Spacer. Metal tube separating the wheel and the drive rim of a wheelchair.

Spasms. A sudden, often violent involuntary contraction of a muscle or a group of muscle.

Spasticity. A state of increase over the normal amount of tension in a muscle.

Spinous process. Piece of bone that protrudes, i.e., in the spine the bones that can be felt down the back.

Strap. Leather or webbing, sewn, riveted, or buckled in a loop.

Supine, supinated. Face up, palm up. Opposite to prone.

Symphysis pubis. Bony part of the base of the abdomen.

Tenodesis. Normal flexion or extension of the relaxed fingers caused by movement of the tendons when extending or flexing the wrist.

Tetraplegic. Some degree of impairment in all four limbs. Also known as quadriplegia.

Thumb web. Web between thumb and first finger.

Tibial tuberosity. Part of the bone just below and in front of the knee joint.

Tipping lever. Protruding bars at rear of the chair. Used by a helper's foot to tip the chair back.

Transfer board. Bridge board, sliding board.

Triceps. Muscle that extends the elbow.

Tridon gear clamp. Hose clamp, adjustable by a screw gear.

Trochanter. Bony prominence at top of thigh bone, hip.

Trolley. A cart, small table on castors, for use in mainly the kitchen.

Ulnar border (of hand). Side of the hand by the little finger.

Index